FIRST EDITION

A LIFE OF WELLNESS:
HEALTH AND FITNESS FOR YOUNG ADULTS

by Daniel Burt

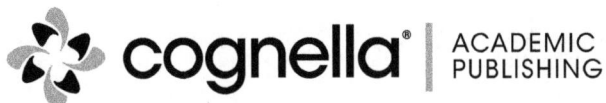

cognella® | ACADEMIC PUBLISHING

Bassim Hamadeh, CEO and Publisher
Kassie Graves, Director of Acquisitions
Jamie Giganti, Senior Managing Editor
Miguel Macias, Senior Graphic Designer
Marissa Applegate, Senior Field Acquisitions Editor
Gem Rabanera, Project Editor
Elizabeth Rowe, Licensing Coordinator
Christian Berk, Associate Editor
Joyce Lue, Interior Designer

Cover image copyright © Depositphotos/lzf.

Printed in the United States of America

ISBN: 978-1-5165-1321-5 (pb) / 978-1-5165-1322-2 (br)

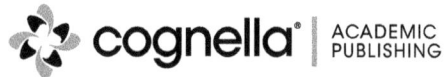

cognella® | ACADEMIC PUBLISHING

CONTENTS

Acknowledgments   xiii

CHAPTER 1   HEALTH AND WELLNESS   **1**

By Daniel and Ashlee Burt

What are Health and Wellness?   1

Dimensions of Wellness   2

Benefits of Wellness   3

Physical Activity vs. Exercise   3

Behavior Management   5

   Behavior Modification   5

Health Belief Model   5

The Transtheoretical Model   6

   Precontemplation   7

   Contemplation   7

   Preparation   7

   Action   7

   Maintenance   7

   Termination/Adoption   7

   Relapse   8

Process of Change   8

   Consciousness Raising   8

   Dramatic Relief   9

   Environmental Reevaluation   9

Social Liberation   9

Self-Reevaluation   9

Self-Liberation   9

Helping Relationships   10

Counter Conditioning   10

Reinforcement Management   10

Stimulus Control   10

Creating Goals Using SMART   10

Specific   11

Measurable   11

Acceptable   11

Realistic   11

Timely   11

Why is it Hard to Change?   12

Values   12

Stress   12

Falsehoods   13

Health Related Components   13

Principles of Training   14

FITT Principles   15

References   16

CHAPTER 2   NUTRITION   **17**

By Ashlee Burt

Nutrition and Health   17

Note the Following Daily Tables   18

Macronutrients   21

Carbohydrates   21

Tips for Choosing Healthy Carbs   24

Protein   25

Fats (Lipids)   29

Carbs, Fats, and Protein Used as Fuel   39

Micronutrients   40

Water 47

Individualizing Your Meal Plans 48

Nutrition Standards 55

Antioxidants 56

Vegetarianism 57

Organic Food Options 57

Athletes and Carb Loading 58

Tips for Eating Healthy in College 59

Know Your Helper's Credentials 60

References 60

CHAPTER 3 BODY COMPOSITION 65

What is meant by Fat and Body Composition? 65

Metabolism 65

So What about "Getting Fat"? 66

Storing Fat: What Causes It 67

Genetics 67

Age 68

Gender 68

Ethnicity 68

Your Lifestyle 68

The Role of Physical Activity 69

Benefits of Physical Activity 69

Concerns about Body Composition and Females 70

How I See Me… 71

Figuring Out Your Body Mass v. Percent Body Fat 72

Body Mass Index 72

Percent Body Fat 73

Skinfold Calipers 73

Hydrostatic Weighing (Underwater Weighing) 74

Bioelectrical Impedance Analysis (BIA) 74

Bod Pod 75

DEXA (Dual-Energy X-ray Absorptiometry)   75
References   76

CHAPTER 4   CARDIORESPIRATORY ENDURANCE   77

How does the Cardiorespiratory System work?   77
Your Heart   77
Your Blood Vessels   79
Your Respiratory System   79
Concepts of the Respiratory System   80
Benefits of Cardiorespiratory Endurance   81
    Physiological Benefits   81
    Self-Esteem and Body Composition 81
    Chronic Illness   82
Creating an Endurance Plan with FITT   82
    Why have a Warm-Up and Cool Down? 84
Assessing Cardiorespiratory Endurance   85
    Common Assessments   85
    Heart Rates   86
    METs   86
Common Safety Concerns   86
    Common Injuries   86
Environmental Concerns   88
    Heat   88
    Cold   89
References   89

CHAPTER 5   DEVELOPING MUSCULAR STRENGTH
AND ENDURANCE   91

Why is it Important?   91
Physiology of Muscles and Training   91
    Muscle Fibers   92
    Types of Fibers   93

Motor Units   94

Benefits of Muscular Strength and Endurance   95

    Performance and Injury   95

    Aging and Health   95

    Quality of Life and Body Composition   96

Types of Strength Training   96

Assessment of Strength Training and Endurance   97

Using FITT Principles   97

Types of Training and Equipment   99

    Concentric and Eccentric Movement   99

    Free Weights   99

    Machines   99

    Resistance Bands   100

    Speed Loading   100

    Kettlebells   100

    Stability Balls   101

    Plyometrics   101

    Pilates   101

Strength Training Safe Practices   102

References   103

CHAPTER 6 FLEXIBILITY   **105**

What is Flexibility and does it matter?   105

Types of Flexibility/Stretching   105

    Static Stretching   106

    Dynamic Stretching   106

    Ballistic Stretching   106

What are Factors in Flexibility?   106

    Muscle Length and Elasticity   106

    Joint Structure   107

    Nervous System Regulation   108

Benefits of Flexibility   108

    Age   109

Lower Back and Joint Issues   110
Assessment and Guidelines   112
   When Should I Stretch?   112
   Using FITT   112
Unique Techniques   113
   Proprioceptive Neuromuscular Facilitation   113
   Active and Passive Stretching   114
Life Tips and Recommendations for Healthy Muscles and Flexibility   115
References   115

CHAPTER 7   ASSESSING AND COPING WITH STRESS   117

By Ashlee Burt

Adaptation to Stress   117
Personality Types   119
Coping with Stress through Exercise and Complementary
Alternative Medicines (CAM)   121
   Physical Activity   121
   Yoga   121
   Tai Chi   122
   Reiki   122
   Progressive Muscle Relaxation   122
   Breathing Exercises (Like Lamaze Classes)   122
   Meditation   123
   Massage Therapy   123
   Acupressure/Acupuncture   123
   Visual/Guided Imagery   123
   Biofeedback   124
   Aromatherapy (Essential Oils & Diffusers)   124
   Herbal Therapy   124
Other Ways to Help Reduce Stress   125
How to Get (and Stay) Motivated!   125
   Tips for Staying Motivated   126

Sleep Consistency Matters 126

    Tips for Better, more Consistent, Sleep 129

References 130

CHAPTER 8   SEXUAL HEALTH   133

By Ashlee Burt

What is Sexuality? 133

Sexual Health 134

Personal Safety and Healthy Relationships 135

What are STI's/STD's? 136

    Chlamydia 136

    Gonorrhea 137

    Human Papilloma Virus (HPV) 137

    Herpes 138

    Pelvic Inflammatory Disease 139

    Syphilis 140

    Trichomoniasis 142

    HIV 142

Responsibility and Sex 143

How to Protect Against STIs and Prevent Unplanned Pregnancy 145

    STI, HIV, and Pregnancy Protection 145

    Contraceptive Methods 148

    Permanent Contraceptive Methods 155

    Miscellaneous Contraceptive Methods 156

    Emergency Contraceptive (EC) Methods 158

    Abstinence 160

References 162

CHAPTER 9   CHRONIC WELLNESS   167

By Kacey DiGiacinto

What is a Chronic Disease? 167

Types and Considerations 167

Cardiovascular Disease 167

Diabetes 170

Cancer Considerations and Preventions 172

Melanoma 174

Breast Cancer 176

Lung Cancer 177

Prevention and Management Techniques 178

The Big Picture 178

Individual Efforts: Looking Back at the Transtheoretical
Model in Action 179

Physical Activity 180

Healthy Eating 180

Alcohol Consumption 181

Tobacco Use 181

Health Screenings 182

Access 182

References 182

CHAPTER 10   ACUTE WELLNESS   **185**

By Kacey DiGiacinto

Common Risk Factors 185

The Nature of Addiction 185

Smoking 185

Smoking and Pregnancy 187

Secondhand Smoke Exposure 187

What's in a Cigarette? 188

What about Other Forms of Tobacco? 189

Alcohol 190

Binge Drinking 191

Underage Drinking 192

What Happens When You Mix Caffeine and Alcohol? 192

Drug Use 193

General Drug Knowledge 193

Hallucinogens or Psychoactive Drugs   194

Over-the-Counter Drugs (OTC)   195

Stimulants and Depressants   195

Sport Drugs   197

   Anabolic Steroids   197

Assessing Behavior and Prevention Planning   197

   Why Should You Quit Using Tobacco?   197

   Do You or Someone You Know Need Help
   With a Drinking Problem?   198

   How Can I Kick a Drug Habit?   198

References   198

Lab 1. Lifestyle Survey and Resting Heart Rate   201

Lab 2. Behavior Modification   205

Lab 3. Food Diary and Estimated Energy and Protein
        Requirement   211

Lab 4. Disease Risk with BMI and Recommended
        Body Weight   217

Lab 5. How Many Calories do I Need per Day?   221

Lab 6. Are You Ready to Begin an Exercise Program?   225

Lab 7. VO$_{2\,Max}$ Using the 1.5-Mile Run   227

Lab 8. Assessing Muscular Strength   231

Lab 9. Assessing Muscular Flexibility   233

Lab 10. Assessing Range of Motion   239

Lab 11. Creating a Personal Fitness Plan   241

Lab 12. How Stressed are You?   245

Lab 13. How at Risk are You for Developing Stress?   249

Lab 14. Alcohol and Addictive Behavior   253

Lab 15. AIDS Awareness   255

Acknowledgments

I want to give a huge thank you to my wife, Ashlee, who has been supportive of my work, even as it poured into our personal life…including on a few vacations; I love you. I want to thank my kids, Aaralyn, Dean, and Xavier for interrupting my work and reminding me to have fun on occasion. I want to thank my parents for being supportive of all the different directions I took in my life, you planned my name with how it would look with a potential doctorate title and on a book…now you know! I also am appreciative to all my mentors over the years, including those I have now, for helping shape who I am as a professional and individual. I want to particularly thank my project editor, Gem, for having the patience and expertise to work with me on this text. To all my students, I appreciate how much I always get to learn from you every year and know that my goal is for you to live long and successful lives, not just get a degree!

1 HEALTH AND WELLNESS

BY DANIEL BURT AND ASHLEE BURT

Chances are pretty good that you may be using this book to take a required course for your major or university. Hopefully, that won't dissuade you from having an interest in a healthier lifestyle. Many people,, especially after their college years, engage in improving their health. A lot of this comes from the fact that the body starts to work against us a little more the closer we get to, and go over the age of 30. Many people get involved with fitness and dieting to improve their health and also to feel better. However, the majority of people are also wanting to just flat out look good physically. While there is nothing wrong with this, it does tend to lead many to use the end result to justify the means; the "whatever works" mentality, which does not take long-term health into account.

People have many beliefs in what they think should make up good fitness and health practices. With the exception of politics and religion, it isn't uncommon to find people's beliefs at odds over the topic and what should be considered "right." How big is this? It is estimated that the Weight Loss industry is $20 billion dollars when books, supplements, diet programs and surgeries are considered. When we discuss who is being targeted in this industry, it is believed that 108 million Americans are on a diet at this moment, and many try to diet 4–5 times a year. The main demographic seems to be that 85% of the clientele is female.[1] You probably have the belief that you know a lot about health and fitness; maybe you have read a lot of articles, or you are (or were) a student-athlete. However, we hope you can take some new knowledge from this text in several, if not all of these sections. Almost every contributor to this text has a PhD in specific fields, and we still do not believe we know everything, and take pleasure in continuing to learn about health and wellness.

WHAT ARE HEALTH AND WELLNESS?

Sometimes these terms are used interchangeably, but they are not exactly the same thing. The traditional term has always been **health**, which we recognize as the overall condition of a person's body and mind, or the absence of injury or illness in a person. What needs to be noted about health is that many things that could alter or effect it may also be outside of your control. This could be seen in the form of aging, or how genetically, things may pass down from your parents. **Wellness**, on the other hand, looks at the concept that we are looking at what YOUR optimum health can be, as considered by the choices that you make. These choices can cause you to increase or decrease the risk of health problems. A person deciding to engage in regular physical fitness for over an hour every day may see the benefits of weight loss, leading to the additional benefits of cancer or diabetes prevention.[1]

DIMENSIONS OF WELLNESS

Researchers placed wellness into six different categories to better understand what factors play a role in our short and long-term health. These are not considered individual and unrelated though, and they interact with each other. The reason these categories exist is so that it is understood that you should not ignore any of them. Since life moves forward and we are constantly altering ours to fit our needs at that time and age, then it is easy to ignore the other aspects that are part of wellness.

Emotional Wellness is how we are able to handle emotional changes. This first category requires us to understand our own emotions, like when we are sad, depressed, or angry. It involves taking the time to address and process the emotions we are experiencing. This could mean facing issues of self-confidence, finding ways to be more optimistic and reduce negativity, being able to discuss our emotions or feelings with others, and developing trusting relationships.

Interpersonal Wellness tends to be defined as our social aspect, or how well we are able to build and continue relationships that are emotionally supportive. This often requires engagement with our surrounding environments, and supporting a helpful cause of some form. It entails being able to reach out to others when you have emotional needs, and having strong communication skills.

Spiritual Wellness does not refer to if you are religious specifically, but if you have some form of guiding belief system that you may prescribe to, or that there are some set of principles that guide your life when things become complicated. People have described it as also turning to things like nature, meditation, and helping others. This usually allows people to help combat the amount of negativity that they may face or deal with in their lives. Often it can be expressed in being compassionate, showing empathy, and placing value through giving to others, or those in need.

Environmental Wellness looks at the area you choose to live in, and what benefits can be gained from it. This can be simply looking at the safety and noise pollution of your surroundings, or the amount of violence that could be involved in the area. For many areas in the world, this comes down to even the simple basic needs for life, involving clean food and water supplies. Choosing to partake in recycling programs and reducing pollution are considered some ways to improve environmental wellness.

We can also be involved in *Intellectual Wellness*, by looking at ways to improve our minds through challenges and adaptations. By being involved in new experiences and choosing to challenge our brains, we often improve our mental capability to problem-solve, by creating or adopting new solutions.

FAQs CHECKS!

I hate my job …

Being satisfied with your job matters…and it matters a lot. It doesn't mean you will be happy all the time, and in research we have discovered that it doesn't usually correlate to making a lot of money or sounding important by having a title like "director." Instead, it usually depends on the following: Do you like your type of work? Do you feel like you have room to grow and improve? And do you have a great relationship with your boss? These things typically let you focus on your job and enjoy it, and since we spend a large amount of our life working, this helps with the negative stress in our lives.

The last and most expected component is *Physical Wellness*, which is looking beyond the terms that were discussed previously. It looks at your capability to take after yourself and your own physical needs. This could be avoiding risky behaviors or engaging in healthy behaviors. This can be seen in a eating a healthy diet, engaging in exercise, avoiding smoking, and getting enough sleep.

BENEFITS OF WELLNESS

Benefits of healthy living tend to be talked about in two forms, acute versus chronic. **Acute** benefits are direct benefits that occur as you engage in healthy behaviors, at that moment. Examples could be eating fruit and vegetables and the benefits your body gains by ingesting vitamins. You could also see acute benefits by going for a run and burning excess calories from this physical activity. **Chronic** benefits are those that relate more to long-term health and the prevention of what we call chronic illnesses. This can be seen in how increased physical activity decreases the likelihood of cancer. Running today may not help prevent it, but engaging in running over the years will help prevent or reduce the likelihood of numerous diseases like cancer, diabetes, and heart disease.

Another consideration is looking at the life we want to live, specifically in terms of quality and quantity. **Quantity of Life** usually refers to the length of our lives, specifically how many years we live. While we are all in agreement that we will all die eventually, how long that takes is another issue. Thanks to modern science and pharmaceutical medicine, we are able to extend life for quite a bit longer then we used to. This comes from finding ways to slow down the effects of disease. However, this does not mean life is back to normal. **Quality of Life** is the other consideration, and it refers to the value we place on the life we are living. While we are living longer at the moment, many individuals are becoming unable to take care of themselves, and are not able to enjoy many things that the younger generation takes for granted. This could be seen in things like feeding yourself, remembering important birthdays, or even just getting out of bed and walking out of your own room. The hope is that as we engage in healthy choices, and work hard to remove the negative behaviors in our lives, that we will not only increase our lifespan in years, but also the quality of our lives in those later years.

PHYSICAL ACTIVITY VS. EXERCISE

People oftentimes think of becoming healthy by altering one thing or another in their lives, usually by changing their diet or by increasing exercise. In reality, it is far more complicated than that, with multiple factors contributing to your health both now and in the long-term. One of the biggest issues is the decrease of **physical activity**. Physical activity is when we engage in physical movement of the body, which causes an increase in calories burned. Lack of physical activity has led us to a **sedentary** lifestyle, which references sitting by its very definition. This is quite serious in the U.S., with a median of 23.5% of Americans reporting zero participation in physical activity during 2013.[2] Since we recognize that our bodies do not respond well to lack of physical activity, and dislike the results, we tend to begin a concept called exercise. **Exercise** is defined as planned, structured, and repetitive, and has as a final or an intermediate objective the improvement or maintenance of physical fitness.[3] While this is physical activity, not all physical activity is exercise. According to the Centers for Disease Control and Prevention (CDC), the top leading causes of death are potentially very preventable: heart disease, cancer, chronic lower respiratory diseases, accidents, and strokes[4].

2013: Percent of adults who engage in no leisure-time physical activity†

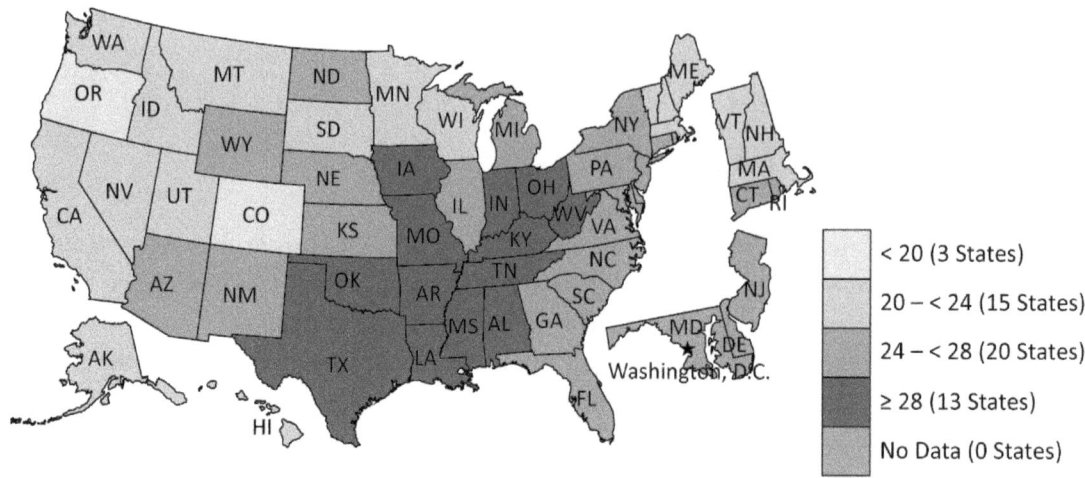

Footnotes

†Respondents were classified as participating in no leisure-time physical activity if they responded "no" to the following question: "During the past month, other than your regular job, did you participate in any physical activities or exercises such as running, calisthenics, golf, gardening, or walking for exercise?" Adults aged ≥ 18 years. Respondents with missing data were excluded.

Figure 1.1: Data reported by the CDC.

FAQs CHECKS!

How much does money play a role in my health?

Money matters quite a bit. Not necessarily the total dollar amount, which I promise you that most people in life feel like they could do with more. Yet, the ability to live within the amount you make and feel confident that your major needs are covered play a huge role in the amount of stress you have and your health. This often goes back to specific issues we all have to learn to deal with. The first is controlling the debt we incur. While debt has become the social norm, it doesn't stop it from being stressful when we constantly have to pay a little bit here and there until we realize we are not getting ahead and it is taking most of our paycheck. This also goes back to having money saved or in reserve, since we all know that stuff just happens and usually costs money. More than once, I had to pay out cash to fix a tire or replace something important, and I had wanted to use the money for something else. Learning good money management techniques and also how to avoid excess debt and create savings goes a long way into relieving that stress. Trying to control the emotions we have towards money is also important; it can buy a lot of stuff, but isn't really the provider of most things we need. Learning to think of money more as a tool, rather than an essential item itself, allows us to be less stressed over the amount we have and focus more on the ability to cover our needs.

BEHAVIOR MANAGEMENT

BEHAVIOR MODIFICATION

Many of us have behaviors we would like to change, stop altogether, or add to our lifestyle. First, we need to understand that many of these behaviors are created or influenced by external factors such as who our peers are, how our parents raised us, the environment we live in, and so forth. We also have behaviors that we choose to incorporate into our life, such as choosing to exercise or choosing to eat out all the time. Other influences are more difficult to control or change, such as having long work hours that don't allow us time to relax and eat healthy meals and exercise. We are also a major multi-tasking society now, and we are constantly on the go with our phones, which we usually keep in our purses or pockets; there's no need to get up and walk to a phone. We choose to park close to stores, use elevators, take escalators, not make time to exercise or eat a well-balanced diet, and all of these things can contribute to an unhealthy lifestyle.

Before changing a behavior, you need to look at factors that determine your health, which includes what your locus-of-control is and your self-efficacy. **Locus-of-control** is how you see your life being controlled; it can be one of two ways, internally or externally. Individuals who believe they have an internal control are more confident and believe that they have the ability to change themselves, or influence the world around them. Those with an external control believe they have no control over events or people that surround them, and in some cases may believe that others control them. Many times those with an external control attribute their successes to chance or luck. **Self-efficacy** is needed for any individual to achieve his or her goal or lifestyle change, and this is having the confidence that you have the ability to perform a certain task. If you have never used equipment at a gym before, you probably lack confidence to go on your own and figure out all the machines. If you feel like you can't do it and have a low self-efficacy, then more than likely you will not go to the gym at all.

There are a variety of health models available to utilize with behavior change. These models are available to help individuals take steps to change unhealthy behaviors to healthy behaviors. Most of the models incorporate goals and objectives. **Goals** are created as a long-term achievement an individual wishes to attain. **Objectives** are created as steps or short-term goals that help a person to slowly make his or her way to an ultimate goal. There are four health theory models that help health educators to develop interventions at the individual level. Below we briefly discuss the Health Belief Model and go into more detail with the Transtheoretical Model. The SMART model is also discussed in terms of a tool to use when creating goals and objectives.

HEALTH BELIEF MODEL

The Health Belief Model helps you realize how susceptible you feel about a health problem, what benefits of avoiding the problem, and what factors play a role in your decision to change or remove that behavior. Factors can include barriers such as money, low self-efficacy, access to information, etc.

The Health Belief Model

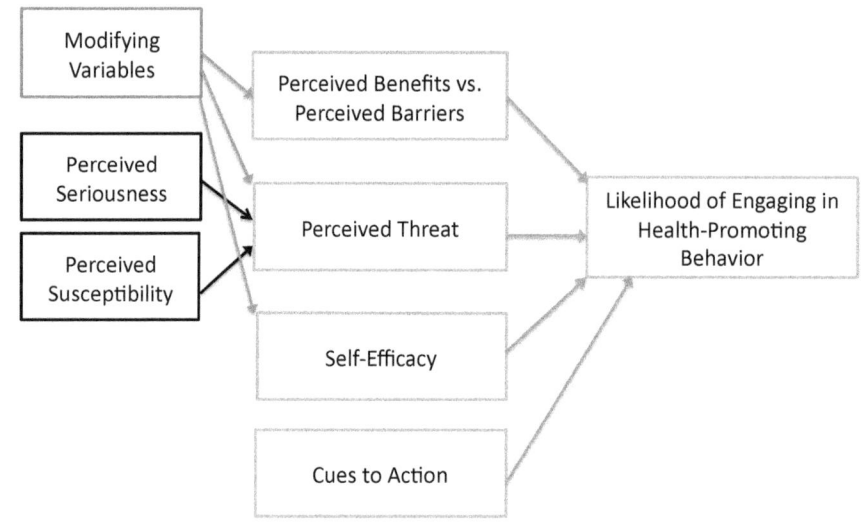

Figure 1.2: Health Belief Model.

THE TRANSTHEORETICAL MODEL

Stages, or the Process of Change, also known as the Transtheoretical Model, is a theory based on progressive and gradual behavior change, mainly intended for health-related behaviors. This model includes six stages and utilizes 10 processes, or behavioral techniques, that help people to change their specific behaviors. After reading about each stage in the model, you will understand how to apply your individual behaviors to their appropriate stages. The goal of using the model is to make a behavior change.[5]

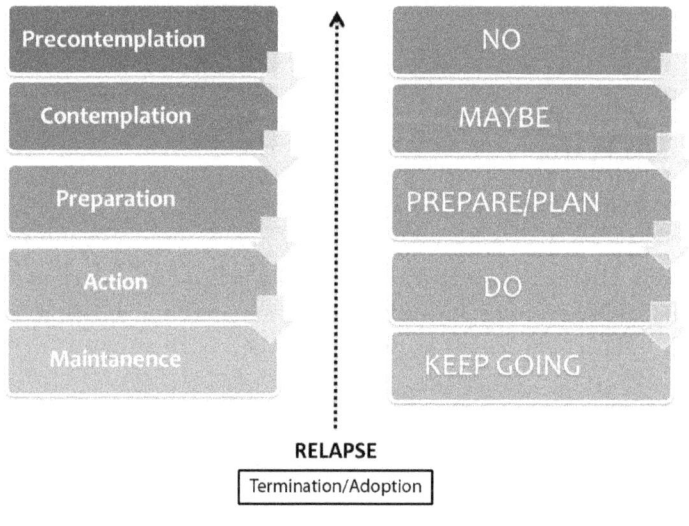

Figure 1.3: Transtheoretical Model.

PRECONTEMPLATION

In this stage people are not thinking about changing, or do not want to change any behavior. Many times those in this stage don't acknowledge having a problem For example, they don't see smoking as a problem, or being physically inactive as a problem. Friends and family may recognize that these people have a problem or behavior that should be changed, but those in this stage dismiss that information. In this stage, they also may try to avoid information about the problem, such as throwing away a brochure on the benefits of quitting smoking. Those in this stage require educating, and in most cases need something that matters enough, or that they value enough to make them want to change and see change as beneficial.

CONTEMPLATION

Once individuals move into the contemplation stage, they have acknowledged their problem or behavior that needs to be changed. They are not necessarily ready to make the change, but at this point they are now looking at the pros and cons of changing their specific behavior. Looking at their pros and cons will allow them to see what will be working against them and for them, when they are finally ready to work on making that change.

PREPARATION

At this point, individuals are now beginning to plan on making their behavior change within the next month. In this stage, people may attempt the new behavior for a few days just to try it out so they know what to expect. Goals and objectives are usually clearly identified during this stage to help prepare for the planning.

ACTION

The action stage is when the CHANGE occurs. This stage ultimately uses the most energy, effort and time to put a plan into action. A person in this stage is now actively working on the change, either by reducing how many cigarettes he or she smokes a day, or starting to walk a mile a day to work up to the guidelines set for those specific behaviors (stop smoking and cardiorespiratory endurance three times a week).

MAINTENANCE

Once people reach this stage, they have maintained their behavior changes for up to five years. They have also followed the specific guidelines for the behavior, such as eating a well-balanced diet, eliminating tobacco products altogether, or participating in cardio three times a week. The main concern in this stage is to focus on keeping the goals the individual has met, to create new goals to continue moving forward, and to continue to avoid relapsing.

TERMINATION/ADOPTION

Individuals will enter this stage once they've maintained their behavior modifications for more than five years. If it was a negative behavior that was changed, for example quitting smoking, then it is considered termination. If it was a positive behavior change, for example maintaining a cardiorespiratory fitness program, then it is considered adoption. There is debate on whether an individual can relapse in this stage or not.

Many health educators believe once people enter this stage, they have terminated or adopted for life and will no longer relapse and therefore leave the model. However, other experts believe relapse can still occur, especially for those removing a negative behavior such as alcoholism, and they believe there will always be a chance to revert back to that lifestyle.

RELAPSE

Relapse occurs when an individual begins the action stage and then stops the change, and therefore reverts back to a previous stage (preparation or contemplation). Relapse can occur at any stage, except the precontemplation stage, and most often occurs during the action stage.

PROCESS OF CHANGE

The stages are there to identify where a person is with a specific behavior. The processes of change are the choices of behavior we engage in under the different stages of the Transtheoretical Model. Note that you can only use certain processes with each stage, and that there are ten of them.

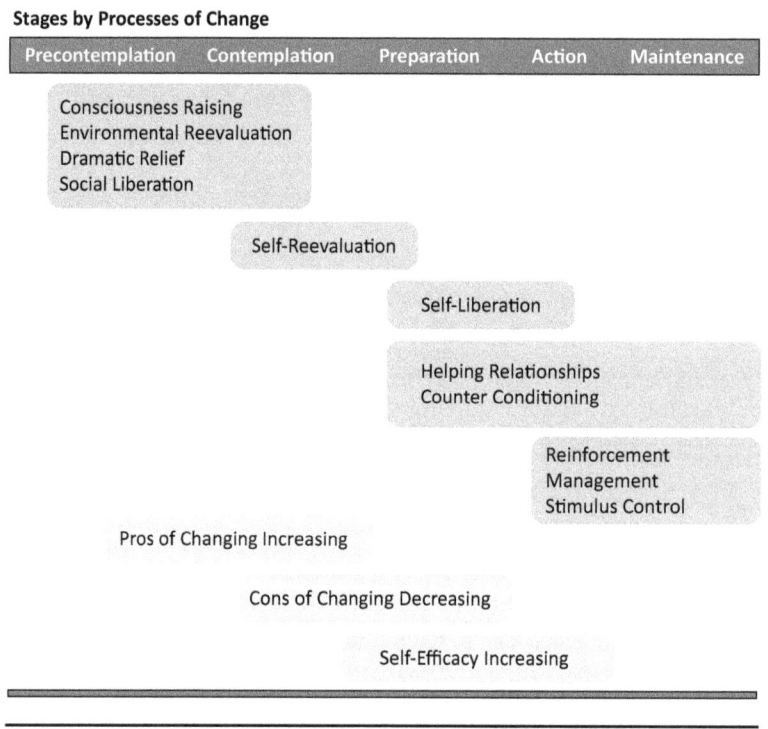

Figure 1.4: Processes of Change.

CONSCIOUSNESS RAISING

This is the first step in making a change, where a person must obtain information about his or her specific problem that would lead to a belief that changing would be beneficial. This could be that you receive a brochure from a physician on why saturated fats are unhealthy, a pamphlet on what smoking does to your body, or a list of benefits you get from aerobic exercise; raising your awareness of the damage or benefits these things cause will make you want to remove that behavior (termination) or add that behavior to your lifestyle (adoption). Due to their close relationship and how quickly people move from one stage to the other, this is located under both the precontemplation and contemplation stages.

DRAMATIC RELIEF

This is oftentimes an emotional response to a serious situation. It creates a sense for change or the need for an intervention. This could be the realization by a man who just suffered a heart attack that he needs a better diet and exercise. It could be a college student finding out that a sexually transmitted disease test is negative, and is now choosing to engage in healthier practices for safer sex. This can occur under both precontemplation and the contemplation stage.

ENVIRONMENTAL REEVALUATION

This is the realization that your health behaviors may have an effect on others around you, and your choice to alter them can be a reflection of that. It may be that know you are out of shape and you choose to engage in exercise to go on a long hiking trip with friends. It could be a father who does not want his children to breathe in secondhand smoke, and so he chooses to quit. This could also be found in both the precontemplation and contemplation stages.

SOCIAL LIBERATION

Social Liberation is a bit unique in that it does not necessarily stem from an individual, as the other processes tend to. It tends to be more of a cultural or social change that occurs. It usually has the goal of making the culture it is in aware of specific behaviors through education or policy changes. Examples of this could be speed bumps, indicating the need to slow down your driving speed, or the placement of non-smoking areas in businesses or restaurants. This tends to be the last process under the dual stages of precontemplation and contemplation.

SELF-REEVALUATION

This is a stage of self-reflection where you examine who you are with or without the behavior. People might see themselves as being a better role model if they drank less alcohol. They may consider how much more attractive they would be to others, and how well they would physically feel if they exercised more often. This stage may fall under contemplation, as well as preparation, since they are likely to make changes by mentally picturing the goals they want and might obtain with their behavior changes.

SELF-LIBERATION

This is individuals having the firm belief that they can make changes in their behavior. It extends beyond just believing to the point that they are choosing to continue that belief even through hard changes that they face and must overcome. This can be someone wanting to quit smoking, but struggling with the fact that every one of their friends and coworkers smoke. Regardless of failing several times, they continue to try and change. This tends to fall under the repeating preparation and action stages of the model. When they plan and engage the plan for change, if they fail, then they repeat the preparation and go into action again.

HELPING RELATIONSHIPS

This process looks at the ability to build strong and supportive social networks to help and encourage you on your behavior change. This could be as easy as finding someone else who wants to be in better physical shape, and the two of you decide to workout together and hold each other accountable for making it to the gym. Due to the fact that this could be started in the planning phase and can continue to be influencing you for years, it falls under three stages. It can be in the preparation, action, and maintenance stages.

COUNTER CONDITIONING

This process works on the concept of providing alternatives, preferably healthy, to the behavior you might be trying to eliminate. This can be seen by people who stress eat or smoke as choosing to go for a walk instead. Sometimes the alternatives are not healthy, but instead, a progressively improved alternative, which can be seen in people choosing to use nicotine gum instead of smoking as they try to quit. Since this can also be planned in advance, it is typically seen in the preparation, action, and maintenance stages.

REINFORCEMENT MANAGEMENT

While this could refer to both positive rewards for good behavior and punishments for negative behaviors, research typically shows that rewards tend to be more effective at behavior change. This could be saving the money from not buying cigarettes for a smoking habit and putting it towards an item you want instead, at two-week, four-week, and eight-week markers. This can also consist of having a good social support network that will remind you how well you are doing, as you progress with healthier behaviors. Reinforcement means something has to actually be done, so it is seen in the action and maintenance stages.

STIMULUS CONTROL

This process looks at what causes, or stimulates, certain behaviors and how to either increase or decrease these behavior triggers. An example could be for a person who tends to snack on junk food, it should be removed from the area. Another could be that they trigger and force themselves to go to the gym by hiring a personal trainer, and setting specific times to be there with them. This tends to focus on the action and maintenance stages.

CREATING GOALS USING SMART

Creating goals using the acronym SMART is not new to health behaviors. It is also found in goal orientation in business, career planning, and pretty much anything that might require a goal to reach.

SPECIFIC

You need to clearly define what you want. People tend to do a better job accomplishing what they want from a project, if they know what specific outcome is desired. It is not enough to say, "be skinny." We need to look at what our current weight is and target specific and reasonable numbers. It could be that "I will reduce my body composition by 5% in six weeks." This specificity also allows us to plan for particular objectives to reach this goal. Examples could be adjusting the amount of trans and saturated fats we are eating, or increasing our cardiorespiratory endurance. These specific objectives should be listed out as goals for us to track, and reflect on, if our goal is not being met.

MEASURABLE

This is not the same as specific; this refers to making the goal and items trackable through numbers. Stating that I plan to have bigger bicep muscles at the end of 16 weeks is not necessarily measurable. That I plan to add two inches to my bicep in 16 weeks creates a number that we can follow. The same can be said when discussing how much weight I may be able to lift in a certain period of time.

ACCEPTABLE

Setting a goal is great, but there has to be some understanding that a goal is usually in some form of framework. Do you have what you need to accomplish it? This could be different types of resources like time, money, equipment, and support. Do not book 4:00 a.m. to be your running time if you're going to bed late due to work, and unable to get up at that time.

REALISTIC

This relates to being acceptable, but realistic goal planning is a bit different. There has to be an understanding of the time it takes to reach some goals. Quitting smoking is great, but rarely can people do it in a few weeks. Many want to see physical results from weightlifting, and while they may be able to lift more in a few weeks, they won't really see permanent size changes in their muscles for eight or so weeks. This means learning about the behavior changes you are going to make, and knowing the reality of what it takes to properly plan your goals and avoid feeling like a failure.

TIMELY

Developed goals should always have deadlines. People tend to take the goal more seriously and stay focused when there is a deadline to reach. It may also work to set several deadlines to check your progress, and plan to reevaluate anything that may or may not be working. Especially for beginners, easier, short-term goals, as long as they are realistic, tend to work better than larger, long-term goals. People feel a sense of accomplishment, and it provides an internal reward when those goals are reached, making shorter goals favored.

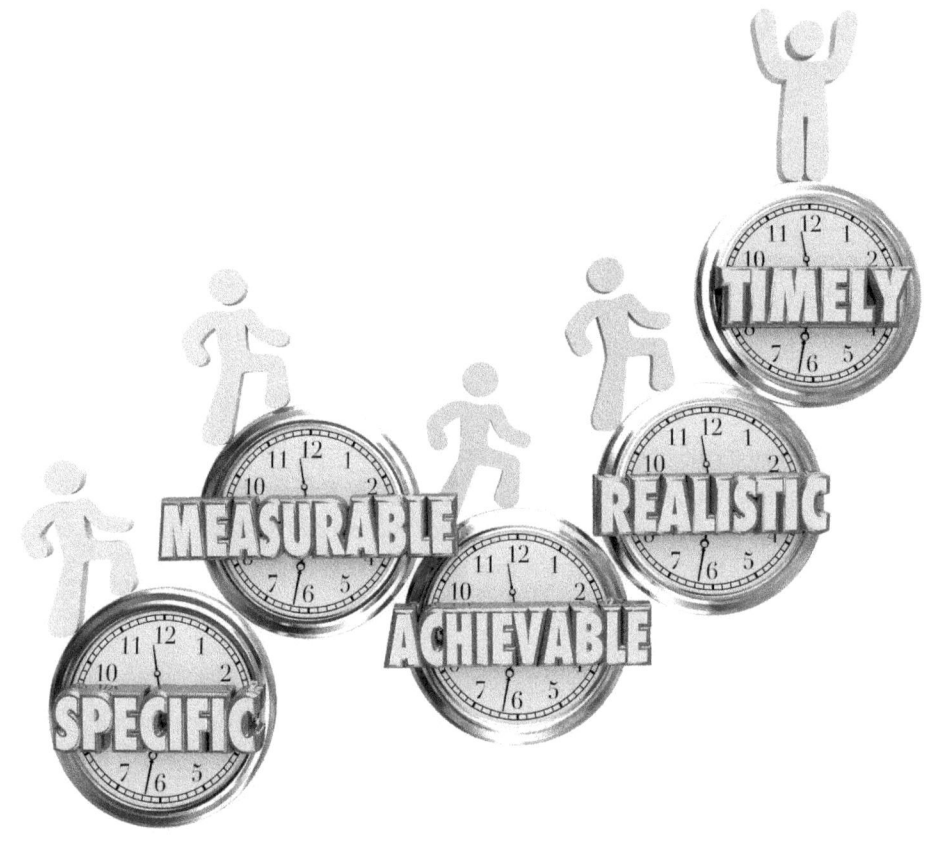

Figure 1.5: Reaching SMART Goals.

WHY IS IT HARD TO CHANGE?

VALUES

People often value the same thing that those around them value, as they are raised to adulthood. While people do not deny the need for better eating habits and increasing physical activity, they do not always consider it a major priority. Sometimes people accept that this is just how they are, because everyone around them is the same and it isn't realistic for them to change. The two greatest ways to combat this is first through education and raising awareness of acute and chronic health. The second is through hooking them into a new "culture" or mindset. Make friends or meet people who are already into what you want to do or become. Although you might feel like the outsider at first, hard work and getting into an encouraging atmosphere, with the same goals goes a long way towards reaching those goals.

STRESS

People struggle with the ability to get things done now more than ever. The more technology we add to make our lives easier, the more work and multitasking we try and take on (to be honest, even I have tried to run and answer emails more than once). This complexity is not only due to us, but also those who surround us: family, friends, and bosses, who know we now have access to instant communication and wonder why it takes us more than five minutes to respond back. Add this to the fact that in most cases we choose options in life that produce results fast, and we are often not patient enough to engage in the time-consuming tasks of actually cooking healthy whole food, or exercising. This constant pull in so many directions can lead us to feel depressed, and easily give up on things we do not see an instant benefit from.

FALSEHOODS

Unfortunately, people tend to delude themselves into thinking many things they do are acceptable at the moment, or that they do engage in moderation. Many people do not track the amount of food they actually eat, but when asked, state that they eat relatively healthily. Many nutritionists have noted that people are usually surprised and shocked when they write out what type and how much bad food they eat. This is typically due to the convenience of unhealthy food, and the good intentions of individuals creating a myth of their behaviors. The same applies to physical activity, with many people in the US stating they get 30 minutes or more of vigorous activity a week, but research has shown that most may get some moderate physical activity, but almost none of them engage in vigorous activity. People also believe that when they are young, that their bodies can handle it, so controlling food and activity are less necessary. However, we are discovering that the way you take care of your body in your 20s has a massive effect on your long-term health, even into your 70s and 80s.

FAQs CHECKS!

How can I increase my daily physical activity?

This comes down to simply being willing to move more, and making daily choices that support that. One example is taking the stairs anytime you are going up a floor or two in a building. Or, you can park the car towards the end of the parking lot instead of circling the lot trying to find the closest space to the door. Dogs tend to have similar health problems as their owners due to similar lifestyles; make a commitment for both of you to get a walk in. This increases the amount of energy needed to meet these demands, and in turn increases caloric expenditure. Since a can of soda is usually 100–160 calories, adding extra movement like this can easily burn several hundred calories more a day.

HEALTH RELATED COMPONENTS

What our bodies need to live a healthy life has been categorized into five components by researchers. This focuses on the acute and chronic needs of the body throughout our life span. There is a chapter dedicated to each of these in the textbook.

Cardiorespiratory Endurance: The ability of the body to perform large-muscle, dynamic exercise for moderate to various intensity levels. This also examines the ability of the body to transfer oxygen-rich blood throughout the body.

Muscular Strength: The amount of force a muscle can produce in a single maximum effort. This looks in detail at the size of the muscle and its importance for daily activity.

Muscular Endurance: The ability for a muscle to resist fatigue from repeated use or from holding the tension in a sustained contraction. This helps with injury prevention, and daily use from work to home.

Body Composition: Looks at your body's make up of fat to fat-free mass (bone, muscle, etc.). It is important to protect against acute injuries and chronic illnesses.

Flexibility: The ability to move the joints through the full range of motion. While of great importance towards joint and muscle health, especially as we age, it is often ignored by even people engaged in regular exercise.

PRINCIPLES OF TRAINING

They key to our bodies being better than they are now, is that they adapt to the various stresses we place on them. Below are four major principles that need to be considered when beginning any type of training so that changes will occur.

Progressive Overload: This principle is the most basic of the principles mentioned, and notes that there has to be additional stress placed on the system we are trying to improve for it to ACTUALLLY improve. Yet, care must be taken to understand the system since too much overload can cause damage, or not allow time for recovery. Too little risk overload also is a problem since it is not providing enough stress for an adaptation to occur. This can be seen when people run on a treadmill for five minutes and call it cardio, or pick up a three-pound weight to do big muscle movements. Each chapter goes over FITT principles to help you understand how to make adaptations (see the FITT explanation below). It is also worth noting that better results come from gradually increasing the stress placed on the body and not trying to make big changes by increasing the weight being lifted, or the distance being ran in large chunks.

Specificity: This principle notes that when you stress certain health components, then those are the areas that will truly benefit. No matter how many bicep curls I do, it will not improve the muscles in my legs, nor will it make me a better runner.

Reverse: The bottom line is that exercise never stops. As soon as you stop trying completely for a reasonable amount to time, usually a few weeks, then you will begin to lose some of your gains. Cardiorespiratory endurance training can leave very quickly if not used for a few weeks, but strength training typically will last longer. This doesn't mean you cannot take a week off once in a while (it is even recommended to occasionally let the body fully rest and recover by doing so), however, it should be included as part of the training plan to do so.

Individuality: Not everyone is the same. This principle notes that there is not a perfect cookie cutter design program that can apply to everyone without adjustments to various parts, like intensity and time. That doesn't mean that people who are so obese that they cannot run, will never run, but instead means that they need to develop a gradual training program that will get them to that point. You will notice that the following FITT principles look at what you CAN do, and work from there towards improvement.

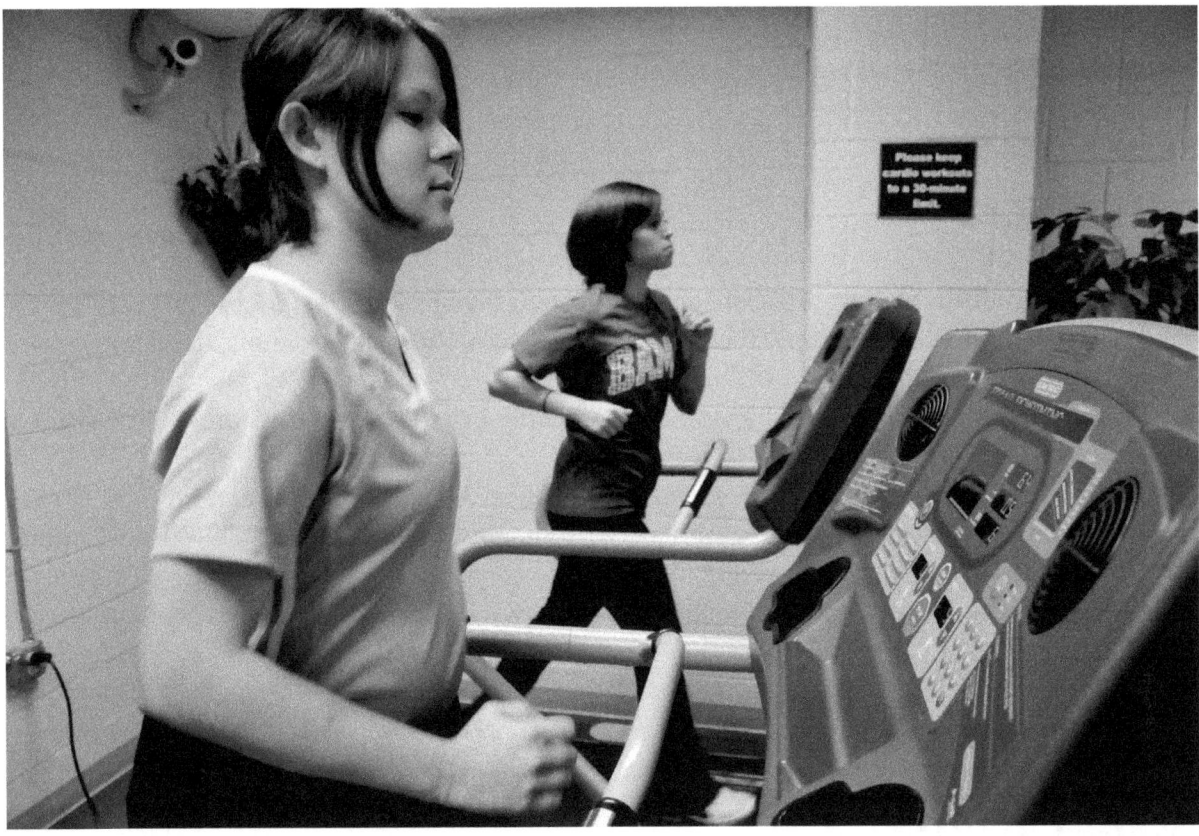
Figure 1.6: US Navy Members Exercise at the Medical Center.

FITT PRINCIPLES

As you read through this text, you will see that each chapter that covers a health related component provides the recommendations for beginning an active involvement with that component. This is done through recommendations of the American College of Sports Medicine (ACSM) and their guidelines, since they are recognized as the foremost professional source on exercise and the average person. This breaks down into a four-letter acronym, FITT, which you will see repeatedly in the chapters.

Frequency: This is how often an activity should occur. Some only place mild strain on the body, like flexibility training, meaning it can be performed almost daily. Others, like muscular strength training, place immense strain, and may risk harm if done too frequently.

Intensity: This is about performing harder than you do on a regular basis so that adaptations can occur. It is looked at differently for each health component, but it can vary depending on your health goals.

Time: Can be looked at in several ways, depending what component we are discussing, but it usually represents how long you are performing an action. As explained later, a 10-minute run is not considered the same as running for 30 minutes.

Type: This can be easy or complex, but it represents what method of activity you are going to use to reach your goals. Those working on cardiorespiratory endurance may choose to walk, run, or even swim to reach their goals.

REFERENCES

1. ABC News. (2012, May 8). "100 Million Dieters, $20 Billion: The Weight-Loss Industry by the Numbers." Retrieved from http://abcnews.go.com/Health/100-million-dieters-20-billion-weight-loss-industry/story?id=16297197.
2. United Health Foundation. "Physical Inactivity in the United States." http://www.americashealthrankings.org/ALL/Sedentary
3. Caspersen, C., Powell, K., and Christenson, G. "Physical Activity, Exercise, and Physical Fitness: Definitions and Distinctions for Health-Related Research. *Public Health Report,* 100, no. 2 (1985): 126–131.
4. Centers for Disease Control and Prevention.. http://www.cdc.gov/nchs/fastats/leading-causes-of-death.htm.
5. Prochaska, J., DiClemente, C., and Norcross, J. "In Search of How People Change: Applications to Addictive Behaviors." *American Psychology,* 47, no. 9 (1992): 1102–14.

IMAGE CREDITS

2 NUTRITION

BY ASHLEE BURT

NUTRITION AND HEALTH

Nutrition is a vital part of our health. It helps give us energy as well as prevent chronic diseases. Knowing what to eat, and how much, is key to having a well-balanced, healthy diet. **Nutrition** can be defined as the scientific study of the relationship between foods and health. **Nutrients** are the substances found in foods that provide us nourishment; each food item has a variety of nutrients in it, and each nutrient does something different for our body, such as help with growth and repair. **Nutrient-dense** is the term we use when a food contains high amounts of vitamins, minerals, and fiber but is absent of or low in saturated fat, sodium, and added sugars. The USDA created the MyPlate to help the general population with a visual understanding of what types of foods and how much of those foods should be on their plate.

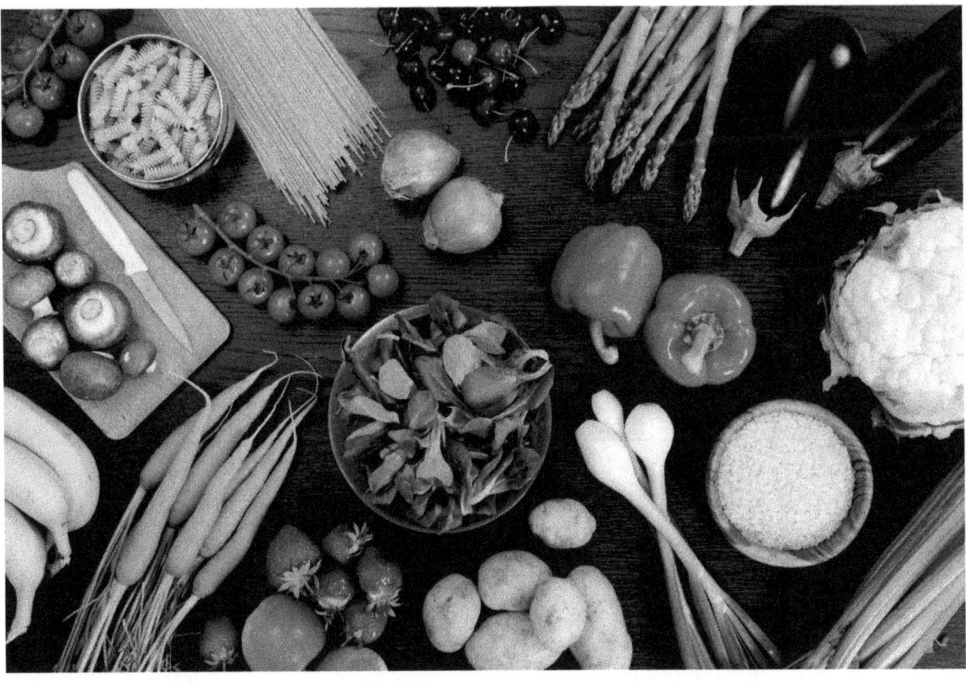

Figure 2.1: Food.

Gender and age both play a role in how much an individual should eat of each food group. Refer to the tables below for each food group recommendation. You may also visit the USDA's website http://www.choosemyplate.gov/MyPlate for fun games, research, tools, and other tables that break down what a serving size is (i.e., one cup of applesauce is equal to one cup of fruit)[1,2].

NOTE THE FOLLOWING DAILY TABLES

Table 2.1: Daily Fruit Table

Daily Recommendation*		
Children	2–3 years old 4–8 years old	1 cup 1 to 1½ cups
Girls	9–13 years old 14–18 years old	1½ cups 1½ cups
Boys	9–13 years old 14–18 years old	1½ cups 2 cups
Women	19–30 years old 31–50 years old 51+ years old	2 cups 1½ cups 1½ cups
Men	19–30 years old 31–50 years old 51+ years old[1]	2 cups 2 cups 2 cups

Table 2.2: Daily Vegetable Table

Daily Recommendation*		
Children	2–3 years old 4–8 years old	1 cup 1½ cups
Girls	9–13 years old 14–18 years old	2 cups 2½ cups[1]
Boys	9–13 years old 14–18 years old	2½ cups 3 cups
Women	19–30 years old 31–50 years old 51+ years old	2½ cups 2½ cups 2 cups
Men	19–30 years old 31–50 years old 51+ years old	3 cups 3 cups 2½ cups[1]

Table 2.3: Daily Grain Table

		Daily Recommendation*	Daily Minimum Amount Of Whole Grains
Children	2–3 years old 4–8 years old	3 ounce equivalents 5 ounce equivalents	1½ ounce equivalents 2½ ounce equivalents
Girls	9–13 years old 14–18 years old	5 ounce equivalents 6 ounce equivalents	3 ounce equivalents 3 ounce equivalents
Boys	9–13 years old 14–18 years old	6 ounce equivalents 8 ounce equivalents	3 ounce equivalents 4 ounce equivalents
Women	19–30 years old 31–50 years old 51+ years old	6 ounce equivalents 6 ounce equivalents 5 ounce equivalents	3 ounce equivalents 3 ounce equivalents 3 ounce equivalents
Men	19–30 years old 31–50 years old 51+ years old	8 ounce equivalents 7 ounce equivalents 6 ounce equivalents	4 ounce equivalents 3½ ounce equivalents 3 ounce equivalents[1]

Table 2.4: Daily Protein Foods Table

Daily Recommendation*		
Children	2–3 years old 4–8 years old	2 ounce equivalents 4 ounce equivalents
Girls	9–13 years old 14–18 years old	5 ounce equivalents 5 ounce equivalents
Boys	9–13 years old 14–18 years old	5 ounce equivalents 6 ½ ounce equivalents
Women	19–30 years old 31–50 years old 51+ years old	5½ ounce equivalents 5 ounce equivalents 5 ounce equivalents
Men	19–30 years old 31–50 years old 51+ years old	6½ ounce equivalents 6 ounce equivalents 5½ ounce equivalents[1]

Table 2.5: Daily Dairy Table

Daily Recommendation					
Children	2–3 years old 4–8 years old	2 cups 2½ cups	**Women**	19–30 years old 31–50 years old 51+ years old	3 cups 3 cups 3 cups
Girls	9–13 years old 14–18 years old	3 cups 3 cups	**Men**	19–30 years old 31–50 years old 51+ years old	3 cups 3 cups 3 cups[1,3]
Boys	9–13 years old 14–18 years old	3 cups 3 cups			

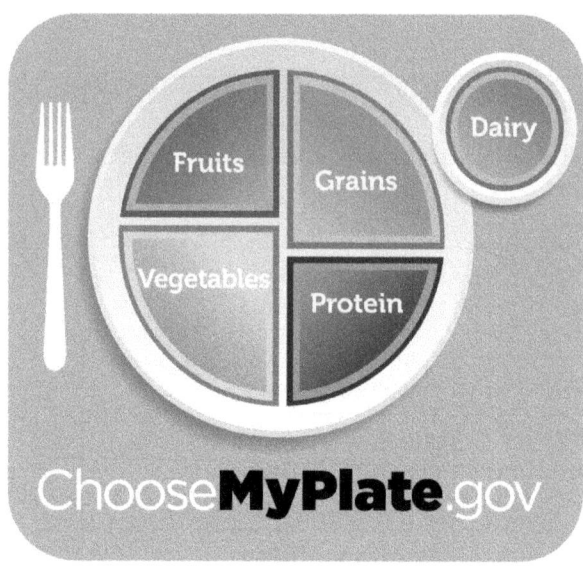

Figure 2.2: Plate.

The U.S. Department of Health and Human Services established a science-based program called Healthy People. Currently, we are on Healthy People 2020; this program creates objectives for improving the overall health of the American people every 10 years. They have over 42 topics with objectives listed within each topic. These topics range from adolescent health, global health, and lesbian, gay, bisexual, and transgender health to items such as public health infrastructure, social determinants of health, and medical product safety. Healthy People is research-based and a great resource for the population to utilize to be aware of what changes are important to live a healthier life. The downside to Healthy People is that the majority of the general population had previously never heard of these initiatives. With the new, updated 2020 initiative, creators changed the framework to be more digital-based and to use tools such as Twitter and LinkedIn to provide updates and therefore reach more interested Americans. The other barrier Healthy People has to deal with is our health system, which does not always allow for these objectives to be adopted and implemented[4].

Before we dive into all the important nutrients, take a look at the table below for a quick glance at the six nutrients we will be discussing.

Table 2.6: Nutrient Types

Carbohydrates	Protein	Fats (Lipids)	Vitamins	Minerals	Water
Main fuel source. Four calories per gram. Consists of single or multiple sugar molecules and provide energy to the body. Two categories: Simple and Complex.	Comprised of amino acids. Four calories per gram. There are 20 total amino acids; nine are essential that must be achieved through diet.	Does not dissolve in water, only in fat. Provides most energy, nine calories per gram. Three main categories: Simple, Compound, and Derived.	Necessary substances found in foods to help with metabolism growth, repair, and development. We require 13 different vitamins.	Substances necessary for body functions, control water and acid-base balance. There are 25 different minerals that our body requires.	Essential nutrient, it is involved in almost all processes and makes up a large portion of our body. Adults require about 11–15 cups a day (from foods and fluids).
Simple Carbs—basic form of carbohydrate, includes glucose, lactose, and sucrose. Refined and processed foods with added sugar.		*Saturated Fats (Simple)*—Found in animal products, should be eaten in small quantities, increases cholesterol.			

(Continued)

Carbohydrates	Protein	Fats (Lipids)	Vitamins	Minerals	Water
Complex Carbs—more complex with longer glucose chains, includes starch, dextrins, glycogen, and fiber. Whole grains, vegetables and legumes.		*Unsaturated Fats (Simple)*—Found in plant foods, eat in larger quantities, decreases cholesterol.			
		Trans Fats (Simple)—Chemically made unsaturated fat, provides no health benefit, only negative effects to body.			
		Poly Omega (Simple)—Essential fats with many health benefits.			
		Lipoprotein (Compound)—Helps transport fats in the blood. Forms the different cholesterol (HDL, LDL, etc.).			

MACRONUTRIENTS

Let's break the word down: macro means large, and we defined what a nutrient is at the beginning of the chapter. Macronutrient is the term we use for nutrients that our bodies require in the largest amounts. These nutrients include carbohydrates, fats (lipids), and protein. We are able to calculate how much energy we receive from these nutrients through counting calories. **Calories** can tell us two things: how much energy we get from a food and how much energy we expel through physical activity.

CARBOHYDRATES

Carbohydrates are one of the main and most important fuel sources our body uses for energy. This basic fuel source is called *glucose*. Our body uses this *glucose* for energy immediately or stores the excess amounts as *glycogen* in the *muscle* and *liver*. For every gram consumed of carbohydrate, you receive four calories from that gram. There are two categories for carbohydrates: *simple and complex*.

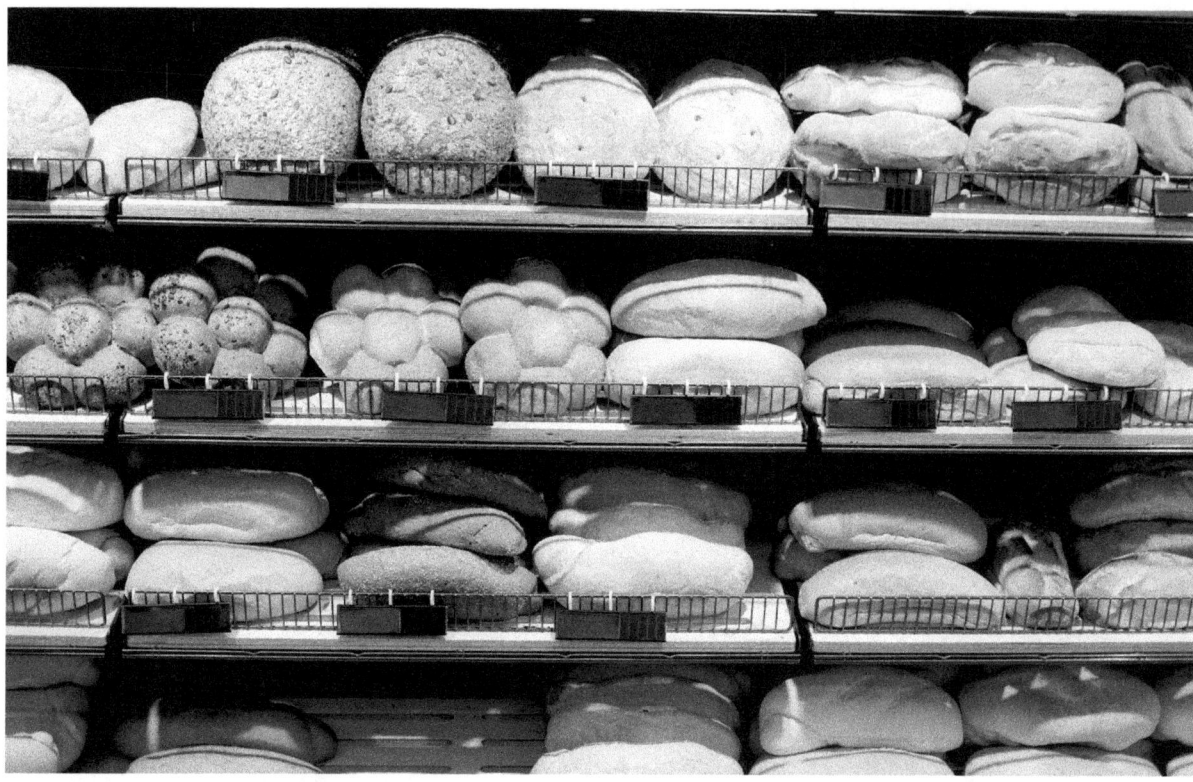

Figure 2.3: Bread.

Simple carbohydrates, known as the "sugars," do not provide a high nutritional value. These carbohydrates often have sugar added after the food has been processed and refined. Some examples include baked goods, candy, and soda. Two categories fall under **simple carbohydrates**, and they include monosaccharides and disaccharides.

Monosaccharides are the most basic and simple form of carbohydrate and include three main types: glucose, fructose, and galactose. Notice that all three end in the suffix **"ose,"** which in this case indicates that these are sugar molecules.

Table 2.7: Types of Carbohydrates

Glucose	Natural sugar obtained through food or broken down from other carbohydrates by the body. Provides energy, excess is stored as **glycogen** in our muscles and liver and can be used for energy later.
Fructose	Natural sugar found in fruits and honey, the body will convert fructose to glucose to be used for energy.
Galactose	Natural sugar found in milk, and like fructose, the body converts it to glucose to be used as energy.
High fructose corn syrup	Process of chemically changing glucose from cornstarch into fructose, therefore making a strong sweetener (found in baked goods, soda, bread, peanut butter, BBQ sauce, ketchup, etc.).

Too much consumption of these basic sugars, which are all broken down by the body into glucose, can lead to filling your **glycogen** stores. If you continue to consume more glucose and your body has not used up your filled **glycogen** stores, then the body will convert this excess glucose into fat to be stored in our **adipose**, or fat, tissue. And keep in mind fat takes longer to burn off as energy than does carbohydrates.

Disaccharides are two monosaccharides linked together. There are three important disaccharides: sucrose, lactose, and maltose. Again, notice these all end in the suffix **"ose,"** and these disaccharides are broken down by the body back into the simple monosaccharide to use glucose for energy.

Sucrose	Glucose + fructose (table sugar)
Lactose	Glucose + galactose (milk)
Maltose	Glucose + glucose (used to create fermented beer)[5]

Complex Carbohydrates are your healthier forms of carbohydrates, whole grains that take the body more time to digest and break down. There are two categories for complex carbohydrates, and they are *polysaccharides* and *fiber*.

Polysaccharides consist of 10 or more monosaccharide chains linked together. There are three types of polysaccharides: starches, dextrins, and glycogen.

Starch	This is a plant's method of storing glucose. When we consume a starchy food, our body will convert the starch into a form we can use for energy, *glucose*.
Dextrin	Dextrins are a byproduct of large starch molecules breaking down, many times through dry heat. They provide a good source of fiber.
Glycogen	The body converts glucose into glycogen to store it. It can also be found in small amounts in meat products, but for the most part, our body creates it. When glucose is depleted and enzymes within our muscles and liver are then released to break apart the glycogen links that we have stored and goes through a process to converting some glycogen back into glucose for energy use.

Fiber comes in two forms: *soluble* and *insoluble* fiber. Within these forms are multiple types of fiber such as cellulose, pectins, and gums. Fiber is also a complex carbohydrate with many health benefits. It helps fill us up without the excessive calories, helps decrease our risk for heart disease as it helps scrape our arteries clean, as well as helps promote bowel movements. Fiber initiates the process of *peristalsis* in our bowels, which is the involuntary, wave-like contractions along the walls of the intestines that forces contents within to move forward, thus producing a bowel movement. On average, it is recommended that men who are 50 years old or younger consume 38 grams of fiber a day and women who are 50 years old or younger consume 25 grams per day. Fiber is mainly found in plant foods such as fruits, vegetables, and legumes, specifically in the skins, seeds, and roots of the foods. Fiber can also be found in whole grain breads and cereals. *Soluble* fiber types can dissolve in water, and when they do, they create a gel-like substance that surrounds food and swells up, kind of like grabbing the leftover food in the body. In doing so, the fiber is able to pull and excrete fats from the body and has been proven to control blood glucose levels and lower cholesterol. *Insoluble* fiber cannot absorb or dissolve in water well, if at all, and therefore moves through our body in almost its original form. We do not digest this fiber, as this is the fiber type that initiates the *peristalsis* and causes softer and bulkier stools. This type of fiber has been shown to lower the risk of colon cancer, as it reduces the time food sits in the intestines and colon. With quick passage, there is less time for the food items to build up and become toxic to the system. Although it seems like fiber only provides positive health benefits, remember you never want too much of anything. Too much fiber can cause bloating and constipation, especially if you aren't drinking fluids, so if you increase your fiber intake, make sure you increase your fluid intake as well[6].

TIPS FOR CHOOSING HEALTHY CARBS

- Choose whole grains: when picking a cold cereal, read the ingredient list; make sure the first ingredient listed is whole grain, and check the sugar amount on the label. If you prefer hot cereal like oatmeal, avoid instant and choose steel-cut oats or old-fashioned oats. In general, look for cereals with at least four grams of fiber and less than eight grams of sugar per serving.
- If you enjoy breads and sandwiches for lunch time, make sure to choose whole grain breads. Again, look at the first ingredient, and make sure it says whole wheat/grain, whole rye, or any other whole grain.
- Oftentimes, breads can be high in sodium; try a different type of whole grain like brown rice, bulgur wheat, or quinoa.
- Avoid juices, as these can be higher in sugars; instead, choose raw, whole fruits, which have more fiber and less sugar compared to juice.
- Beans and legumes (i.e., chickpeas) are an excellent carbohydrate source in comparison to potatoes. These carbs are complex and therefore digested slower by the body, and these options also provide some protein[7,8,9,10,11]!

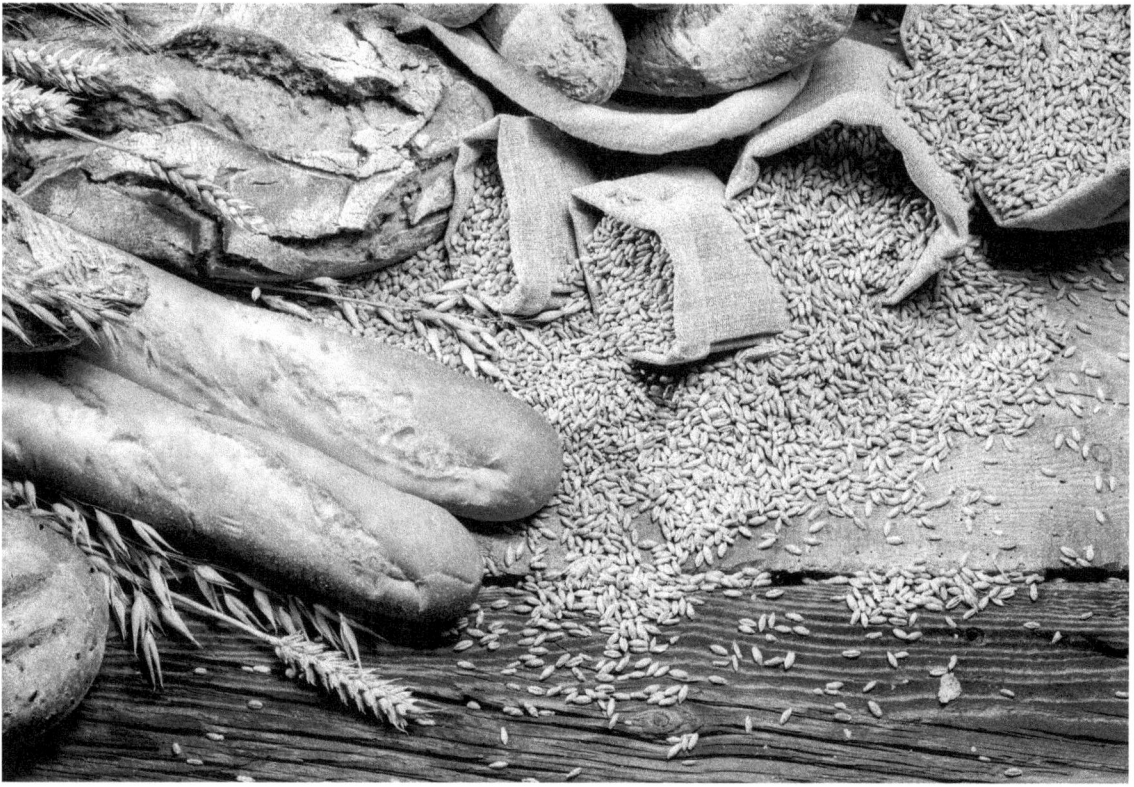

Figure 2.4: Whole Grains.

The table below provides some examples of healthy carbohydrate and fiber options. These foods are high in complex carbohydrates and fiber but low in fats and sugars, which make them great options.

Table 2.8: Food by Carbohydrates and Fiber

Food	Serving Size	Grams of Carbs	Grams of Fiber	Total Calories
Apple	1 medium	22	5	80
Barley	100 grams	175	6	193
Canned Pinto Beans	1 cup	37	11	206
Lentils	1 cup, raw	122	21	675
Steel-Cut Oatmeal	1 cup	108	16	600
Spinach	1 cup, raw	1	1	7
Spaghetti Squash	1 cup, baked	10	2	42
Sweet Potato	1, raw	26	4	112
Whole Wheat Bread	1 slice (1 oz)	13	2	70
Zucchini	1 large, raw	9	4	46[12,13]

FAQs CHECK!

Research on plant consumption and heart disease...

Repeatedly, research shows that diet is one of the major keys to long-term health and prevention of major health "events," an example being a stroke or a heart attack. The average American diet is unfortunately absent of many essential vitamins and minerals, and generally, we eat a lot of refined and processed foods instead of fruits and vegetables. Yet studies have shown that not only can we slow heart disease, but a strong plant-based diet can even reverse it. In a study of 198 people with heart disease, 177 were able to stick to a plant-heavy diet for over four years. Only one of them had an event, in this case a stroke, but of the 21 people who had quit the diet, 13 of them had some form of an event. Another study found a major difference when comparing the American Heart Association's recommended diet to a plant-heavy Mediterranean diet, with the Mediterranean diet showing 70% less heart attacks and death[53].

PROTEIN

Protein is a necessary nutrient that has a variety of functions in our body. They are comprised of thousands of smaller cell units that we call *amino acids*. Similar to carbohydrates, for every gram of protein consumed, you receive four calories from that gram. There are a total of 20 different amino acids that can combine with one another to create a protein. Of these 20 amino acids, nine of them are *essential* amino acids, ones that we can only obtain through our diet, whereas the remaining 11 are *non-essential* and can be created in our body. A protein that includes all nine essential amino acids is referred to as a "*complete protein*" or "higher-quality protein." If a food item is missing one or more of the nine essential amino acids, it is then called an "*incomplete protein*" or "lower-quality protein." The main food sources to find complete proteins are in animal products (meats, milk, dairy, and meat alternatives). Because the majority of sources with high amounts of protein come mainly from animal products, consumers must be careful, as animal products also increase your blood cholesterol levels since many of them contain saturated fat (discussed later).

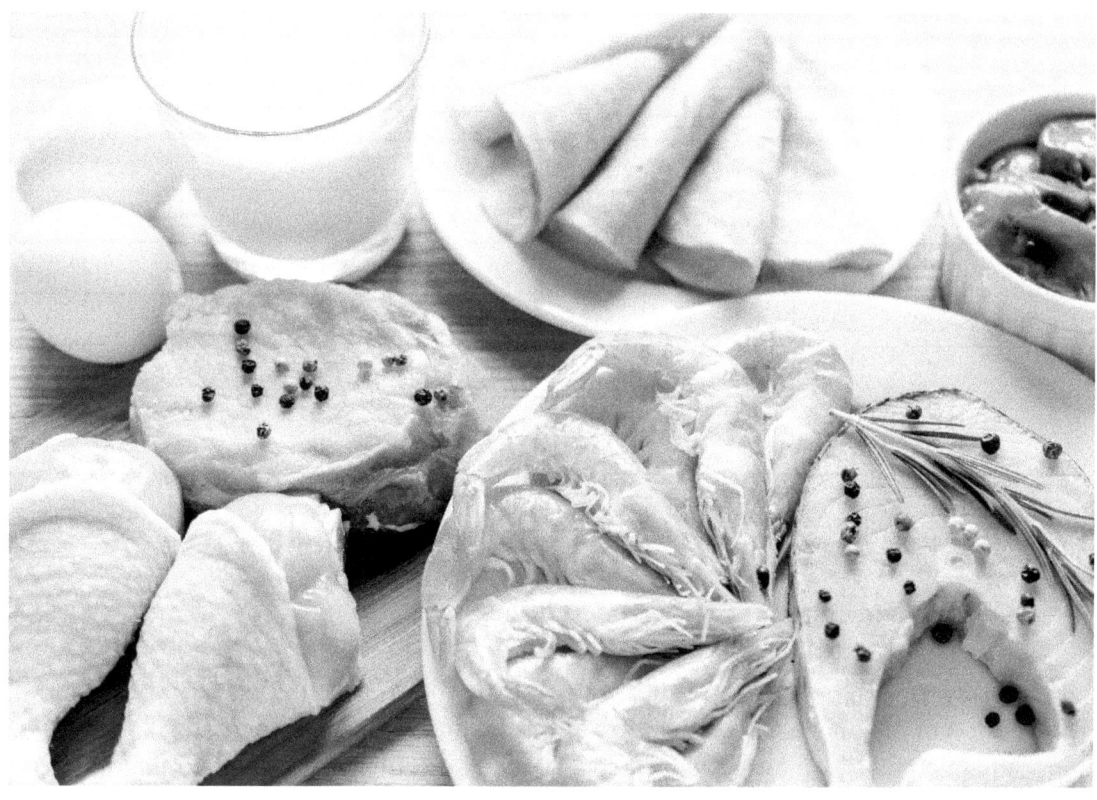

Figure 2.5: Proteins.

There are multiple types of proteins (see table below). Some of the key functions proteins provide include building and repairing our muscle, tissues, internal organs, skin, hair, nails, and bones, boosting our immune system, controlling our blood sugar, transporting molecules, helping with digestion, and helping with synthesizing new molecules such as red blood cells. Protein can also be used to provide our body with energy; however, this only occurs when our body does not have sufficient carbohydrates available to use as fuel. Protein can be converted to glucose, fat, or excreted through the kidneys. Overconsumption of protein should not occur long term. Increasing your protein intake can be beneficial in losing weight and helping you feel full. However, sometimes these high-protein, low-carb diets can lead to other nutritional deficiencies, increase your risk of heart disease due to the increased fat intake from animal products, and if you have kidney disease, it may make it worse, as the kidneys already have a more difficult time processing out the waste products. There is still not enough significant research to clearly identify the risks of a high-protein diet (Martin, Armstrong and Rodriguez, 2005)[15,16,17].

Table 2.9: Types of Protein

Enzymes	Causes chemical reactions within the body; for example, pepsin (a digestive enzyme that helps break down proteins in food)
Antibodies	Produced by your immune system to fight and remove infections
DNA-associated	Regulates chromosomal structure during cell division
Contractile	Proteins such as actin and myosin that help with muscle contraction and movement
Structural	Collagen is an example of a structural protein that helps support our body's connective tissues
Hormone	Help control body functions; for example, insulin controls our body's uptake of glucose
Transport	Hemoglobin is a protein molecule that helps transport oxygen throughout our blood[14]

The table below provides some examples of healthy protein options that are high in protein but low in fat or mostly a healthy fat (i.e., nuts). Be careful with some items, as they can have high amounts of sodium. Always try to avoid processed meats, fried foods, shortening, etc.

Table 2.10: Protein-based foods

Food	Serving Size	Grams of Protein	Total Calories
Pinto Beans	1 cup	12	206
Black Beans, boiled	1 cup	15.2	240
Broccoli	1 cup	3	31
Bulgur, cooked	1 cup	5.6	151
Chickpeas, boiled	1 cup	14.5	269
Cod	3 oz.	18	104
Cottage Cheese (low sodium and fat)	½ cup	12	90
Dried Lentils	¼ cup	13	160
Edamame	½ cup	8	100
Eggs	1 large	6	72
Greek Yogurt	1 container (5.3 oz)	15	90
Lean Beef (97%)	3 oz.	17	98
Lentils, boiled	1 cup	17.9	230
Nuts (Almonds)	½ cup	15	414
Peanut Butter	2 tablespoons	7	190
Quinoa	½ cup	4	111

(Continued)

Food	Serving Size	Grams of Protein	Total Calories
Skinless Poultry	3 oz. breast	13	107
Spinach, boiled	1 cup	5	41
Soy Milk	8 oz.	11	127
Tempeh	½ cup	15	160
Tofu	½ cup	10	88
Whey Protein	1 scoop	25	150
Whole-Wheat Bread	1 slice	3	70
Yellowfin Tuna	3 oz.	20	115

Table 2.11: Recommended Protein Intakes

Lifestyle	Grams per lb of Body Weight
Sedentary adult	0.4 (i.e., 140 lbs = 56 grams/day)
Recreational exerciser, adult	0.5–0.7
Endurance athlete	0.6–0.7
Growing teenage athlete	0.7–0.9
Adult building muscle mass	0.7–0.8
Athlete restricting calories	0.8–0.9
Avg. protein intake of male endurance athlete	0.5–0.9
Avg. protein intake of female endurance athlete	0.5–0.8 (i.e., 140 lbs = 70g – 112g)

FAQs CHECK!

High-Protein Diets and Research?

The current trend for those trying to lose weight while still needing calories to exercise is to exchange the carbohydrates and fats usually eaten with protein. This is common not only among power lifters and bodybuilders, but also the average person and seen in diets like the Atkins and South Beach diets. This allows for the individual to lose the excess nutrients that are not used as fuel instead of storing them. However, a study of over 7,000 men and women showed an association between protein substituting carbohydrates in a diet and a 59% increase in risk of premature death. Other studies have specifically noted that high and/or excessive protein usage can lead to cancer, osteoporosis, and heart-related diseases. While this is not a clear cause and effect, researchers note that more scientific studies need to be conducted in this area[15,52].

FATS (LIPIDS)

Out of all the macronutrients, fats are the most concentrated energy source, as they provide us with nine calories per gram of fat consumed. We need fat for multiple reasons: it provides warmth, helps absorb shock if we fall, and helps transport certain nutrients throughout our body. Fat also allows us to store certain vitamins (A, D, E, and K) known as the fat-soluble vitamins. Cholesterol is a form of fat we will be discussing in this section; there are two forms of cholesterol that are most important when talking about cholesterol levels. HDL is considered the healthy cholesterol, and we want to have higher amounts of this type; LDL is the negative cholesterol, and our goal is to have lower levels of this type in our blood. There are three categories that fall under fats: simple, compound, and derived fats.

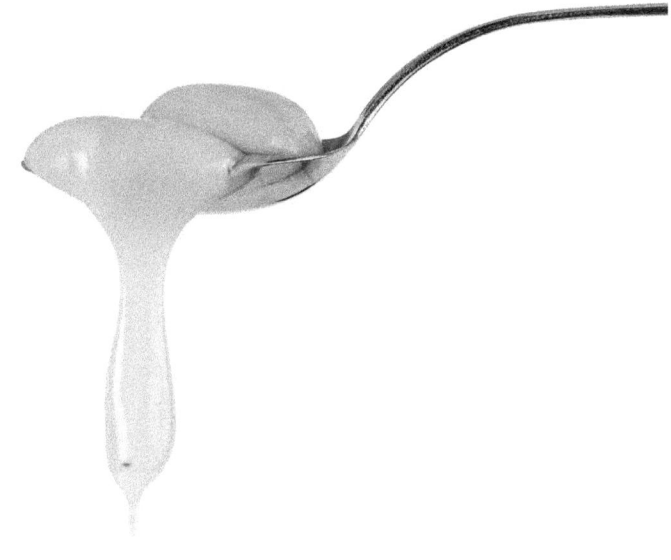

Figure 2.6: Egg yolk contains lipids that provide energy.

Simple fats include saturated and unsaturated fats, trans fatty acids, and polyunsaturated essential omega fatty acids. Unsaturated fats break down into two categories: monounsaturated and polyunsaturated. Simple fats are considered monoglycerides, diglycerides, or triglycerides depending on how many fatty acid chains are attached to the glyceride molecule.

Saturated fats are primarily found in animal products (meats, dairy, etc.) and are considered the unhealthy fat. These types of fats increase the bad cholesterol, or LDL. Saturated fats are fat molecules without double bonds between carbon molecules because they are instead saturated with hydrogen molecules. These fats also generally do not melt at room temperature. The American Heart Association recommends that only five to six percent of an individual's diet consist of saturated fat, so for example, a person on a 2,000 calorie diet should only consume approximately 13 grams of saturated fat a day[19].

Unsaturated fats are mainly of plant origin, specifically in oils, and considered the healthy fat choice. Some unsaturated fat types are also found in fish. These fats are healthy because they help lower the LDL cholesterol from the blood by stimulating the liver to release enzymes that remove this cholesterol. Unsaturated fats break down into two categories: monounsaturated fatty acids (MUFA) and polyunsaturated fatty acids (PUFA). Monounsaturated fatty acids mainly consist of omega-3s, whereas polyunsaturated fatty acids consist of omega-6s and omega-9s. Keep in mind, some oils can consist of both mono- and polyunsaturated fats, but in the table below, they are categorized as to which fatty acid they have more of.

Table 2.12: List of MUFA & PUFA

MUFA	PUFA
Avocado Oil	Almonds
Avocados	Corn Oil
Canola Oil	Fish
Cashews	Grapeseed Oil
Olive Oil	Pecans
Peanut Oil	Safflower Oil
Peanuts	Soybean Oil
Rice Bran Oil	Sunflower Oil
Sesame Oil[20]	

According to the American Heart Association, you should choose oils that contain less than four grams of saturated fat per tablespoon and definitely avoid any partially hydrogenated (trans fats) oils. Some of the above oils come as blended oils, oftentimes called "vegetable oil"; these oils, even in the form of a cooking spray, are also healthy choices. Canola oil is especially healthy for our body; it has the closest requirement of fatty acids that our body needs that increase our cardiac health. Canola oil contains omega-3 fatty acids that also neutralize a substance called fibrinogen. Fibrinogen is a compound found in our blood that has been shown to increase clot formation (thrombosis) as well as inflammation[21].

Trans fats are created through a hydrogenation process. The purpose of this process is to increase shelf life of a food item as well as change semi-soft products into something more solid so they are easily spread. The way this is done is by adding a hydrogen molecule to either a monounsaturated fatty acid or a polyunsaturated fatty acid, which changes up the chain and creates a trans fatty acid. This process of changing a MUFA or PUFA is called partial hydrogenation. Trans fats are generally not naturally occurring (except in small amounts in meat and dairy); it is a chemical process that we do to make this fat. Therefore, these fats serve absolutely no health benefit to us and are not required in any amount by our body. In fact, these fats can potentially be even worse for your body than consuming saturated fats. Why is that? Because while saturated fats INCREASE your LDL, or bad cholesterol, trans fats INCREASE your LDL as well as DECREASE your HDL (good cholesterol). They have also been shown to increase your risk of blood clot formation. Avoid purchasing food items that list *partially hydrogenation* or *trans fatty acids* on the label. However, understand that the USDA (United States Department of Agriculture)/FDA (Food and Drug Administration) only require a food label to report any trans fats if the amount per serving is 0.5 grams or more. You may find a product with the claim on the front of the bag "0 grams trans fat!" Keep in mind that there may still be some traces—0.4 or fewer grams per serving—in that item. You must always check the ingredient list to look for any partially hydrogenated oils that may have been used. In past years, the Mayo Clinic gave the recommendation to not consume more than two grams of trans fat a day. So, if you are consuming a product that claims zero grams but really has 0.4 grams per serving and you eat four servings, then you are almost at the daily recommendation for trans fat. But as of June 16th, 2015, the FDA took action against trans fatty acids. There have been an abundance of studies showing the damage trans fats have on our health, specifically our cardiovascular system. Therefore, the FDA has officially declared that partially hydrogenated oils (PHOs) are not generally recognized as safe (GRAS), and food manufacturing companies will have three years to remove all PHOs from their products. This action is expected to have a positive impact on our nation's coronary heart disease dilemma as well as prevent heart attacks. The FDA does remind consumers, though, that small amounts of trans fats do occur naturally in small amounts of meat and dairy products[22,23,24].

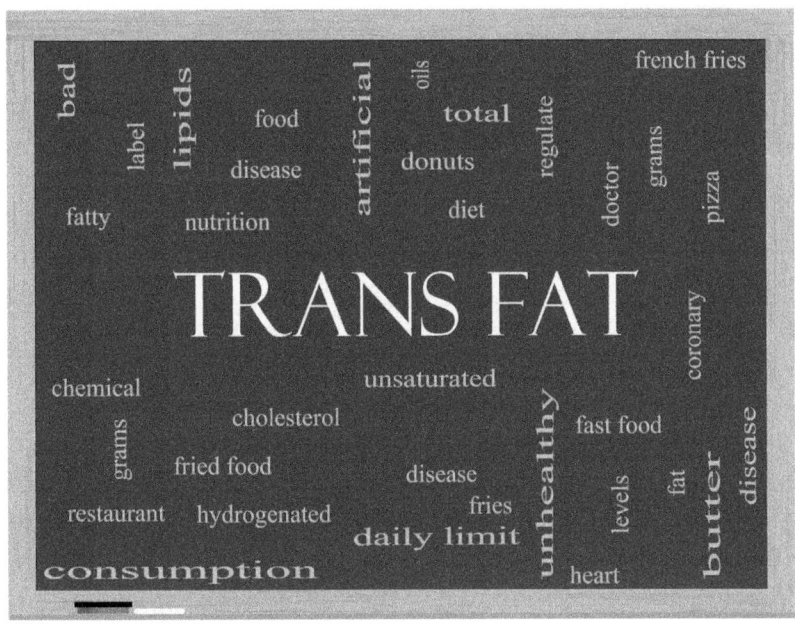

Figure 2.7: Transfat.

Table 2.13: Examples of Foods with Trans Fats

Cakes (store bought)
Coffee creamers
Cookies (store bought)
Crackers (store bought)
Ready-to-use frostings
Refrigerated dough products (biscuits and cinnamon rolls)
Some microwave popcorn
Stick margarines

Butter or margarine? This may have been a topic of debate among your friends or family; let's take a look at the differences. Refer to the adapted FDA table below to compare the differences.

Table 2.14: Comparing Margarine to Butter

Serving Size = 1 Tbsp (14g)					
Product	Calories	Total Fat g	Saturated Fat g	Trans Fat g	Combined Saturated and Trans Fats g	Cholesterol mg
Margarine, 80% fat, stick	100	11	2	3	5	0
Butter	100	11	7	0	7	30
Margarine, 60% fat, tub	80	9	1.5	0	1.5	0
Margarine, 70% fat, stick	90	10	2	2.5	4.5	0

There are also butter spreads available with options such as made with canola oil. After looking at the above table, you may be thinking, "Butter is the worst option because it has the highest combined saturated and trans fats!" But stop and think about what we already discussed. Although it has the highest combined, note that all seven are from saturated fat only. What did we just discuss about trans fats? There is absolutely no health benefit, and in fact, they are more damaging than saturated fats; hence, the FDA has made the decision to pull them off the market altogether. However, in this case, the 60% fat margarine tub would be the best option, as it only has 1.5 grams of saturated fat and zero grams of trans fat. Always read the ingredient list, do not just look at the label. In doing so, you would see the stick of butter only has cream and salt, whereas the margarine sticks would maybe have soybean oil listed first, and then partially hydrogenated oil, with a lot of items listed in parentheses after that[25].

Polyunsaturated Omega Fatty Acids have three classifications: omega-3, 6, and 9. Omega-3 and omega-6 fatty acids are most important to us, as we can only obtain these essential fats through our diet, whereas omega-9s can be synthesized in our body from other foods we consume. Omega-3 fatty acids have been shown to be the most beneficial to our health in a variety of ways, such as decreasing triglyceride levels and inflammation, decreasing our risk of blood clots, decreasing cholesterol levels, as well as helping control high blood pressure. Some of the best sources of fish with hefty amounts of omega-3s include mackerel, salmon, and herring. Flaxseeds also contain omega-3s, and more and more research is showing the many health benefits flaxseeds have to offer. Flaxseeds also contain anti-oxidants (discussed later in this chapter) and both soluble and insoluble fiber, and they reduce your LDL (bad cholesterol). Flaxseeds should be ground up for access to the nutrients inside the hard outer shell. Flaxseed is great because it can be used on and in almost anything and doesn't carry a flavor. It can

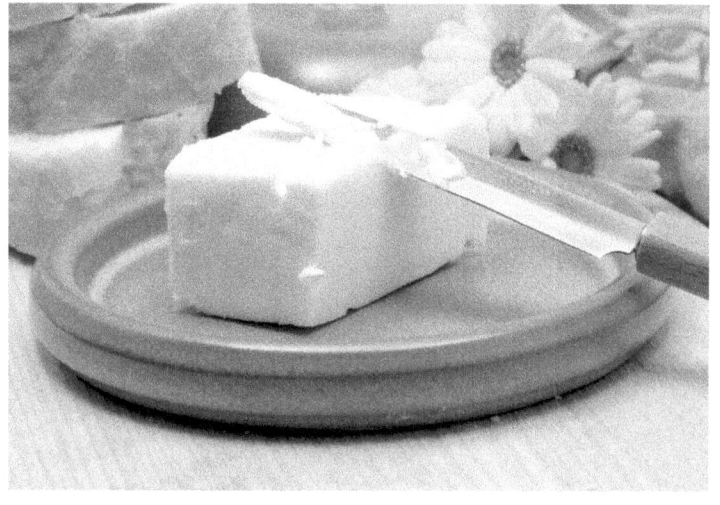

Figure 2.8: Butter.

be mixed in with yogurt, sprinkled in cereal or on toast, added into baked goods such as cookies, muffins, and pancakes, as well as added to salads and salad dressings.

Compound fats are simple fats that combine with another chemical. Some examples include phospholipids (phosphorus group is attached), glycolipids (carbohydrate attaches), and lipoproteins (protein attaches). Of these three, lipoproteins are one of the most important that we are going to discuss. These lipoproteins are necessary to transport fats (like cholesterol, which is a waxy substance) throughout our blood and body. Lipoproteins come in many forms, such as HDL (healthy cholesterol) and LDL (bad cholesterol). There are other types out there as well, such as VLDL and chylomicrons, but they're not discussed in this chapter. Our bodies need some cholesterol for certain functions such as the formation of cell membranes, the creation of hormones, Vitamin D and additional substances that assist with digestion.

LDL cholesterol increases development of **atherosclerosis**, or hardening of the arteries. It does so by contributing to plaque buildup, which is a thick, hard deposit from the bad cholesterol that has stuck to the arteries for some time. In doing so, it builds up, clogs the artery, and makes the artery rigid and less flexible. If the buildup narrows or almost blocks the artery, blood can pool in that area and form a clot that can also block blood flow or go through and can result in a heart attack or a stroke. Peripheral artery disease is a condition when plaque builds up in the arteries that supply blood to the legs, therefore affecting circulation to the legs.

HDL, on the other hand, does the opposite of LDL—it helps remove the LDL from the arteries. When it scrapes or picks up the LDL, it carries it back to the liver to be broken down and excreted from the body. Higher levels of HDL have been shown to protect against heart attacks and strokes.

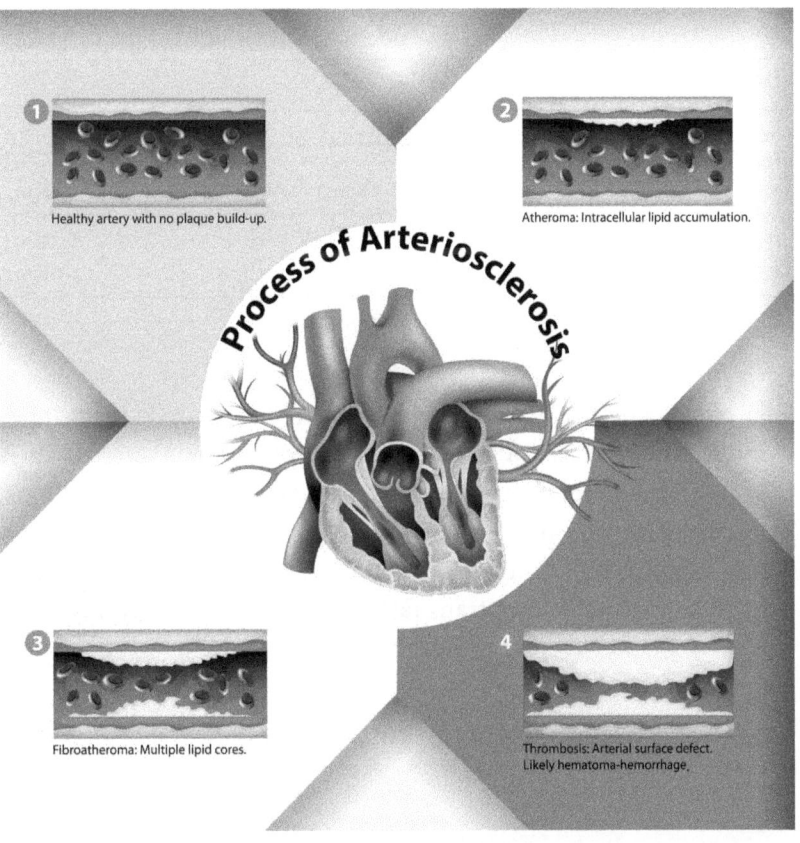

Figure 2.9: Hardening.

Your total cholesterol level includes triglycerides (formed from other fats we eat—saturated and trans fats), HDL, and LDL. It is recommended healthy adults keep their total cholesterol level below 200, and those who are at higher risk due to having coronary heart disease, diabetes, or have more than two risk factors should keep their total cholesterol level less than 180. To give you an idea of how much cholesterol is in a food item, one large boiled egg has approximately 187 mg of cholesterol. Some studies have also shown that lifestyle affects your triglyceride levels, such as being overweight, being physically inactive, and cigarette smoking. In many cases, individuals can adjust their lifestyle and see a drop in their triglyceride levels. The important thing is eating a well-balanced diet. As we previously discussed in this chapter, a variety of foods help reduce LDL. Please see the table below for a list of food items with LDL, HDL, and triglycerides. Keep in mind, avoiding foods with saturated, trans fats, and high cholesterol (as we have already discussed) will significantly help control and/or decrease your LDL and triglyceride levels. By eating foods high in soluble fiber, you will also help to decrease your LDL[26,27,28,29,30].

Table 2.15: A Look at HDL and LDL

HDL	LDL & Triglycerides
Apples	Cakes (store bought)
Avocados	Cheese
Beans and Legumes	Cookies (store bought)
Fish	Cottage Cheese
Flaxseed	Crackers (store bought)
Nuts (walnuts, almonds, pecans, etc.)	Ice Cream
Oatmeal	Margarine
Olive Oil	Processed Foods (sausage, hot dogs, cold cuts, etc.)
Whey Protein (studies have shown it lowers LDL and total cholesterol as a supplement)	Red Meats
Whole Grains	Sour Cream

Derived fats are a combination of a simple and compound fat bonded together. One of the most important types of derived fat is sterols. Although these do not contain any fatty acid chains, they are still considered a lipid, as they are not soluble in water. The most common sterol most everyone knows of is chole*sterol*. As discussed previously, there are two main types of cholesterol we are concerned with: the "bad," LDL, and the "good," HDL. Cholesterol is found in foods, and our bodies also manufacture cholesterol by breaking down saturated fats, trans fats, as well as refined carbohydrates.

Table 2.16: Food, Fat, and Calories

Food	Serving Size	Grams of Fat	Total Calories
2% milk	1 cup	5	121
Almonds	¼ cup	19	211
Apple	1	0	81
Avocado	½ cup	11	121
Bacon (pork)	1 slice	3	36
Blackberries	½ cup	0	37
Broccoli	½ cup	0	26
Carrots	½ cup	0	35
Chicken breast, skin removed	1 medium	3	161
Coleslaw with regular mayo	½ cup	21	211
Corn dog	1	25	341
Grilled ham and cheese Sandwich	1	21	392
Guacamole	¼ cup	8	93
Hot dog on bun, plain	1	15	258
Hot dog on bun, with chili and cheese	1	25	396
Hummus with olive oil	¼ cup	21	276
Lean ground beef (96% lean)	3 oz	3	122
Personal pan supreme pizza, Pizza Hut	1	49	944
Reese's peanut butter cup	1.6 oz. pkg. of 2	14	222
Regular cream cheese	2 Tbsp	10	101
Regular ground beef (80% lean)	3 oz	19	260
Scrambled eggs	2 medium	10	150
Turkey sub sandwich, Arby's	1	22	495[31]

Table 2.17: Energy Systems

Key terminology	
Anaerobic	Exercise that does not need oxygen to produce ATP
Aerobic	Exercise that does need oxygen to produce ATP
ADP (adenosine diphosphate)	Chemical compound comprised of adenosine and two phosphate groups
ATP (adenosine triphosphate)	Chemical compound comprised of adenosine and three phosphates to provide body immediate energy

Energy systems are the main component to providing our bodies with energy so we may be active. There are three energy systems we will discuss, and how much energy you need and what activity you are doing will determine which energy system(s) your body will utilize. The three systems are ATP-PC (sometimes listed as ATP-CP, ATP-PCr, or Phosphagen System), Glycolytic, and Oxidative. If you are participating in an activity that requires more energy, then the body will initiate each system as needed to make sure there is a continuous supply of energy. Understand that just because the body is using the Glycolytic or Oxidative Systems does not mean the previous systems stop. Previous systems continue to provide ATP (energy), it is just not enough ATP for the activity you may be doing, and therefore, the other systems engage to provide more ATP as needed. Recall the nutrients that can be used to provide us energy, the macronutrients: carbohydrates (glucose/glycogen), fats (fatty acids), and protein (amino acids). Also remember that if glucose is not used immediately for ATP (energy), it is then stored as glycogen in our muscles and liver. Excess fat that is not used for energy also gets stored. In this case, excess fatty acids will be stored in our adipose tissue as body fat, and protein, which really shouldn't be used as an energy source, as we will discuss later, is broken down into amino acids to be used in the body for things such as growth and repair or excreted out due to protein being rarely stored.

The *ATP-PC* system, or adenosine triphosphate-phosphocreatine, provides energy for muscle contraction immediately and does not require any oxygen to do so. Therefore, this system is anaerobic in nature. This system can provide energy for quick bursts for approximately eight to 10 seconds. Some activity examples include throwing a baseball, jumping, short sprint, weightlifting heavy resistance for approximately three reps, football, and gymnastics. This system is primarily utilizing stored ATP as the source for fuel. Our body stores very small amounts of ATP and phosphocreatine for quick access

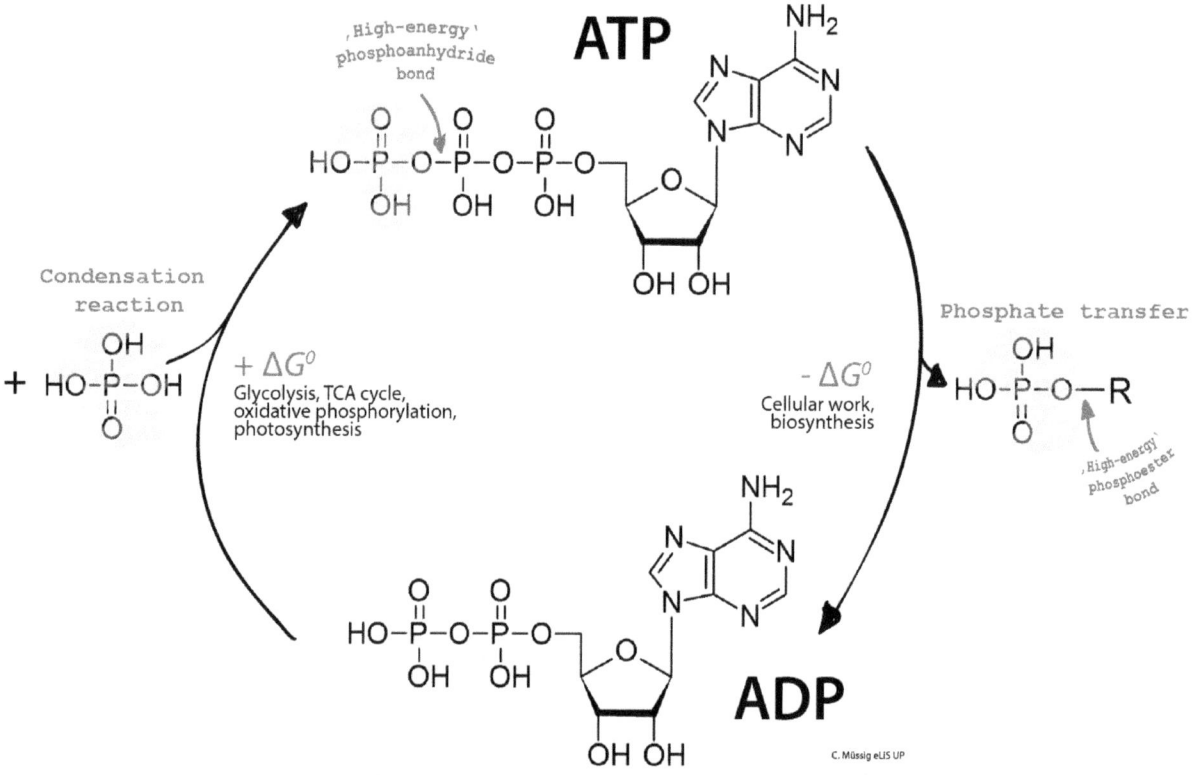

Figure 2.10: ATP System.

for energy. This system constantly rebuilds itself so long as it has phosphocreatine to do so. There is an enzyme called *ATPase* that acts on the ATP to separate the phosphorus; the splitting of the phosphate bond creates the energy we need. After the split, we are then left with ADP (adenosine diphosphate) and a phosphate. The way this system rebuilds is through the process of *Phosphorylation*. Another enzyme, called *Creatine Kinase*, brings the phosphate and creatine molecules together, creating the PC. This PC (phosphocreatine) then binds to the ADP we have left over to recreate a new ATP, and then the process repeats. The ATP-PC system can create energy at a rate of approximately 36 calories per minute.

If the body requires more energy than can be provided from the ATP-PC system, the next system is initiated, the *Glycolytic System*. This system can provide us energy for approximately one to three minutes. For the most part, the Glycolytic System is also anaerobic. This system can be broken down into fast and slow glycolysis, but for the purpose of this textbook, we will only discuss the basics of the system as a whole. When we enter this system, our body now utilizes carbohydrates (glucose and glycogen) as the main source for fuel/energy. There are a couple of processes that occur depending on what compound our body is breaking down for energy. *Glycolysis* occurs when our body breaks glucose down into ATP for energy. *Glycogenolysis* occurs when our body takes the stored glycogen from our muscles or liver to break down into glucose to then move on to the process of *Glycolysis*. Toward the end of this system, a byproduct called *pyruvic acid* is created. Remember, this system is generally anaerobic, and if our activity stops at the end of this system, the *pyruvic acid* will be changed into *lactic acid*, which builds up in our muscles and causes muscle fatigue. This system creates energy at approximately 16 calories per minute. Some activity examples include 200-yard run, one to two minutes in MMA, tennis, field hockey, short-distance swimming, and other stop-and-go sports. Now, this system does turn aerobic (with oxygen) if our activity continues on. In this case, once oxygen enters our system, instead of the *pyruvic acid* turning into *lactic acid*, it will turn into *Acetyl CoA (co-enzyme A)* and the lactic acid will be burned out. Our body will then move on to also using the *Oxidative System* as more energy is needed.

In the *Oxidative System*, our body is now utilizing oxygen to transform substances, such as carbohydrates, fats, and protein, into energy. This system is aerobic, and if our body has an oxygen deficit, then we cannot obtain the energy we require, which will cause exhaustion and a severe reduction in our activity intensity. When this system is activated, we are participating in physical activity that is continuously using large muscle groups for an extended period of time. Some examples include cross-country skiing, long-distance running or swimming, long-distance cycling, etc. It is estimated this system creates 10 calories per minute. In this system, energy can be created in three different ways: Kreb's Cycle, or Citric Acid Cycle, Electron Transport Chain (ETC), and Beta Oxidation (discussed later). When Acetyl CoA and glucose enter the Krebs Cycle, they go through a chain of reactions, and the outcome is ATP production (see table below, 2.18, to see how many ATP are created per system). Because this process causes acid buildup (extra hydrogen), there are two important byproducts that come into play: FAD/FADH and NAD/NADH. The acid/hydrogen binds with these byproducts and is then sent through the Electron Transport Chain (ETC), where it undergoes more chemical reactions, and the outcome provides us with even more ATP. The ETC provides the most ATP out of all processes (see table below). The Oxidative System allows an individual to endure longer activities without fatiguing out. Recall, fats give us nine calories per gram, so this is where they are providing us with more energy when we need it.

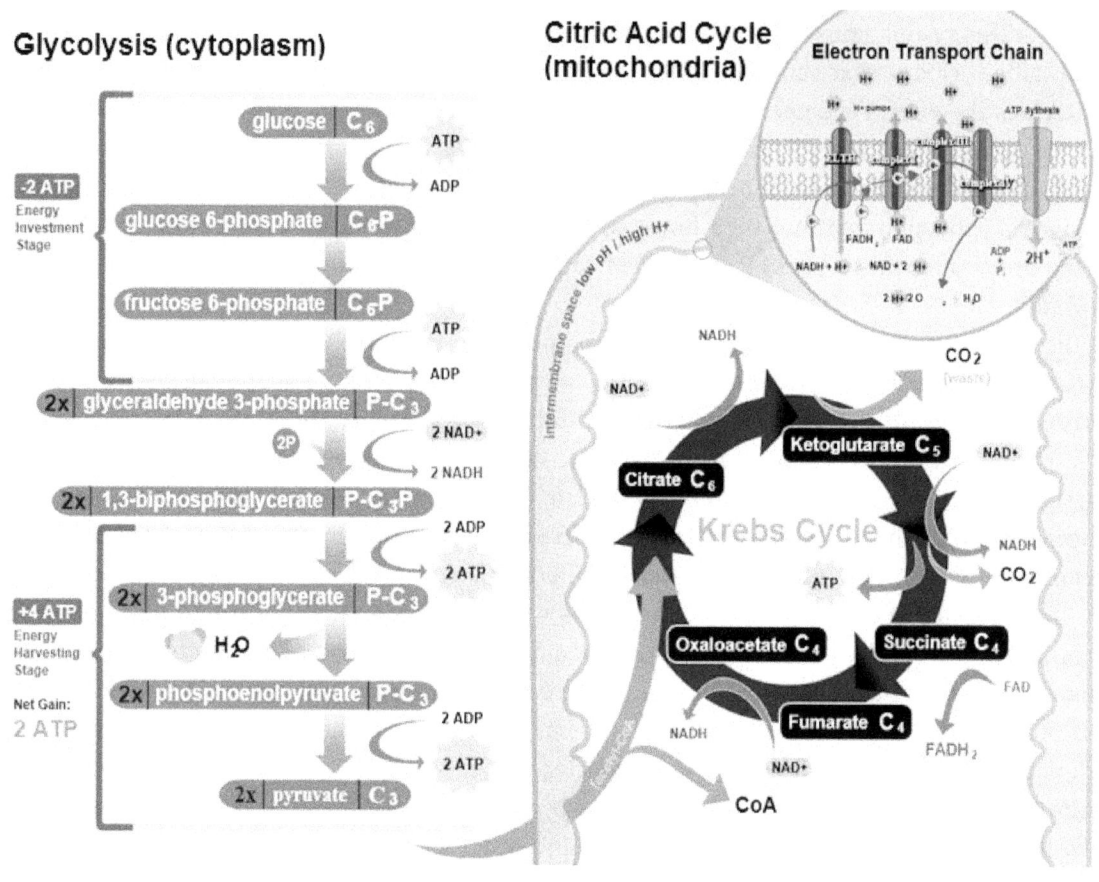

Figure 2.11: Glycolysis and the Kreb's Cycle.

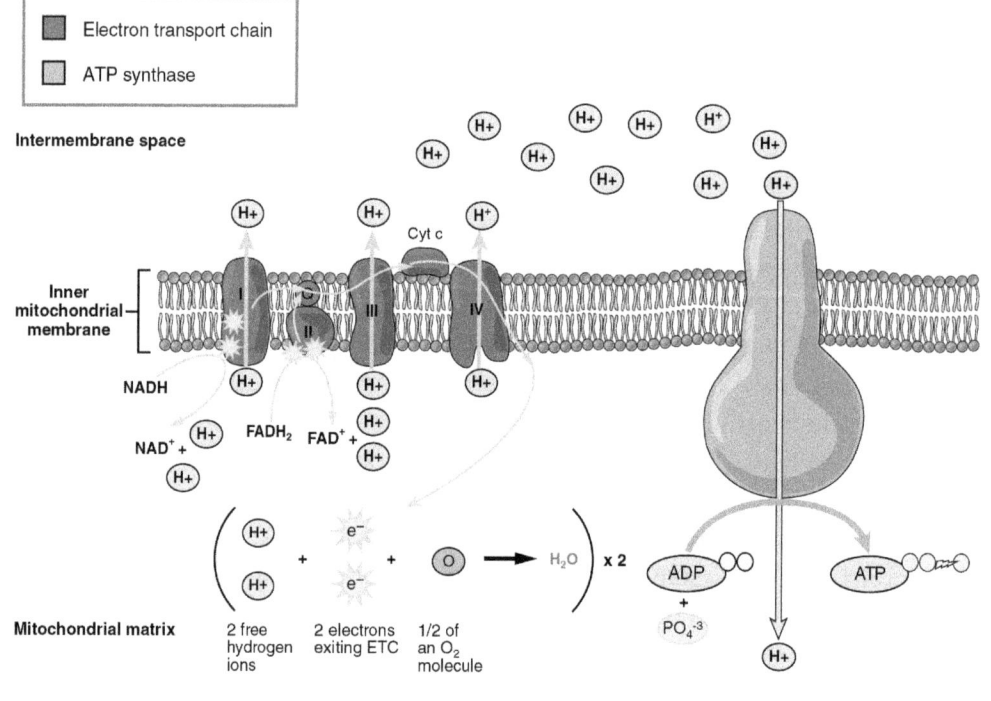

Figure 2.12: Electron Transport Chain.

Table 2.18: Energy Systems and ATP Production

System	Number of ATP Produced	Reason
ATP-PC	N/A	Since this is reclaiming ATP that was recently used, nothing "new" is produced.
Glycolytic	2	A highly involved process of glucose breakdown, transforming and creating few ATP.
Kreb's Cycle (Citric Acid)	2	Introducing oxygen into the glycolytic system grants a few more ATP.
Electron Transport Chain (ETC)	34	Through the re-oxidation (recycling) of the leftover 10 NADH and two FADH from previous work.

Table 2.19: Sport and Percentage of Energy Use

Sport	ATP-PC	Anaerobic Glycolytic	Aerobic
Basketball	60%	20%	20%
Field events (shotput, discus, javelin)	90%	10%	0%
Golf swing	95%	5%	0%
Gymnastics	80%	15%	5%
Hockey	50%	20%	30%
Rowing	20%	30%	50%
Running (distance)	10%	20%	70%
Skiing	33%	33%	33%
Soccer	50%	20%	30%
Swimming (50m freestyle)	40%	55%	5%
Tennis	70%	20%	10%

CARBS, FATS, AND PROTEIN USED AS FUEL

In general, carbohydrates (glucose/glycogen) are the main fuel source used for energy when our body is performing anaerobically (mainly in the glycolytic system). Each individual is different, but it takes approximately 15–20 minutes of being physically active before you start burning fat. Once you have used up all your glucose and glycogen for energy first, your body will switch over to burning fat. Protein is not, and should not, be a main source for fuel. This usually occurs in an emergency; for example, those with eating disorders or certain conditions will experience muscle wasting as the body pulls protein from the muscles to use as fuel because there is no glucose or fat available. Protein can also act as a fuel source for those on a decreased carb diet; however, they usually have increased their protein intake to fulfill their energy needs.

When moving into the Oxidative System, the Glycolytic System becomes aerobic: it uses the glucose/glycogen from the carbs we consume and changes them into Acetyl Coa. This substance then goes through changes as it circles through the Kreb's Cycle, or Citric Acid Cycle, and is then sent through the Electron Transport Chain (ETC) to create plenty of ATP. Once we have used up all of our glucose and glycogen stores, our body moves on to our stored fats. This is done through a process called lipolysis, where triglycerides are broken down into free fatty acids and glycerol. These free fatty acids are then sent through a process called beta oxidation, which changes them into Acetyl CoA, where it enters back into the Krebs Cycle and continues through the oxidative system just like glucose would. Protein goes through a process called gluconeogenesis, which means synthesis of new glucose from non-carbohydrate substances. The liver and kidneys help in this process to change protein into glucose. In some cases, it is converted into other sources, such as Acetyl CoA; however, protein does not supply energy at the same level that carbohydrates and fats do for us[34,35,36].

FAQs CHECK!

Will Protein Make Me Fat?

Some individuals become concerned that the protein they eat in excess of their immediate needs will be turned into glucose by spontaneous gluconeogenesis discussed earlier. Just because protein CAN be turned into glucose doesn't mean it WILL be turned into glucose. Gluconeogenesis is actually a very slow process, and the body tends to stay stable and has to be under pretty extreme conditions to use protein as a fuel source at high rates. In fact, most studies show that if you have an excess of protein in the system, it will not be turned into additional fuel unless the fuel is actually needed … not before. Therefore, it rarely will be stored and risk ever turning into fat [32,33].

MICRONUTRIENTS

Vitamins and minerals make up the micronutrients, as these are required by our body in small amounts. Don't underestimate the need for these substances, though; vitamins and minerals play many crucial roles in the functioning of our body. You can have toxic or deficient syndromes if you have too much or not enough of specific vitamins and minerals, which we will discuss some later in this section.

Vitamins help in utilizing carbohydrates, fats, and proteins, as well as other functions such as growth and releasing energy from food. Some vitamins we can only obtain through our diet, whereas others we can create in our body—for example, Vitamin D after sun exposure to our skin. Vitamins A, D, E, and K are fat-soluble vitamins, which means when these vitamins are ingested, our body can absorb and store excess and use later as needed. The B and C vitamins are water-soluble—we use what our body needs, and the rest is excreted through urination. Since the B and C vitamins are not stored, we must obtain these from our diet daily. Refer to Table 2.20 for a list of vitamins, sources of them as well as functions and signs of deficiency or excess.

Table 2.20: Vitamins

Fat-Soluble Vitamins					
	Recommended Daily Intake (RDI)	**Major Sources**	**Major Functions**	**Signs of Deficiency**	**Signs of Excess**
Vitamin A	Males 19–50: 900 mcg RAE Females 19–50: 700 mcg RAE	Cheese, milk, eggs, liver, spinach, dark leafy greens, deep orange fruits (cantaloupes)	Antioxidant, provides healthy bones, teeth, skin, and hair. Maintains inner mucous membranes and helps with immunity. Provides adequate vision	Night blindness, cracks in teeth, dry skin, higher risk to infections	Hair loss, skin rashes, liver failure, bone abnormalities
Vitamin D	Males and Females 19–50: 15 mcg	Sunlight exposure, fortified milk, eggs, liver, tuna, salmon	Mineralization of bone and teeth and needed for calcium and phosphorous absorption	Rickets (bowing of legs), fractures, soft bones, joint pain, muscle spasms	Increased blood calcium level, excessive thirst, kidney stones, headaches, nausea
Vitamin E	Males and Females 14+: 15 mg	Polyunsaturated plant oils/ vegetable oils, green and yellow leafy vegetables, whole grains, nuts, wheat germ	Antioxidant, stabilizes cell membranes, regulates oxidation reactions	Breakdown of red blood cells, anemia, leg cramps	Blurred vision, changes effect of anticlotting medications
Vitamin K	Males and Females 19+: 90 mcg	Green leafy vegetables, cabbage, peas, potatoes, cauliflower, soybeans, vegetable oils	Needed for blood clotting	Hemorrhage	Interferes with anticlotting medications
Water-Soluble Vitamins					
	Recommended Daily Intake (RDI)	**Major Sources**	**Major Functions**	**Signs of Deficiency**	**Signs of Excess**
Vitamin B$_1$ (Thiamin)	Males 14+: 1.2 mg Females 19+: 1.1 mg	Whole grains, legumes, liver, pork, fish, poultry, nuts	Helps utilize carbohydrates, supports normal appetite and nervous system function	Nausea, confusion, loss of appetite, enlarged heart, muscle spasms	None known

(Continued)

Water-Soluble Vitamins					
	Recommended Daily Intake (RDI)	**Major Sources**	**Major Functions**	**Signs of Deficiency**	**Signs of Excess**
Vitamin B$_2$ (Riboflavin)	Males 14+: 1.3 mg Females 19+: 1.1 mg	Eggs, milk, leafy green vegetables, whole grains, lean meats	Helps release energy from carbohydrates, fats, and proteins. Provides normal growth, vision, and skin health	Magenta tongue, corners of the mouth are cracked, impaired vision, skin rash/inflammation	None known
Vitamin B$_6$ (Pyridoxine)	Males 14–50: 1.3 mg Females 19–50: 1.3 mg	Whole grains, meats, potatoes, soy products, fish, legumes	Metabolizes fatty acids and proteins and helps with red blood cell formation	Anemia, muscle spasms, nausea, depression	Impaired memory, irritability, headaches, loss of reflexes
Vitamin B$_{12}$	Males and Females 14+: 2.4 mcg	Meat, poultry, fish, eggs, milk, cheese, liver	Synthesizes new red blood cells, helps with growth, and functioning of nervous system and digestive tract	Anemia, weakness, disorientation, fatigue, nervous system degeneration	None known
Vitamin C (Ascorbic Acid)	Males 19+: 90 mg Females 19+: 75 mg Smokers: +35 mg more	Citrus fruits, dark green vegetables, peppers, cantaloupe, strawberries, mangoes, tomatoes	Antioxidant, forms collagenous tissue (strengthens blood vessel walls), provides protection against infection, helps absorb iron, and restores vitamin E to active form	Bleeding gums, frequent infections, loose teeth, slow-healing wounds, hemorrhaging, joint pain, fragility	Diarrhea, abdominal cramps, nausea, rashes, fatigue
Niacin	Males 14+: 16 mg Females 14+: 14 mg	Whole grains, liver, meat, poultry, fish, nuts, dried beans and peas	Helps metabolize energy from carbohydrates, fats, and proteins. Also helps form hormones and nervous system substances	Black smooth tongue, loss of appetite, confusion, depression, weakness, diarrhea, weight loss	Nausea, vomiting, sweating, blurred vision, liver damage, impaired glucose tolerance

(Continued)

Water-Soluble Vitamins					
	Recommended Daily Intake (RDI)	**Major Sources**	**Major Functions**	**Signs of Deficiency**	**Signs of Excess**
Folic Acid (Folate)	Males and Females 19+: 400 mcg	Leafy green vegetables, legumes, liver, whole grains, whole grain cereals, dried beans	Helps create new cells and helps form red blood cells	Anemia, increased risk for infections, smooth red tongue, depression, confusion	Hides vitamin B_{12} deficiency
Pantothenic Acid	Males and Females 14+: 5 mg	Natural foods such as liver, kidney, yeast, milk, nuts, eggs, green leafy vegetables	Helps metabolize carbohydrates and fats	Low blood sugar, vomiting, depression, leg cramps, insomnia, fatigue, nausea, headaches	None known
Biotin	Males and Females 19+: 30 mcg	Natural foods such as liver, kidney, yeast, milk, nuts, dark green vegetables	Required for metabolizing carbohydrates and manufacturing fatty acids	Muscle pain, depression, loss of appetite, nausea, inflammation of the skin	None known

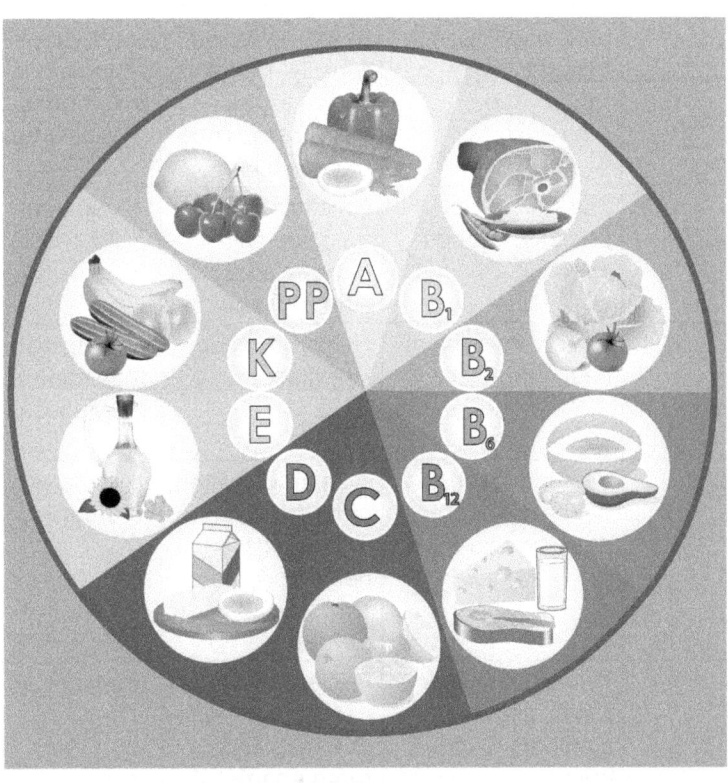

Figure 2.13: Vitamin and Related Foods.

Minerals also play a vital role in a variety of body functions. They are especially important in helping our bodies maintain homeostasis, or internal stability, with our water and acid-base balance. Minerals are substances usually found in the hard parts throughout our body such as bones, teeth, and nails. Some other functions include blood clotting, controlling our heart rhythm, and regulation of our nervous and muscular impulses. Let's discuss a couple of select minerals and their importance. Magnesium helps stabilize the structure of ATP (energy), as well as helps with synthesizing other substances such as protein, fatty acids, and glucose into ATP. Magnesium also plays a large role in our muscular contraction by helping it to relax (calcium is the stimulator/contractor). Toxicity or large/excess doses of magnesium can cause a sedative effect. This is why some people choose to consume or purchase magnesium tablets to take at bedtime to help them sleep!

Phosphorous is another example of a mineral we need; this substance binds with creatine to make more ATP (energy), if you recall when we discussed this phosphocreatine earlier in the energy system section. Also, zinc helps in synthesizing and degrading our macronutrients, so if you are lacking micronutrients, it could potentially affect the rest of your body's functions, including its ability to use your macronutrients properly[36,37].

Refer to Table 2.21 for a list of minerals, sources of them as well as functions and signs of deficiency or excess.

Table 2.21: Minerals

Minerals	Recommended Daily Intake (RDI)	Major Sources	Major Functions	Signs of Deficiency	Signs of Excess
Calcium	Males and Females 19–50: 1,000 mg	Milk, yogurt, tofu, green leafy vegetables, dried beans/legumes, salmon, tofu, oysters	Essential for strong bones and teeth, helps with muscle, nerve, and heartbeat activity, helps with blood clotting	Weak bones or bone loss (osteoporosis), bone pain and/or fractures, muscle cramps	Calcium deposits in kidneys, constipation, decreased absorption of other minerals
Chloride	Males and Females 14–50: 2.3 g	Soy sauce, salt, processed foods	Helps maintain fluid and acid-base balance, aids in digestion	Doesn't normally occur	Vomiting
Chromium	Males 19–50: 35 mcg Females 19–50: 25 mcg	Liver, whole grains, beer, wine	Helps the body use glucose	Unstable glucose control, weight loss	None known
Copper	Males and Females 19+: 900 mcg	Seafood, beans, whole grains, drinking water	Aids in formation of hemoglobin and collagen, helps body absorb iron and use oxygen	Anemia, growth retardation	If nonfood source is consumed in excess: diarrhea, vomiting, liver disease
Fluoride	Males 18+: 4 mg Females 14+: 3 mg	Fluoridated water, foods, and beverages, tea, shrimp, crab	Prevent tooth decay, component of bones and tooth enamel	Tooth decay	Brittle bones, mottled teeth, vomiting, diarrhea

(Continued)

Minerals	Recommended Daily Intake (RDI)	Major Sources	Major Functions	Signs of Deficiency	Signs of Excess
Iodine	Males and Females 14+: 150 mcg	Seaweed, seafood, iodized salt, bread	Part of thyroid hormones to regulate energy production and growth	Goiter, cretinism in newborns	Decreased thyroid function, pimples, goiter
Iron	Males 19–50: 8 mg Females 19–50: 18 mg	Red meats, organ meats, legumes, nuts, eggs, green leafy vegetables	Helps transport oxygen, major component of hemoglobin, also helps with energy metabolism	Anemia, fatigue, weakness, pale appearance, reduced attention span	Abdominal pain, vomiting, organ damage, blue coloring of skin, shock
Magnesium	Males 19–30: 400 mg Females 19–30: 310 mg	Whole grains, dark green vegetables, nuts, seafood, chocolate, cocoa	Helps with bone growth and maintenance, nerve activity, temperature regulation, energy and protein formation, immune function	Weakness, stunted growth in children, muscle spasms, irregular heartbeat, sleeplessness, personality changes, hallucinations	If nonfood source is consumed in excess: dehydration, diarrhea, acid-base (pH) imbalance
Manganese	Males 19–30: 2.3 mg Females 19–30: 1.8 mg	Whole grains, tea, nuts, dried beans, coffee	Help form body fat and bone	Unlikely to occur	Muscle spasms, infertility in men, disrupt nervous system activity
Molybdenum	Males and Females 19–50: 45 mcg	Dark green vegetables, milk, dried beans, grains, liver	Helps transfer oxygen	None known	None known
Phosphorous	Males and Females 18+: 700 mg	Milk, eggs, fish, legumes, milk, whole grains, meats, dried beans and peas	Essential for bone and teeth formation, helps metabolize energy and maintains cell membranes	Impaired growth, bone pain, muscle weakness, fractures, weight loss	Calcification of soft tissues, especially in kidneys
Potassium	Males and Females 19+: 4.7 g	Bananas, legumes, whole grains, legumes, orange juice, dried fruits, potatoes	Helps maintain fluid, acid-base balances, required for muscle and nerve activity, essential for heart action	Irregular heartbeat (dysrhythmia), nausea, weakness, confusion, paralysis	Heart attack, vomiting, irregular heartbeat, muscle weakness
Selenium	Males and Females 19–50: 55 mcg	Seafood, meats, whole grains, eggs	Antioxidant in conjunction with vitamin E, regulates thyroid hormone	Possibility of hair loss and nail loss, muscle pain, anemia, heart failure, possible deterioration of heart muscle	Weakness, skin rash, garlic or metallic breath

(Continued)

Minerals	Recommended Daily Intake (RDI)	Major Sources	Major Functions	Signs of Deficiency	Signs of Excess
Sodium	Males and Females: Limit to 2,300 mg/day With HTN: Limit 1,500 mg/day	Processed foods, table salt, meats, soy sauce	Required to maintain fluid and acid-base balance in body, transmits nerve impulses, heart action	Unlikely to occur—possibly muscle cramps, poor appetite	High blood pressure, edema (swelling)
Sulfate	N/A	Protein-containing foods	Helps stabilize protein shape, component of specific amino acids	Unlikely to occur	None known
Zinc	Males 14+: 11 mg Females 19+: 8 mg	Meats, seafood, poultry, shellfish, whole grains, nuts, milk	Component of insulin, hormones, and enzymes, helps transport vitamin A	Slow-healing wounds, loss of appetite, growth failure, skin problems	Impaired immunity, reduces copper and iron absorption, fatigue, metallic taste

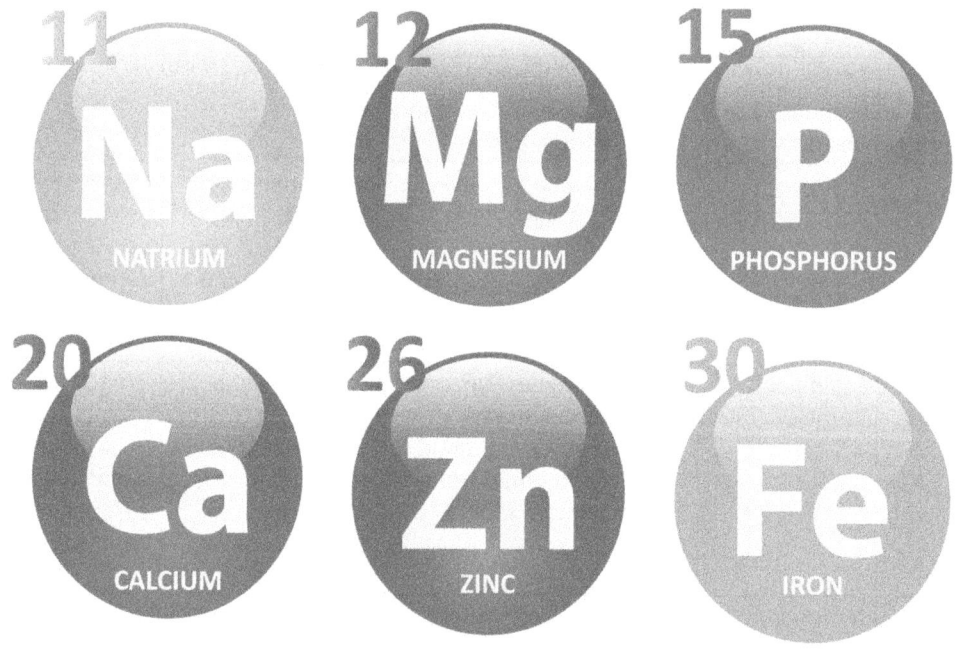

Figure 2.14: Minerals.

WATER

Water is not necessarily categorized as a "macro" or "micro"; however, it is one of the most essential nutrients that we must consume on a daily basis. Water provides a variety of functions, including absorbing nutrients, digesting foods, excreting waste, lubricating our joints, preventing dehydration, and keeping us cool. If an adult loses approximately 20% of their body's water, then death is possible. Each individual will have a different amount of water makeup in their body (anywhere from 45–85% of total body weight) depending on their weight and gender. In an adult female who weighs approximately 130 pounds, her body is about 50% water; this includes intracellular and extracellular water. In a male who weighs 150 pounds, his body is approximately 54% water. In most cases, men will have a higher percentage of water weight than women due to the higher amount of muscle mass. Almost all reactions that take place within our body require water; therefore, we need to constantly replace what is lost and used. The daily recommended intake is about three liters for men and 2.2 liters for women. We should consume water through liquid sources, but almost all foods also contain water. Keep in mind caffeinated drinks act as a diuretic and increase the amount you excrete, which can quickly lead to dehydration. Generally speaking, you should not wait until you become thirsty to start drinking fluids, as by this point you may have already lost too much[38,39].

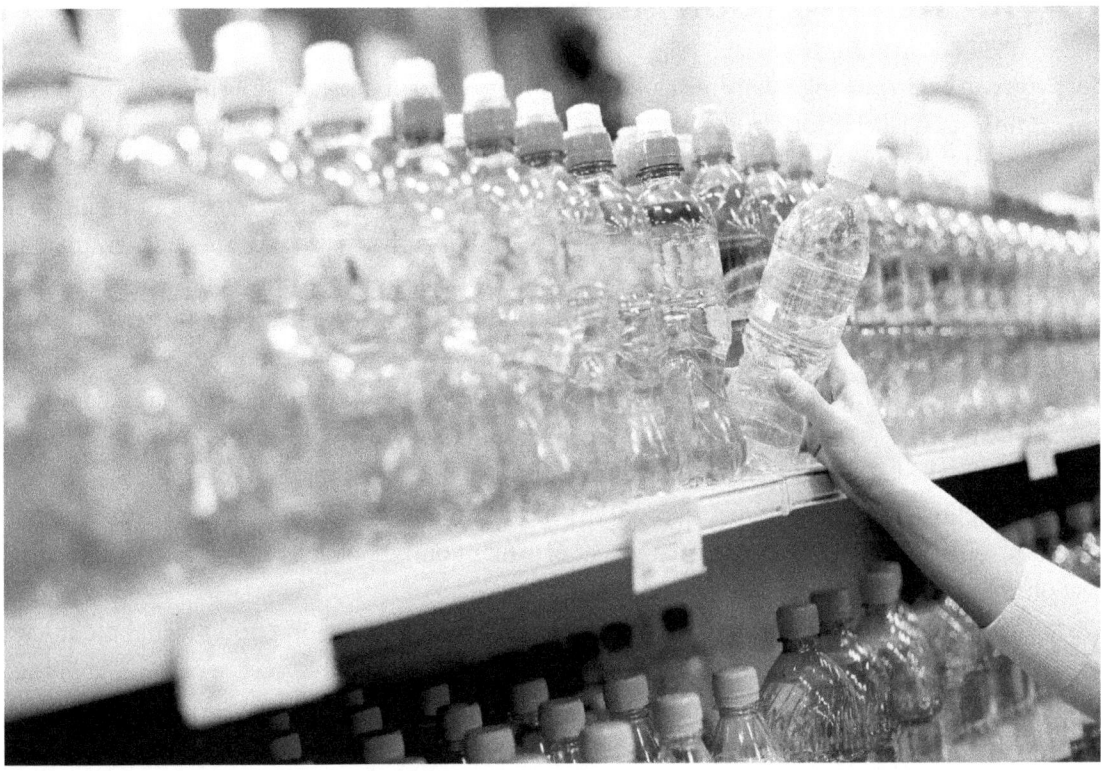

Figure 2.15: Water.

INDIVIDUALIZING YOUR MEAL PLANS

Before you can begin making a daily meal plan, you first need to understand how to read a food label. Refer to the sample food label below. Notice at the very top of the label, it tells you what is considered a serving size; in this case, one cup is one serving size. The second line is telling you how many single servings are in this entire container. You will see that there are two one-cup servings in this container. Moving to the next line down, you will see "amount per serving"; all the numbers that fall under this header are telling you how much you are getting if you eat only one serving (one cup). So if you only eat the one cup, you will be getting a total of 250 calories. If you choose to eat the whole container, you will be eating two cups, and your calorie intake will instead be 500 calories. You will do the same for all the other nutrient amounts listed beneath this. When reading a food label, you want to look for low amounts of saturated fats, cholesterol, and hopefully no trans fats. Look for sources with higher amounts of protein, fiber, and complex carbohydrates. After reviewing the label, you then need to read the ingredient list; although it may be low in fat and seem like a good option for carbohydrates, that doesn't mean it is a whole grain complex carbohydrate option. Make sure you avoid things like "enriched wheat or white flour." Look first for ingredients that say whole wheat or grain, etc[40].

Another important aspect to creating your meal plan is to keep a daily food journal for at least three days. The purpose of the journal is to help you keep track to make sure you are obtaining all the macro and micronutrients your body requires as well as meeting your caloric needs. You will get a chance to practice this with the lab assignment in the back of this book.

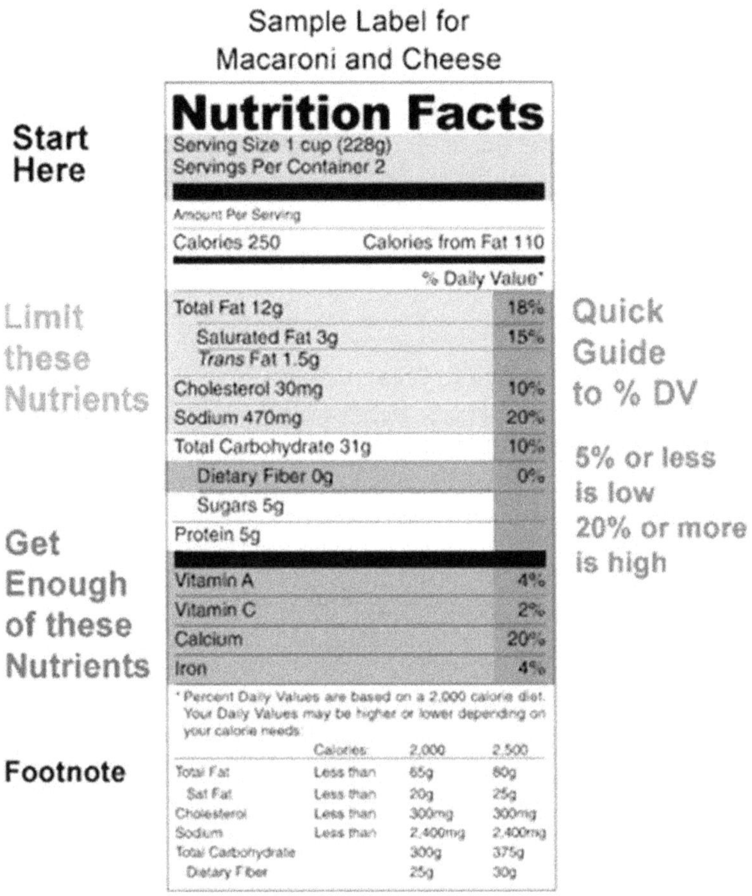

Start Here

Nutrition Facts
Serving Size 1 cup (228g)
Servings Per Container 2

Amount Per Serving

Calories 250   Calories from Fat 110

% Daily Value*

Limit these Nutrients

Total Fat 12g	18%
Saturated Fat 3g	15%
Trans Fat 1.5g	
Cholesterol 30mg	10%
Sodium 470mg	20%
Total Carbohydrate 31g	10%
Dietary Fiber 0g	0%
Sugars 5g	
Protein 5g	

Quick Guide to % DV

5% or less
is low
20% or more
is high

Get Enough of these Nutrients

Vitamin A	4%
Vitamin C	2%
Calcium	20%
Iron	4%

* Percent Daily Values are based on a 2,000 calorie diet. Your Daily Values may be higher or lower depending on your calorie needs.

		Calories:	2,000	2,500
Total Fat	Less than		65g	80g
Sat Fat	Less than		20g	25g
Cholesterol	Less than		300mg	300mg
Sodium	Less than		2,400mg	2,400mg
Total Carbohydrate			300g	375g
Dietary Fiber			25g	30g

Footnote

Figure 2.16: How to read a Nutrition Label.

FAQs CHECK!

Nutrition Journals and Technology

Many people and research studies support reports that keeping a food diary or journal tends to lead to making healthier food choices, increasing one's acute and chronic health. To that end, many people would carry a notebook and write down everything they could, read as many nutritional labels as possible, and try to track their macro and micronutrients while adding up calories. It could be quite time-consuming. Now with technology, this has become extremely easy and even more accurate. Apps, like the highly used MyFitnessPal, allow you to type in items manually or use the search function for common items or items from restaurants. They also allow for a barcode scan on most food items to place all nutritional values into the app, allowing you to track everything. Apps can even track your steps per day or allow you to enter your workout. This lets you get an understanding of how the calorie exchange works on a day-to-day basis and make healthier choices[59].

When you are making food choices, either cooking at home or eating out, keep in mind portion control. Over the past 20 years, portion sizes have increased tremendously. Oftentimes, main entrees ordered at restaurants contain two or more servings and could be shared. Many Americans, though, see these new portions as a normal size to have at any time; this act is called portion distortion. For example, when eating a chicken breast, we really only require about three ounces of meat; however, you know when you purchase chicken breast from the grocery store, the majority of the time the meat options are much larger than three ounces. Refer to the table below to compare and contrast portion sizes and their respective calorie amounts from 20 years ago to today[41].

Table 2.22: Portions and Calories 20 Years Ago to Present Day

	20 Years Ago		Today	
	Portion	Calories	Portion	Calories
Bagel	3" diameter	140	6" diameter	350
Cheeseburger	1	333	1	590
Spaghetti with meatballs	1 cup sauce 3 small meatballs	500	2 cups sauce 3 large meatballs	1,020
Soda	6.5 ounces	82	20 ounces	250
Blueberry muffin	1.5 ounces	210	5 ounces	500

Our body does a great job at adapting to what it needs. For example, if we are not consuming enough calories, our body will adjust our metabolism to maintain the set point our body has established of controlling fat stored and appetite. The basal metabolic rate is the rate at which our body requires the lowest amount of calorie intake and is still able to sustain life. Your body knows itself and knows how to regulate its weight. Although you may be thinking, "why does my body not store enough fat" or "why does mine store too much," think of it as an individual mechanism where some have higher settings and some have lower settings. If you choose to diet or restrict calories and not support a lifestyle change where you are still providing the calories your body needs but with healthier choices, then your body may react and trigger your appetite, as it thinks it's in starvation mode[42,43].

Table 2.23: Current and Recommended Energy Intake Percentages

Current Macronutrient Percentage Intake of Americans as of 2012		
	Men	Women
Carbohydrate	48.1%	50.8%
Protein	16%	15.5%
Fat	33%	32.8%
Saturated Fat	10.6%	10.6%

(*Continued*)

Recommended Macronutrient Intake Percentage of American Adults as of 2002	
Carbohydrate	45–65%
Protein	10–35%
Fat	20–35%
Polyunsaturated fat	5–10%
Cholesterol, Trans Fats, and Saturated Fats	Should be kept as low as possible (i.e., lower than 7%)
Sugar	Up to 25%

Before you dive into doing your food diary and making your meal plans, you should also know what your estimated energy requirement (EER) is. This is a calculation based on your height, weight, and age, and it tells you how many calories you should be consuming per day to maintain your current weight and to be able to function (exercise not included). Find the formula below:

For Men: $\qquad$ EER $= 663 - (9.53 \times \text{Age}) + (15.91 \times \text{body weight}) + (539.6 \times \text{height})$
For Women: $\qquad$ EER $= 354 - (6.91 \times \text{Age}) + (9.36 \times \text{body weight}) + (726 \times \text{height})$

Prior to plugging in your data, you must first convert your weight from pounds to kilograms. To do this, take your weight and divide it by 2.2046. For example: 130 lbs $\rightarrow$ 58.97 kg. Second, you must convert your height from inches to meters by multiplying by .0254. For example: 5'4" $\rightarrow 5 \times 12 = 60 + 4 = 64$ inches. Therefore, $64 \times .0254 = 1.63$ m. Then, make sure you utilize the correct formula depending on whether you're male or female; see the example below:

$354 - (6.91 \times 19) + (9.36 \times 58.97) + (726 \times 1.63)$
$354 - 131.29 + 551.96 + 1183.38 = 1,958.05$ calories required per day to maintain current weight.

Keep in mind, if you are participating in an exercise program, sports, or physically active, then your EER will be higher. Also, if you are physically active and you want to lose weight, then it will more than likely be lower. You will have the opportunity to apply this when you complete your lab.

After you know your EER, you may want to go a step further and figure out how many carbohydrates, fats, and proteins you want to consume on a daily basis. Let's look at carbohydrates first.

Remember, when choosing your carbohydrates, you want to choose whole grain complex carbs that are high in fiber. For individuals who participate in a general fitness program, it is recommended they make their diet approximately 45%–55% (3–5 g/kg/day) carbohydrates. If the individual participates in a higher-intensity fitness program, then they may choose to go up to 60%–70% (5–8 g/kg/day). Let's say we participate in general fitness and want our diet to consist of 55% carbohydrates. We will calculate how many grams that is by using the 5 g/kg/day. Our weight is 58.97 kg; multiplied by five, it tells us we need to eat at least 294.85 grams of carbohydrates a day. We can also change this into calories because we know that we receive four calories per gram of carbohydrates. We have 294.85 grams, so we will multiple this by four and see that 1,179.40 of our calories need to come from complex carbohydrates.

Moving on to protein, for general fitness, the recommended intake can be 10%–15% (0.5–1 g/kg/day) and for resistance training athletes can be as high as 1.2–2 g/kg/day; however, the American College for Sports Medicine (ACSM) does not recommend anything above 0.8 g/kg/day. For our example, we will say we want our diet to consist of 15% protein. We will take our weight in kilograms again, 58.97, and multiply by one; therefore, we need to consume 58.97 grams of protein per day. To convert this amount into calories, we will do the same thing we did for carbohydrates. We know from earlier that there are four calories for every gram of protein. We want to consume 58.97 grams a day; therefore, 235.88 calories from our diet should be from protein.

Last, we still need to consume fats, but choose healthy, unsaturated, plant-based fats. Approximately 20%–35% of your diet should be from fats—anywhere from 0.3–1.5 g/kg/day. We are going to go with about 30% of our diet from fat. We will use our weight of 58.97 kilograms again, and we will go with 1 g/kg/day; therefore, we should be consuming 58.97 grams of fat per day. To convert to calories, recall that fat is different and provides nine calories per gram of fat. So instead, we will multiply the grams of fat, 58.97, by nine, and we see that 530.73 of our calories should come from healthy fats per day.

Let's break it down. Here were our choices:

- Carbs at 55%, 5 g/kg/day, 294.85 grams of carbs to be consumed per day, which is equal to 1,179.40 calories from carbohydrates for the day.
- Protein at 15%, 1 g/kg/day, 58.97 grams of protein to be consumed per day, which is equal to 235.88 calories from protein for the day.
- Fats at about 30%, 1 g/kg/day, 58.97 grams of fat to be consumed per day, which is equal to 530.73 calories from fat per day.
- If you add up all the calories from carbohydrates, protein, and fat, you will see your total daily calorie intake would be 1,946.01. This is very close to our EER of 1,958.05.

Below, you will find example meal plans for two weeks provided by the USDA. Keep in mind that any time you see a grain, always choose a whole wheat or whole grain option. Try to avoid using any salt or butter if possible. This meal plan is based on a 2,000 calorie diet; you will need to make adjustments to carbohydrate and protein intake as well as total calories depending on your EER and whether or not you are physically active[44,45,46].

SAMPLE 2-WEEK MENUS

	DAY 1	DAY 2	DAY 3	DAY 4
BREAKFAST	Peanut Butter Raisin Oatmeal: *1 cup cooked oatmeal* *1 Tbsp peanut butter* *¼ cup raisins* Beverage: 1 cup orange juice	Cereal with Fruit: *1 cup toasted oat cereal* *1 medium banana* *¼ cup lowfat milk* 1 hard-cooked egg Beverage: Water, coffee, tea	Scrambled Eggs: *2 eggs* *2 Tbsp lowfat milk* *1 tsp vegetable oil* 2 turkey sausage links 1 slice whole-wheat toast *½ tsp tub margarine* *1 tsp jelly* Beverage: 1 cup apple juice	**Banana Walnut Oatmeal** 1 large orange Beverage: 1 cup lowfat milk
LUNCH	Tuna-Cucumber Wrap: *1 8" flour tortilla* *3 oz tuna (canned in water)* *2 Tbsp mayonnaise* *5 cucumber sticks* *¼ cup lowfat vanilla yogurt* Beverage: 1 cup lowfat milk	Green Salad with **Honey Lemon Chicken:** *1 cup romaine lettuce* *3 oz sliced Honey Lemon Chicken** *3 slices tomato* *5 slices cucumber* *2 Tbsp vinaigrette dressing*** *1 slice whole-wheat bread* *½ tsp tub margarine* **1 Chocolate Chip Yogurt Cookie*** Beverage: 1 cup lowfat milk	**One Pan Spaghetti*** Side Salad: *1 cup romaine lettuce* *3 medium slices tomato* *5 slices cucumber* *1 Tbsp vinaigrette dressing*** *1 slice whole-wheat bread* *½ tsp tub margarine* Beverage: 1 cup lowfat milk	Green Salad with Tuna: *1 cup romaine lettuce* *3 oz tuna (canned in water)* *¼ cup sliced carrots* *2 Tbsp vinaigrette dressing*** *1 slices whole-wheat bread* *1 tsp tub margarine* **Shake-A-Pudding*** Beverage: 1 cup lowfat milk
DINNER	**Honey Lemon Chicken*** **Brown Rice Pilaf** 1 cup peas and corn: *½ cup corn (frozen)* *½ cup green peas (frozen)* *1 tsp tub margarine* **1 Chocolate Chip Yogurt Cookie*** Beverage: 1 cup lowfat milk	**One Pan Spaghetti*** *(Includes ground beef and tomato sauce)* *½ cup steamed broccoli (frozen)* *½ tsp tub margarine* 1 white roll *1 tsp tub margarine* **Shake-A-Pudding*** Beverage: 1 cup lowfat milk	**Polenta with Pepper and Cheese** *(includes black or kidney beans)* 1 cup cooked green beans (frozen) *1 tsp tub margarine* **1 Chocolate Chip Yogurt Cookie*** Beverage: 1 cup lowfat milk	**Marinated Beef** Mashed potatoes: *1 cup cooked potatoes* *1 Tbsp lowfat milk* *2 tsp tub margarine* 1 cup mixed vegetables (frozen) *1 tsp tub margarine* Beverage: Water, coffee, tea
SNACKS	Carrot Sticks with Dip: *½ cup carrot sticks* *2 Tbsp hummus* 6 whole-grain crackers	Popcorn (3 cups popped) *2 Tbsp kernels* *1 tsp vegetable oil* 1 large orange	Pretzels and Dip *½ cup pretzels* *1 Tbsp hummus* 1 medium banana	**Banana Bread*** *½ tsp tub margarine* 1 cup grapes

Figure 2.17a: Week menu page 1.

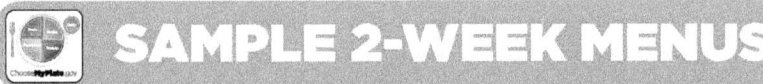

	DAY 5	DAY 6	DAY 7	DAY 8
BREAKFAST	Open-faced Egg and Tomato on an English Muffin *2 eggs, fried in 1 tsp oil* *1 English muffin, toasted* *2 medium slices tomato* *¼ cup cheddar cheese, shredded* Beverage: 1 cup apple juice	**Scrambled Tofu** Burrito *1 serving Scrambled Tofu* *1 8" flour tortilla* *¼ cup black beans (canned)* *2 Tbsp salsa* Beverage: 1 cup lowfat milk	**Fantastic French Toast** *1 Tbsp pancake syrup* *1 tsp tub margarine* *Dash of cinnamon (optional)* 1 medium banana Beverage: 1 cup orange juice	Raisin Oatmeal: *1 cup cooked oatmeal* *1 Tbsp raisins* 1 medium banana *1 Tbsp peanut butter* Beverage: 1 cup lowfat milk
LUNCH	Peanut Butter and Banana Sandwich: *2 slices whole-wheat bread* *2 Tbsp peanut butter* *1 medium banana* ½ cup celery sticks Beverage: 1 cup lowfat milk	**Crunchy Chicken Salad** Sandwich: *2 slices whole-wheat bread* *¾ cup Crunchy Chicken Salad* *1 romaine lettuce leaf* ½ cup carrot sticks *1 Tbsp Ranch dressing* 1 large orange Beverage: 1 cup lowfat milk	**Lentil Stew*** 1 cup brown rice 1 slice whole-wheat bread *½ tsp tub margarine* Beverage: 1 cup lowfat milk	Tuna Sandwich: *2 slices whole-wheat bread* *3 oz tuna (canned in water)* *2 Tbsp mayonnaise* *2 medium slices tomato* *1 romaine lettuce leaf* 10 cucumber slices *1 Tbsp Ranch dressing* Beverage: 1 cup lowfat milk
DINNER	**Mouth-Watering Oven-Fried Fish** **Couscous with Peas and Onions** 1 cup green beans (frozen) 1 white roll *1 tsp tub margarine* Beverage: Water, coffee, tea	**Lentil Stew*** 1 cup brown rice ½ cup broccoli (frozen) *½ tsp tub margarine* ½ cup canned pears Beverage: Water, coffee, tea	Pan-fried Pork Chop (5 oz raw chop with bone) 1 medium baked potato *2 Tbsp margarine* Cabbage slaw *½ cup shredded green cabbage* *1 Tbsp vinaigrette dressing*** Beverage: 1 cup apple juice	**Red Hot Fusilli Pasta** *2 Tbsp shredded Parmesan cheese* ½ cup green peas (frozen) *½ tsp tub margarine* 1 white roll *1 tsp tub margarine* **Apple Cinnamon Bar*** Beverage: Water, coffee, tea
SNACKS	**Banana Bread*** *½ tsp tub margarine* 1 cup lowfat milk	Yogurt Parfait: *¾ cup lowfat vanilla yogurt* *¼ cup toasted oat cereal* *1 Tbsp chopped nuts* *1 Tbsp raisins*	**Banana Bread*** *½ tsp tub margarine* 1 cup lowfat milk	1 large orange 2 graham crackers 1 cup lowfat milk

Figure 2.17b: Week menu page 2.

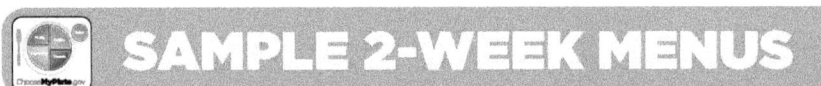

	DAY 9	DAY 10	DAY 11	DAY 12
BREAKFAST	Sausage Omelet: *2 eggs* *2 Tbsp lowfat milk* *1 tsp vegetable oil* *1 turkey sausage link, diced* *¼ cup cheddar cheese, shredded* *½ cup hash brown potatoes (frozen)* *Cooked in 1 tsp vegetable oil* Beverage: 1 cup orange juice	Cold Cereal: *1 cup toasted oat cereal* *1 medium banana* *¾ cup lowfat milk* 1 slice whole-wheat toast *1 Tbsp peanut butter* Beverage: Water, coffee, tea	**Breakfast Burrito with Salsa** 1 slice whole-wheat toast *½ tsp tub margarine* *1 tsp jelly* Beverage: 1 cup apple juice	1 cup toasted oat cereal *¾ cup lowfat milk* Scrambled Egg with Salsa: *1 egg* *1 Tbsp lowfat milk* *½ tsp vegetable oil* *1 Tbsp salsa* Beverage: 1 cup apple juice
LUNCH	Peanut Butter and Jelly Sandwich: *2 slices whole-wheat bread* *2 Tbsp peanut butter* *2 tsp jelly* 1 cup sliced apple *½ cup carrot sticks* 1 Tbsp Ranch dressing Beverage: 1 cup lowfat milk	Green Salad with Salmon: *1 cup romaine lettuce* *3 oz salmon (canned)* *2 medium slices tomato* *4 slices cucumber* *2 Tbsp vinaigrette dressing*** 6 whole-grain crackers Beverage: 1 cup lowfat milk	Roast Beef Sandwich: *2 slices whole-wheat bread* *2 oz lean roast beef (deli meat)* *2 slices tomato* *1 romaine lettuce leaf* *1 Tbsp mayonnaise* ½ cup carrot sticks 1 cup sliced apple *1 Tbsp peanut butter* Beverage: Water, coffee, tea	**White Chili*** Side Salad: *¾ cup romaine lettuce* *¼ cup chopped carrot* *1 Tbsp vinaigrette dressing*** 1 slice whole-wheat bread *½ tsp tub margarine* Beverage: 1 cup lowfat milk
DINNER	**Quick Tuna Casserole** ½ cup green beans (frozen) *½ tsp tub margarine* 1 white roll *1 tsp tub margarine* **Apple Cinnamon Bar*** Beverage: Water, coffee, tea	**Honey Mustard Pork Chops** 1 medium baked potato *1 tsp tub margarine* ½ cup shredded green cabbage *Sauteed in ½ tsp vegetable oil* 1 white roll *1 tsp tub margarine* **2 Applesauce Cookies*** Beverage: Water, coffee, tea	**White Chili*** **Herbed Vegetables** 1 small sweet potato, baked *½ tsp tub margarine* ½ cup chocolate pudding (prepared from a dry mix) Beverage: 1 cup lowfat milk	**Misickquatash** (Indian Succotash with ground beef) Mashed potatoes: *1 cup cooked potatoes* *1 Tbsp lowfat milk* *2 tsp tub margarine* 1 slice whole-wheat bread *½ tsp tub margarine* Beverage: 1 cup lowfat milk
SNACKS	Peanut Butter on Banana: *1 medium banana* *1 Tbsp peanut butter* 1 cup lowfat milk	2 graham crackers 1 cup lowfat milk	**Apple Cinnamon Bar*** 1 cup lowfat milk	**2 Applesauce Cookies*** ½ cup canned pineapple chunks

Figure 2.17c: Week menu page 3.

SAMPLE 2-WEEK MENUS

	DAY 13	DAY 14
BREAKFAST	**Banana Walnut Oatmeal** 1 hard-boiled egg Beverage: 1 cup orange juice	**Perfect Pumpkin Pancakes** *2 Tbsp pancake syrup* 1 turkey sausage link 1 medium banana Beverage: 1 cup apple juice
LUNCH	**Tofu Salad** Sandwich: *2 slices whole-wheat bread* *¾ cup* ***Tofu Salad*** *2 slices tomato* *1 romaine lettuce leaf* ½ cup carrot sticks *1 Tbsp Ranch dressing* **Apple Cinnamon Bar*** Beverage: 1 cup lowfat milk	**Easy Red Beans and Rice*** *¼ cup cheddar cheese, shredded* Side Salad: *¾ cup romaine lettuce* *4 slices cucumber* *¼ cup chopped carrot* *1 Tbsp vinaigrette dressing*** 1 slice whole-wheat bread *½ tsp tub margarine* Beverage: 1 cup lowfat milk
DINNER	**Easy Red Beans and Rice*** *¼ cup cheddar cheese, shredded* **Lemon Spinach** 1 large orange Beverage: 1 cup lowfat milk	**Manly Muffin Meatloaf** Mashed potatoes: *1 cup cooked potatoes* *1 Tbsp lowfat milk* *2 tsp tub margarine* ½ cup green peas (frozen) *½ tsp tub margarine* Beverage: 1 cup lowfat milk
SNACKS	Yogurt Parfait: *¾ cup lowfat vanilla yogurt* *¼ cup toasted oat cereal* *1 Tbsp chopped nuts* *1 Tbsp raisins*	Popcorn (3 cups popped) *2 Tbsp kernels* *1 tsp vegetable oil* **Yogurt Pop**

* Bolded recipes are from the SNAP-Ed Recipe Finder, and those with a star make 8 or more servings. These recipes are used two or more times in these menus. Prepare the entire recipe on the first day it appears and eat the remaining portions as noted on the following days.

**Homemade vinaigrette salad dressing. To make about 4 Tbsp of the dressing, mix:
- 3 Tbsp vegetable oil (canola, olive, soybean, etc.)
- 1 Tbsp vinegar (cider, wine, or balsamic)
- ¼ tsp mustard (yellow, Dijon, or brown)
- ¼ tsp sugar
- Optional: black pepper, dried herbs to taste

Notes:
- Italicized foods are part of the dish or food that precedes it.
- Unless indicated, all beverages are unsweetened.
- To keep sodium amounts within recommended limit, use salt only as specified in recipes, not in cooking other foods or at the table.
- Be sure to follow food safety guidelines when preparing and cooking food. Tips for keeping food safe can be found at www.foodsafety.gov.

Figure 2.17d: Week menu page 4.

Average Food Group and Nutrient Content

Average Food Group Content of Menus		
Food Group	**Goal***	**Average Daily Amount in Menus**
Grains	6 ounces	6 ounces
Whole Grains	≥3 ounces	3 ½ ounces
Refined Grains	≤3 ounces	2 ½ ounces
Vegetables	2 ½ cups	2 ½ cups
Dark Green	1 ½ cups/week	1 ¾ cups
Red & Orange	5 ½ cups/week	5 ¼ cups
Beans & Peas	1 ½ cups/week	1 ¾ cups
Starchy	5 cups/week	5 cups
Other	4 cups/week	3 ¾ cups
Fruits	2 cups	2 ¼ cups
Whole Fruit	No Specific Goal	1 ½ cups
Fruit Juice	No Specific Goal	¾ cups
Dairy	3 cups	3 cups
Milk & Yogurt	3 cups	2 ¾ cups
Cheese	No Specific Goal	¼ cups
Protein Foods	5 ½ ounces	5 ½ ounces
Seafood	8 ounces/week	8 ½ ounces/week
Meat, Poultry & Eggs	No Specific Goal	3 ounces
Nuts, Seeds & Soy	No Specific Goal	1 ½ ounces
Oils	6 teaspoons	6 teaspoons
	Limit*	**Average Daily Amount in Menus**
Total Calories	2000 Calories	1948 Calories
Empty Calories**	≤258 Calories	233 Calories
Solid Fats	No Specific Goal	143 Calories
Added Sugars	No Specific Goal	90 Calories

*Food group goals and limits are the amounts in the 2,000 calorie USDA Food Pattern (http://www.cnpp.usda.gov/USDAFoodPatterns.htm).

**Empty Calories are calories from food components such as added sugars and solid fats that provide little nutritional value. Empty Calories are part of Total Calories.

Figure 2.17e: Avg food group and nutrient content page 1.

Average Nutrient Content of Menus		
Nutrients	Goal*	Average Daily Amount in Menus
Macronutrients		
Protein (g)**	46 g	93 g
Protein (% Calories)**	10 - 35% Calories	19 % Calories
Carbohydrate (g)**	130 g	261 g
Carbohydrate (% Calories)**	45 - 65% Calories	54% Calories
Dietary Fiber	25 g	27 g
Total Fat	20 - 35% Calories	30% Calories
Saturated Fat	<10% Calories	8% Calories
Monounsaturated Fat	No Daily Goal or Limit	11% Calories
Polyunsaturated Fat	No Daily Goal or Limit	8% Calories
Linoleic Acid (g)**	12 g	15 g
Linoleic Acid (% Calories)**	5 - 10% Calories	7% Calories
α-Linoleic Acid (g)**	1.1 g	2.5 g
α-Linoleic Acid (% Calories)**	0.6 - 1.2% Calories	1.1% Calories
Omega 3 - EPA	No Daily Goal or Limit	63 mg
Omega 3 - DHA	No Daily Goal or Limit	133 mg
Cholesterol	<300 mg	291 mg
Minerals		
Calcium	1000 mg	1339 mg
Potassium	4700 mg	3859 mg
Sodium	<2300 mg	2197 mg
Copper	900 µg	1491 µg
Iron	18 mg	14 mg
Magnesium	320 mg	405 mg
Phosphorus	700 mg	1721 mg
Selenium	55 µg	138 µg
Zinc	8 mg	12 mg
Vitamins		
Vitamin A	700 µg RAE	1140 µg RAE
Vitamin B6	1.3 mg	2.7 mg
Vitamin B12	2.4 µg	6.9 µg
Vitamin C	75 mg	130 mg
Vitamin D	15 µg	11 µg
Vitamin E	15 mg AT	9 mg AT
Vitamin K	90 µg	115 µg
Folate	400 µg DFE	501 µg DFE
Thiamin	1.2 mg	1.6 mg
Riboflavin	1.2 mg	2.6 mg
Niacin	14 mg	24 mg
Choline	425 mg	423 mg

*Goals are recommended intakes for a 20- to 35-year-old woman consuming about 2,000 calories per day.

** Nutrients that appear twice (**protein, carbohydrate, linoleic acid,** and **α-linolenic acid**) have two separate recommendations: (1) Amount eaten (in grams) compared to your minimum recommended intake and (2) Percent of Calories eaten from that nutrient compared to the recommended range.

Figure 2.17f: Avg food group and nutrient content page 2.

NUTRITION STANDARDS

The Food and Nutrition Board (FNB) and Institute of Medicine (IOM) developed nutrient recommendations for the United States and Canada. In conjunction with these organizations, the U.S. Department of Agriculture (USDA) and Department of Health and Human Services (DHHS) also share responsibility in issuing dietary recommendations. They created what's called the *Dietary Reference Intake* (DRI), which is the overall umbrella term that includes specific types of nutrient recommendations. These include the following: Recommended Dietary Allowance (RDA), Adequate Intake (AI), Estimated Average Requirement (EAR), and Tolerable Upper Intake Level (UL).

The recommended dietary allowance (RDA) is the average daily dietary nutrient intake level that is sufficient to meet the nutrient requirements of almost all healthy individuals (97% to 98%) depending on their age and gender.

The adequate intake is the recommended average daily intake level based on observed or experimentally determined estimates of nutrient intake by a group (or groups) of healthy people. The AI is used when a recommended dietary allowance (RDA) cannot be used.

The estimated average requirement (EAR) is the average daily nutrient intake level that is estimated to meet the requirement of half the healthy population, again depending on their age and gender.

The tolerable upper intake level tells an individual the highest average daily nutrient intake they can consume that does not pose any risk of adverse health effects. This works for almost all individuals in the general population. If an individual consumes above their UL, their risk of adverse health effects may increase.

We also have the daily values (DV), which is a reference found on food labels to help consumers in selecting a healthy diet. It consists of two sets of values: the daily reference values (DRVs), which are expressed as percentages, and the reference daily intakes (RDIs). The daily reference values is a set of food labeling that references values for fat, saturated fat, cholesterol, total carbohydrates, protein, dietary fiber, sodium, and potassium. The reference daily intake is a set of references for vitamins and minerals on food labels[47].

ANTIOXIDANTS

Antioxidants are substances that can be found naturally occurring in certain foods that help prevent free radicals from forming and therefore preventing cell damage in the body. Free radicals are substances that form through oxidation, and these byproducts damage cells in our body. Recall back to the energy system section, and remember that when we need more ATP, our body begins utilizing oxygen to transform carbohydrates and fats into energy; during this process, byproducts are also created, and those are the free radicals. Free radicals can also be obtained through pollution, smoking, radiation, and stress. When these substances damage our cells, research has shown it can cause conditions such as cardiovascular disease, emphysema, cancer, premature aging, and many others. Research has also shown that our body naturally has its own defense system to neutralize the free radicals, but when they are produced at a faster rate, our natural defense is not enough. We have also found through research that physically fit individuals have a better defense system against free radicals. Antioxidant-rich foods are mainly fruits and vegetables; the problem Americans face is that we are currently not eating enough fruits and vegetables on a daily basis. The most looked-at antioxidants include Vitamin C, E, beta-carotene, and selenium.

Some food examples high in antioxidants include blueberries, blackberries, cranberries, acai berries, goji berries, artichoke, kidney beans, pecans, dark chocolate, and cilantro. There have also been antioxidant supplements available over the counter; however, a research study published in the *Journal of the American Medical Association* showed that antioxidant supplements may actually increase the risk of death. Needless to say, there is not enough research in regards to antioxidant supplements, so they should be considered with caution.

VEGETARIANISM

Key terminology	
Vegan	Individual who does not eat any food that comes from an animal (no meat or dairy)
Semivegetarian	Individual does not eat red meat, but eats fish and poultry in addition to milk products and eggs
Ovovegetarian	Individual allows eggs in their diet
Lactovegetarian	Individual allows foods from the milk group in their diet
Ovolactovegetarian	An individual who includes dairy products and eggs in their diet

There have been many debates as to whether a vegan diet is safe and healthy, especially in children. An estimated consumption of 54.3 pounds of beef, 92.1 pounds of chicken, and 50.4 pounds of pork was determined in 2016 by the USDA. These amounts are in reference to per person, per year. We will not go into the history or debate of the topic, but we will discuss research studies conducted in regards to living a vegetarian lifestyle.

Research conducted by Harvard found that high consumption of red meat potentially increases the risk of heart disease by 50% among women with type 2 diabetes. Another researcher, Dr. Ornish, completed an experimental study that showed a decrease of heart disease in those who were on a vegetarian diet, incorporated aerobic exercise, quit smoking, and received stress management training. There are many other studies that show the vegetarian, or plant-based, diet lifestyle has many health benefits, including lowering cholesterol, reducing obesity, reducing heart disease and the incidences of breast, colon, and prostate cancer, as well as helping lower and control blood pressure[55,56,57,58].

ORGANIC FOOD OPTIONS

There are a variety of food options to choose from in a majority of stores, from vendors, to type of food, to whether or not you want organic, hormone-free, etc. Organic foods are foods that must meet specific criteria that are set by the USDA. So what is the difference between a conventionally grown orange or apple to one that is organic? Both may look ripe and provide the same vitamins and contain no fat, cholesterol, or salt, so how do you know which one you should choose? Organic means more than one thing; it's the way a farmer grows and processes their products. This includes how they process and/or grow fruits, grains, vegetables, dairy products, and meat. The main goal of organic farming is to conserve soil and water and to reduce pollution. Some examples include using natural fertilizer and crop rotation, using fewer pesticides, and not using any food additives. There is still not enough research to clearly state whether an organic food option is more nutritious than a conventional food option. However, this does not include the processes used to make the foods, which may have negative effects on our health and environment.

- Choose a variety of foods from different sources. This will expose you to multiple nutrients and reduce your risk of consuming the same single pesticide.
- Always try to purchase fruits and vegetables when they are in season; this is when they are the most fresh and least expensive. It is always a great idea to check for a local farmers market as well.

- Always read the label. Even if it is labeled organic it may still contain high amounts of sugar, salt, fat, or calories.
- Always wash and scrub your fruits and vegetables under running water. This helps remove bacteria, dirt, and some of the chemicals used, such as pesticides, from the surface.
- Try to eat a majority of fruits and vegetables raw—that means no peeling, baking, steaming, boiling, or grilling—to get the most of all the nutrients.

ATHLETES AND CARB LOADING

Physically active people require the same basic nutrients as anyone else; however, an athlete who competes has an increased energy requirement. Typically, athletes do not require more protein unless they are active in intense strength training. Complex carbohydrates are the key nutrient for a competitive athlete, along with fats (choosing the right kind). Fat provides more energy per weight and helps replenish intramuscular fat stores. As an athlete or a physically active person, when you eat plays a big role in how your exercise goes. If you eat just prior to exercising, you may feel nauseous, bloated, fatigued, or have abdominal cramping or diarrhea. However, if you choose to not eat at all and go to work out, then you may feel dizzy, weak, extremely fatigued, and nauseous and possibly faint. The best way to prepare for your exercise is to eat three to four hours prior to working out.

Many athletes may choose to carb load, which is basically eating enough complex carbohydrates to completely fill any empty spots that hold glycogen. This idea is that when they go to compete, their glycogen stores are filled up, similar to an extra tank of gas, to keep them fueled for the duration of the competition along with the energy they consume the night before and day of and any fat they have available to keep them going even longer. Athletes should keep in mind that carb loading takes practice. It isn't something you can do for the first time right before a competition. It can take months to train your body to carb load. You more than likely will feel full and bloated when starting out, and your body won't know exactly what to do except be sluggish. Muscles need approximately two days to replace glycogen stores, so you can see how carb loading just the night before does not work. Generally, carb loading is used for competitions that are going to last 90 or more minutes.

Sport nutritionist Nancy Clark provides a nine-step plan to carb loading. See below for the steps:

1. **Carb load daily**—Doing so daily will slowly build up your glycogen stores and prevent them from depletion (e.g., 100 lbs → 300–500 g/day, 175 lbs → 525–875 g/day).
2. **Taper your training**—Intense training should be completed about three weeks prior to competition so you have time to heal. If two to four pounds of water weight is gained, then carb loading was completed successfully.
3. **Eat enough protein**—Endurance athletes usually burn some protein, so it is recommended they consume an additional two servings a day.
4. **Do not fat load**—You need more carbs than fat; if you overeat fat, then you run out of room for carb calories. For example, skip the butter, sour cream, and jelly and instead eat another plain slice of whole grain toast or baked potato.
5. **Choose fiber-rich foods**—Remember, complex carbs provide higher amounts of fiber and will keep your GI system clean. If you eat too many processed carbohydrates such as white bread, pasta, etc., then you may feel bloated and/or constipated. If diarrhea is a concern from a high fiber diet, then avoid these foods just prior to a competition.

6. **Plan mealtimes**—Make sure you incorporate snacks throughout your day. Also, the day before the competition, you may make breakfast or lunch your largest meal of the day rather than dinner so your body has time to process everything. You want to stop as little as possible for bathroom breaks during the competition.

7. **Drink extra fluids**—Avoid alcohol, as this will dehydrate you. Don't overhydrate, as this may just increase your bathroom time during the competition. On competition day, it is recommended an athlete drink about two to three glasses of water two hours prior to the event so the body has time to excrete any excess. Then, they should drink another cup about five to 10 minutes before the competition to make sure they are fully hydrated.

8. **Chose foods wisely**—Avoid alcohol, avoid processed, refined carbs, do not eat new foods that your body isn't familiar with, and avoid eating just fruit to prevent diarrhea.

9. **Eat breakfast daily**—Breakfast is important in supplying energy for the day, preventing nausea due to hunger and helping maintain blood sugar levels[48].

TIPS FOR EATING HEALTHY IN COLLEGE

As a young adult living on a college campus, it can be difficult, and sometimes even feel impossible, to make healthy food choices. Besides the fact that you are now finally living on your own, food consumption also depends on whether you have access to cook at home and know how to cook, and whether you can financially afford certain foods. Oftentimes, students use money as the main reason for not eating healthy; however, choosing healthier options does not always need to cost more. Some examples include choosing whole wheat every time it is an option in the dining hall, or asking the staff whether they can make it available; asking for larger portions of vegetables and fruits; asking for gravies and sauces on the side and limiting your overall intake of these, as they are high in sodium; avoiding cream-based soups and instead choosing broth-based; loading up on dark green leafy vegetables when eating from the salad bar and avoiding bacon, mayonnaise, and asking for dressing on the side; and choosing to eat fruit as a dessert rather than a baked good. Most of these options are available at dining halls on college campuses. If you are financially able, choose to pre-pack snack bags of healthy foods to use throughout the week as you are "on the go" between classes or work. Pick a day to buy what you need and to spend time bagging the foods. Then keep the bags in a basket or in your pantry for you to grab each day as needed. Some healthy options include fresh or dried fruit, granola bars, raw fresh veggies like baby carrots, whole wheat fig bars, plain popcorn, low-fat crackers, or low-fat yogurt cups.

There are many other ways to help control weight when living on campus that don't all involve a cost; many times, it's just about discipline. Some of these include:

- Eating slower to give your body time to absorb and release the hormone that makes you feel full. If you eat too fast, your body can't respond quickly enough, and you don't realize you were already full. Try to avoid eating while studying, doing homework, watching TV, or sitting at the computer. It's easy to "snack" and end up eating a whole bag of chips. Instead, control your portion by grabbing a handful and placing in a bowl and not going back for more once the bowl is empty.

- Always try to choose a wide variety of colors in your foods. From fruits to vegetables, choose yellows, greens, dark green, reds, purples, and whites; they all contain different nutrients that our bodies require. French fries do not constitute a vegetable intake, as they are high in saturated fats, and many times trans fats, and offer little to no nutritional value.

- Always eat breakfast. This is the meal that provides you the energy you need to get through your day. Skipping breakfast oftentimes leads to grabbing a quick unhealthy snack mid-morning due to hunger.
- Pick healthy snacks a majority of the time (whole grains, fruits, vegetables).
- Drink water over soda; this will cut down your sugar intake.
- Observe and control your portion sizes. It is better to eat smaller portions and incorporate more small meals or snack times throughout the day. Always read the food labels to know how many servings are in the package so you know exactly what your intake is[49].

KNOW YOUR HELPER'S CREDENTIALS

If you are looking for help on meal planning, calorie counting, or being educated on how to make proper choices for a condition you may have (i.e., heart disease), there are certified individuals who went to school to specifically do this. Before you dive in searching for someone to help you, you should understand the differences in titles you may come across. You may come across two different titles: "nutritionist" or "registered dietician." One of the major differences between the two is the legal restrictions that they carry. Nutritionists who become registered with the Commission on Dietetic Registration (CDR) may legally declare themselves as a registered dietician. Nutritionists are not as protected under the law and are usually free from government regulation. In fact, some states do not require licensing, and therefore, almost anyone can make the claim that they are a "nutritionist." Always ask to see the individual's credentials and professional affiliations. Most often, choosing a registered dietician is the better option, as they have obtained a bachelor's degree, which has to be accredited through the Dietetics' Accreditation Council for Education in Nutrition and Dietetics (ACEND), and have received specialized training as well as completed an internship in their field prior to taking and passing a certification exam. They are also usually a member of the American Dietetic Association. In some cases, a nutritionist may have just had to pay their dues to an obscure organization and received a diploma. Also, some states do not require any educational background for nutritionists, just some formal coursework in nutrition-related subjects to qualify for employment[50,51].

REFERENCES

1. USDA (2016). Build a Healthy Eating Style. Retrieved from http://www.choose myplate.gov/MyPlate
2. Merriam-Webster (2016). Nutrition. Retrieved from http://www.merriam-webster.com/dictionary/nutrition
3. USDA (2016). NUTRITION (NUTRIENT DENSITY). Retrieved from http://www.choosemyplate.gov/nutrition-nutrient-density
4. Fielding JE, Kumanyika S, & Manderscheid RW. (2013) A perspective on the development of the Healthy People 2020 Framework for improving U.S. population health. *Public Health Reviews*; 35 Retrieved from http://www.publichealthreviews.eu/upload/pdf_files/13/00_Fielding.pdf
5. Wise Geek (2016). What is Maltose? Retrieved from http://www.wisegeek.org/what-is-maltose.htm
6. MyFoodDiary (2016). Soluble & Insoluble Fiber: What is the Difference? Retrieved from https://www.myfooddiary.com/resources/ask_the_expert/soluble_insoluble_fiber.asp

7. Harvard School of Public Health (2016). Carbohydrates. Retrieved from https://www.hsph.harvard.edu/nutritionsource/carbohydrates/

8. MedlinePlus (2016). Carbohydrates. Retrieved from https://medlineplus.gov/carbohydrates.html

9. Oldways Whole Grain Council (2016). Whole Grains from A to Z. Retrieved from http://wholegrainscouncil.org/whole-grains-101/whole-grains-a-to-z

10. MyFoodDiary (2016). Soluble & Insoluble Fiber: What is the Difference? Retrieved from https://www.myfooddiary.com/resources/ask_the_expert/soluble_insoluble_fiber.asp

11. Merriam-Webster (2016). Peristalses. Retrieved from http://www.merriam-webster.com/dictionary/peristalses

12. MyFitnessPal (2016). Nutritional Labels. Retrieved from www.myfitnesspal.com

13. NutritionMD (2016). Making Sense of Food. Retrieved from http://www.nutritionmd.org/nutrition_tips/nutrition_tips_understand_foods/carbs_versus.html

14. Science Learning (2011). Role of Proteins in the Body. Retrieved from http://sciencelearn.org.nz/Contexts/Uniquely-Me/Science-Ideas-and-Concepts/Role-of-proteins-in-the-body

15. Physicians Committee for Responsible Medicine (n.d.) The Protein Myth. Retrieved from http://www.pcrm.org/health/diets/vegdiets/how-can-i-get-enough-protein-the-protein-myth

16. Martin, W., Armstrong, L., & Rodriguez, N. (2005). Dietary protein intake and renal function. *Nutr. Metab. (London), 2*(25). Retrieved from http://www.ncbi.nlm.nih.gov/pmc/articles/PMC1262767/

17. Zeratsky, K. (2015). Are high protein diets safe for weight loss. Retrieved from http://www.mayoclinic.org/healthy-lifestyle/nutrition-and-healthy-eating/expert-answers/high-protein-diets/faq-20058207

19. American Heart Association (2016). Saturated Fats. Retrieved from http://www.heart.org/HEARTORG/HealthyLiving/HealthyEating/Nutrition/Saturated-Fats_UCM_301110_Article.jsp#.V6n6IpX6s5s

20. American Heart Association (2016). Healthy Cooking Oils. Retrieved from http://www.heart.org/HEARTORG/HealthyLiving/HealthyEating/SimpleCookingwithHeart/Healthy-Cooking-Oils_UCM_445179_Article.jsp#.V6tbvFsrKUk

21. American Heart Association (2016). Know Your Fats. Retrieved from http://www.heart.org/HEARTORG/Conditions/Cholesterol/PreventionTreatmentofHighCholesterol/Know-Your-Fats_UCM_305628_Article.jsp#.V6n96pX6s5s

22. U.S. Food and Drug Administration (2015). FDA cuts Trans Fat in Processed Food. Retrieved from http://www.fda.gov/ForConsumers/ConsumerUpdates/ucm372915.htm

23. U.S. Food and Drug Administration (2015). The FDA takes step to remove artificial trans fats in processed foods. Retrieved from http://www.fda.gov/NewsEvents/Newsroom/PressAnnouncements/ucm451237.htm

24. U.S. Food and Drug Administration (2016). Talking About *Trans* Fat: What You Need to Know. Retrieved from http://www.fda.gov/Food/IngredientsPackagingLabeling/LabelingNutrition/ucm079609.htm

25. U.S. Food and Drug Administration (2015). *Trans* Fat Now Listed With Saturated Fat and Cholesterol. Retrieved from http://www.fda.gov/Food/IngredientsPackagingLabeling/LabelingNutrition/ucm274590.htm

26. Mayo Clinic (2015). Cholesterol: Top foods to improve your numbers. Retrieved from http://www.mayoclinic.org/diseases-conditions/high-blood-cholesterol/in-depth/cholesterol/art-20045192?pg=2

27. University of Washington. (n.d.). Cholesterol, Lipoproteins, and the Liver. Retrieved from https://courses.washington.edu/conj/bess/cholesterol/liver.html

28. Greger, M. (2016). Egg Consumption and LDL Cholesterol Size. Retrieved from http://nutritionfacts.org/2016/04/28/egg-consumption-and-ldl-cholesterol-size/

29. John Muir Health (2016). Cholesterol (Lipids) Retrieved from https://www.johnmuirhealth.com/health-education/health-wellness/heart-disease-risk-factors/cholesterol-lipids.html

30. American Heart Association (2016). Good Vs. Bad Cholesterol. Retrieved from http://www.heart.org/HEARTORG/Conditions/Cholesterol/AboutCholesterol/Good-vs-Bad-Cholesterol_UCM_305561_Article.jsp#.V6yEKJX6s5s

31. National Institute of Health (2016). Retrieved from https://www.niddk.nih.gov/…programs/…/gp_fatcal.pdf

32. The Ketogenic diet for health (n.d.) Retrieved from http://www.ketotic.org/2012/08/if-you-eat-excess-protein-does-it-turn.html

33. Schutz, Y. (2011). Protein turnover, ureagenesis and gluconeogenesis. *International Journal of Vitamin Nutritional Research*. 81(2–3), 101–7. Retrieved from http://www.ncbi.nlm.nih.gov/pubmed/22139560

34. Kelso, T. (n.d.). Understanding energy systems: ATP-PC, glycolytic, Oxidative, oh my!. Retrieved from http://breakingmuscle.com/health-medicine/understanding-energy-systems-atp-pc-glycolytic-and-oxidative-oh-my

35. PT Direct. (2016). Energy systems in action. Retrieved from http://www.ptdirect.com/training-design/anatomy-and-physiology/the-energy-systems-2013-an-overview

36. Institute of Medicine (US) Panel on Micronutrients. (2001). Dietary Reference Intakes for Vitamin A, Vitamin K, Arsenic, Boron, Chromium, Copper, Iodine, Iron, Manganese, Molybdenum, Nickel, Silicon, Vanadium, and Zinc. Retrieved from https://www.ncbi.nlm.nih.gov/pubmed/25057538?_ga=1.7707890.1758414987.1470235408

37. MedlinePlus (2016). Retrieved from https://vsearch.nlm.nih.gov/vivisimo/cgi-bin/query-meta?v%3Aproject=medlineplus&v%3Asources=medlineplus-bundle&query=Sulfate+in+diet

38. Mahan, L. K., Escott-Stump, S. (2008). Krause's Food & Nutrition Therapy (12th Ed.) St. Louis, Missouri: Saunders ElSevier.

39. Kravitz, L. (n.d.) Water: the science of nature's most important nutrient. Retrieved from https://www.unm.edu/~lkravitz/Article%20folder/WaterUNM.html

40. U.S. Food and Drug Administration (2015). Trans fats now listed with saturated fats and cholesterol. Retrieved from http://www.fda.gov/Food/IngredientsPackagingLabeling/LabelingNutrition/ucm274590.htm

42. Centers for Disease Control and Prevention. (2015). Mean macronutrient intake among adults aged 20 and over. Retrieved from http://www.cdc.gov/nchs/data/hus/hus15.pdf#056

43. Centers for Disease Control and Prevention. (2016). Diet/Nutrition. Retrieved from http://www.cdc.gov/nchs/fastats/diet.htm

44. The National Academies of Science, Engineering, and Medicine. (2002). Dietary Reference Intakes for Energy, Carbohydrate, Fiber, Fat, Fatty Acids, Cholesterol, Protein, and Amino Acids. Retrieved from http://nationalacademies.org/hmd/Reports/2002/Dietary-Reference-Intakes-for-Energy-Carbohydrate-Fiber-Fat-Fatty-Acids-Cholesterol-Protein-and-Amino-Acids.aspx

45. Institute of Medicine (2005) Dietary Reference Intakes for Energy, Carbohydrate, Fiber, Fat, Fatty Acids, Cholesterol, Protein, and Amino Acids (Macronutrients) Retrieved from http://www.nap.edu/read/10490/chapter/1

46. U.S. Department of Agriculture (2016). Sample Menus https://www.choosemyplate.gov/budget-sample-two-week-menus

47. U.S. Department of Agriculture (2016). Interactive DRI Glossary. Retrieved from https://fnic.nal.usda.gov/interactive-dri-glossary

48. Clark, N. (2008). Nancy Clark's sports nutrition guidebook (4th Ed.). Champaign, IL.: Human Kinetics.

50. NutritionEd.org (2016). Distinguishing between a dietitian and nutritionist. Retrieved from http://www.nutritioned.org/dietitian-vs-nutritionist.html

51. Hales, D. (2013). An invitation to health: Build your future (15th ed.). Belmont, CA: Wadsworth Cengage Learning.

52. Rienberg, S. (2015). This diet may be dangerous for those with heart disease risk. Retrieved from http://www.webmd.com/heart/news/20150508/high-protein-diet-may-be-dangerous-for-those-at-risk-of-heart-disease#1

53. Harvard School of Public Health (2014). Halt heart disease with a plant-base oil-free diet. http://www.health.harvard.edu/heart-health/halt-heart-disease-with-a-plant-based-oil-free-diet-

54. DiLonardo, M. (2014). Can you drink too much water? Retrieved from http://www.webmd.com/fitness-exercise/features/water-intoxication#1

55. Ornish, D., Scherwitz, L., Billings, J., Gould, L., Merritt, T., SParler, S., Armstrong, W., Ports, T., Kirkeeide, R., & Hogeboom, C. (1998). Intensive Lifestyle Changes for Reversal of Coronary Heart Disease. *JAMA 280*(23):2001–2007. Doi:10.1001/jama.280.23.2001.

56. Qi, L., van Dam, R., Rexrode, K., & Hu, F. (2007). Heme Iron From Diet as a Risk Factor for Coronary Heart Disease in Women With Type 2 Diabetes. *Diabetes Care 30*(1): 101–106.

57. Down to Earth. (2016). Retrieved from https://www.downtoearth.org/go-veggie/top-10-reasons

58. ProCon.org (2016). Retrieved from http://vegetarian.procon.org/

59. MyFitnessPal. (2016). Retrieved from https://www.myfitnesspal.com/

IMAGE CREDITS

Fig. 2.1: Copyright © Depositphotos/sumners.

Fig. 2.2: USDA, https://www.choosemyplate.gov/myplate-graphic-resources. Copyright in the Public Domain.

Fig. 2.3: Copyright © Depositphotos/darknula.

Fig. 2.4: Copyright © Depositphotos/Shaiith79.

Fig. 2.5: Copyright © Depositphotos/alex9500.

Fig. 2.6: Copyright © Depositphotos/vojislav.

Fig. 2.7: Copyright © Depositphotos/mybaitshop.

Fig. 2.8: Copyright © Depositphotos/llepet.

Fig. 2.9: Copyright © Depositphotos/blueringmedia.

Fig. 2.10: Copyright © Muessig (CC BY-SA 3.0) at https://commons.wikimedia.org/wiki/File:ADP_ATP_cycle.png.

3 BODY COMPOSITION

WHAT IS MEANT BY FAT AND BODY COMPOSITION?

One of the common methods used by professionals to determine the health of an individual is the amount of a person that is made up of fat and fat-free mass. The human body is made up of a variety of parts that qualify as fat-free mass; muscles, ligaments, the brain, additional internal organs, water, etc. Although it tends to get a bad reputation due to the amount of concern over society's recent weight gains, **essential fat** is needed for the human body to properly function. This is typically about 8–12% in adult females and 3–5% in adult males. Keep in mind there are some things discussed later in this chapter that explain why the "average" numbers do not fit everyone. The reason for females having more essential fat is due to extra fat-depositing sites naturally occurring in the body (i.e., uterus, breasts, etc.).

The body stores this in cells dedicated to fat storage, and this is also known as **adipose tissue**. Fat storage can also be found in various locations on the body, such as **subcutaneous fat** (i.e., under the skin) and **visceral fat** (i.e., around internal organs). It is worth noting that visceral fat is considered more dangerous for your health then subcutaneous fat, because it surrounds vital organs, like your heart. The amount of fat cells you carry on your body is determined by your genetics, and you do not increase or decrease the number of cells by eating or exercising. Instead, you alter the size of the fat cell and how much it stores.. There are other factors that can play a role in the amount of fat being stored per cell, for example:

- Metabolism
- Gender
- Age
- Diet
- Activity level

METABOLISM

Your body operates on certain requirements to maintain its existence and function. The process takes calories to produce energy for the body's ability to operate. For your general existence and functioning with your body at rest, this process is called **Resting Metabolic Rate (RMR)**. Alterations to this can be found in respiration rate (i.e., how hard you breathe), your heart rate, your temperature, and your physical activity. Increasing these (for example through exercise) tends to cause a temporary increase in your body's metabolic rate, and burns more calories. Some people are born with higher resting metabolic rates. Due to this, they tend to burn more calories, and then, in turn, are able to eat more. An important way to increase resting metabolic rate is through increased muscle mass. The more musculature on the body, the more calories the body requires. The process of building muscle can also increase the resting metabolic rate, meaning even if you haven't made new muscle gain, just performing resistance training can help increase the burn of calories (although not near the amount of cardiovascular work). This is also why it is important for those who are doing heavy exercise (and trying to gain more muscles) to increase the amount of healthy and appropriate food being consumed.

SO WHAT ABOUT "GETTING FAT"?

Breaking down what makes us "fat" is usually, but not always, due to excessive calorie intake. This means that we are eating more calories than we are typically using throughout the day. As this continues, our bodies tend to store the extra calories in case we need them later. A pound of fat on the human body directly relates to 3,500 calories to burn, so no wonder it takes so long to make it come off! Another way to look at it is:

140 calories (average per soda) × 365 days = 51,100 calories per year = 14.6 pounds of waste.

This means even one soda a day, or similar wasted calorie intake, can make a huge difference on calories being over the required needs. Recognizing caloric needs and knowing what our body requires to function, as well as being active, is extremely important to proper fat maintenance and health. We look at having too much fat in the terms of **overweight** and **obesity.** Overweight is defined as the total weight of our body above the recommended weight for good health. The national weight recommendation is created by surveying very large populations. In the reports for 2014, 68.5% of adult Americans were considered overweight, more than double what it was 30 years ago. Obesity is the term used when a person is severely overweight, and it is considered a major negative factor in a person's health. Over 34% of adults in America are considered obese[1]. This raises major concerns not only for the health of Americans, but also for the health costs of the country, and paying for the side effects of being overweight and obese.

The physical consequences of being overweight or obese are:

- Diabetes
- Heart disease
- Stroke
- Dyslipidemia (e.g., high blood cholesterol and triglycerides)
- High blood pressure
- Metabolic syndrome
- Liver disease
- Gallbladder disease
- Kidney disease
- Asthma
- Sleep apnea
- Arthritis
- Chronic back pain
- Mobility limitations
- Some types of cancer
- Reproductive complications (e.g., irregular menses, infertility)
- Pregnancy-related complications (e.g., birth defects, gestational diabetes, preeclampsia)
- Poor health-related quality of life
- Increased all-cause mortality
- Decreased life expectancy
- Increased risk of hospitalization[1]

The potential psychological consequences of being overweight and obese are:

- Depression
- Anxiety
- Substance use disorders
- Social discrimination and stigmatization
- Employer discrimination (e.g., hiring prejudice, lower wages)
- Work impairment
- Time away from work
- Disruption of work, family, and social life[2]

Unfortunately, the issues of being overweight and obese are not just restricted to adults in American society, but have also grown among children and adolescents. It is reported that over 31% of children and adolescents are considered overweight, and over 16% are considered obese in this country. This has caused concern over the issues of children becoming unhealthy and at risk for major illness at this age, as well as concern for the cost on the country for healthcare in caring for individuals from early ages into late adulthood for what is a preventable disease[1]. Much of this can be looked at as an increase in the last 30 years. From 1980 to 2012, it is reported that 12- to 19-year olds in the US went from 5% to 21% in obesity. Younger children did not fare any better during that same time period with 6- to 11-year olds going from obesity levels of 7% to 18%[4].

FAQs CHECK!

Does a great looking body = being healthy or fit?

Unfortunately, looking good does not always equate to being healthy. Again, the culture that surrounds our health tends to be very supportive of how we look, but not necessarily healthy. Athletes and naturally thin people (being young at 18 helps) may be great to look at, but depending on what else they choose to do, they may actually be unhealthy. Professional athletes are famous for needing to make a change in their lifestyles once they retire, although their bodies are designed and maintained for their sport, they typically are not good for long-term health. Even bodybuilders who are fanatical about food and exercise, typically cut parts of their lifestyle that are more healthy to focus on their goals of maximizing gains. None of these actions have proven to move someone into a longer life or even a healthier one; however, it is worth noting that doing SOMETHING is better than doing NOTHING!

STORING FAT: WHAT CAUSES IT

GENETICS

Unfortunately, the genes given to you by your parents are the ones you are stuck with. They also determine your natural tendencies in your metabolic rate, as well as how your body reacts to physical activity, exercise, and what you eat. As stated earlier, different body types explained in Chapter 1 can explain how genetics apply. It is believed that genetics can contribute as much as 50% in your body's reaction to the factors mentioned above. The problem with a lot of the research in this area is that it is hard to separate the genetics from the exercise and eating behaviors learned within your family. Currently, researchers are working hard to assess and discover genes to better understand how our bodies develop differently, and why they react the way they do. Among all the genes researchers have discovered, we currently have been looking at an altered gene that controls insulin and in certain cases (about 1 out of 10 individuals), can cause them to build up excess fat. Other genes being discovered cause fat to be more likely to be stored in different areas of the body. For example, one person may store in the pectoral region and someone else in the thighs. However, recent research has suggested that a person engaged in regular physical activity has a tendency to negate many of these genes and can cause them to have little to no effect.

AGE

Age plays an odd part in the conversation of body composition. Typically we are less active as we age and our resting metabolic rate also slows down. This often leads to an increase in body fat as we get older. Even worse is that if we do not engage in physical activity and exercise during our younger years before middle age (and even in our middle age years), then this decline in metabolic rate happens more quickly and severely. This then can lead to increased health risks with the extra increase of body composition.

GENDER

Being male and female does play a role in one's body composition. Oftentimes, males will burn more calories than females, due to having a higher metabolic rate, and usually that means they can eat more. Keep in mind these are also based on age and maturity. Typically, in the infant and early stages the amount of fat tends to be the same, although males tend to weigh a bit more, making female infants having a larger percentage of fat. Early childhood tends to contain many similarities until around the age of six. Then females begin to see a rise in body fat levels, but puberty is usually when the largest amount of change occurs. Additional changes oftentimes occur due to childbirth, causing an increase in body fat composition.

ETHNICITY

When we look at the big picture of health, it should be reasonable to expect that outside of age and gender, there should not be changes across various ethnicities. However, medical research has indicated that there are some different averages in weight and body composition. Additional research is ongoing to fully understand this, and how much culture plays a role versus actual ethnicity. The largest obesity rates are among the African-American community (47%). This is followed by Hispanics (42%), Caucasians (32%), and Asian-Americans (10%).[3] This again creates issues, since it means that some ethnicities are potentially susceptible to health risks. It is worth noting that government agencies have also linked this to socioeconomic status.[4]

YOUR LIFESTYLE

Regardless of genetics, ethnicity, and gender, the choice of lifestyle often makes a difference. Although physical activity and exercise and how you eat do play a major role, the importance of sleep and stress in body composition cannot be overstated. Sleeping for short amounts of time has consistently been linked with higher body fat and visceral fat. Sleep is also able to keep us rested and better energized; otherwise, our body starves for energy and increases our appetite. Besides making us feel the need to snack more often, it also has been linked to inconsistent insulin levels, and creates a risk in diabetes. Stress also causes issues. Oftentimes, work and home life cause psychological stress, and has been associated in increased calorie intake (stress eating), weight gain, and visceral fat gain. The biggest threat again is diabetes. This is due to your body producing more glucose from the liver when stressed so that you have access to what the body thinks is "needed" energy. This constant increased dumping of glucose into the blood stream causes repeated insulin spikes until your body gets used to it, and you become diabetic.

FAQs CHECK!

Male Gut v. Female Hips

Body "shape" is often discussed when referring to where fat is stored. There is usually a general "apple" shape for men, and a "pear" shape for women. This especially begins to be more noticeable after puberty. We also know that this does alter as women go through menopause, as their bodies usually become more apple shaped. The "pear" shape is linked to the rise and fall of estrogen levels, with the drop of estrogen causing a women to be less "pear" shaped. However, this is a health problem since an "apple" shape is connected with more visceral fat and, as stated before, that equates to more health risks.

THE ROLE OF PHYSICAL ACTIVITY

Although nutrition plays an important role in controlling weight gain and obesity, it is discussed in another chapter. The role that physical activity plays in controlling the increasing weight gain in the country is enormous. Research indicates that 50% of adult Americans state that they get two and a half hours of moderate physical activity and exercise per week. About 31% get about 5 hours a week, but 26% of adults report that they do not get any physical activity at all. In fact, it is reported that the amount of adults meeting the minimum aerobic and muscular strength guidelines is 20%.[5] This isn't unique to adults though, as only about 27% of adolescents in the US are physically active daily. If we are wondering if these adolescence have free time, over 32% report watching TV for more than 3 hours a day.

Physical activity may not be a priority for many in this country, as seen by the health statistics, but it should be. Any physical activity has health benefits even on a moderate scale, and even if the individual is obese.

BENEFITS OF PHYSICAL ACTIVITY

- Build and maintain bone and muscle
- Reduce obesity and chronic diseases (diabetes, cholesterol levels, heart conditions, colon cancer)
- Reduce depression, anxiety, and improve psychological well-being
- Improve academic achievement in the classroom[6]

Although physical activity does not always respond immediately the same way in every individual, some will show weight loss immediately, while others will only after a significant amount of time has passed. Even though we have mentioned the health benefits of physical activity besides weight loss, the weight loss is usually the main goal for many. When reaching certain levels of physical activity, it allows you to burn significant enough calories to alter the calorie intake and outtake. This increase of calories burned, and the more physically active you are, the more calories you will burn and the more weight you will lose. Interestingly, the more body fat an individual has, the more calories an individual will burn during physical activity! Even better is that when combined with an appropriate reduction of, calories, there is an even greater weight loss, as there is a shift to burning more calories than are consumed. This creates a negative calorie total and causes the body to take it from spare calories stored in the body. This doesn't always mean it will show on the scale. A reminder is that 3,500 calories make up a pound. So running a few miles for a few days and burning a total of 2,000 calories may not show when you net weigh yourself, but it is happening over time, and over time, it will begin to show.

FAQs CHECK

Can I spot reduce?

The concept of spot reducing is the attempt to target specific areas of fat, your stomach for example, by performing exercise that targets those areas. The truth we have found in research is that the only thing that does is burn calories in general, based on the amount of exercise you perform. The risk (and this is only visual) of doing a lot of sit ups to reduce abdominal fat is that you might gain your six pack, but you may not lose the fat and you might have a larger belly to show for it, as the muscle pushes the fat forwards. The truth boils down to the fact that you need to burn more calories than you consume, as demonstrated in chapter 2, and cardio is often the way to go.

CONCERNS ABOUT BODY COMPOSITION AND FEMALES

With our society's continued emphasis on ultra-thin and extreme visual musculature as the model for health and fitness, there have been obsessions on achieving this look. Much of this focuses around females and what society feels is an optimal body or look by being extremely thin. This blend of extreme thinness, combined by exercise can lead to what is known as the **female athlete triad**. The triad consists of three separate problems, often to the point of disorder, that create many health problems. The first part often noted is excessive exercise combined with abnormal or disordered eating habits. This is where there is a restriction on calorie intake and nutritional needs are not being met for the amount of physical activity or exercise that is being performed. Oftentimes, this is extreme to the point of either a disorder or borderline disorder, with the female engaging in bulimia, where they purge or vomit their food after eating it, or anorexia, where they restrict calories to the extreme of barely eating. Unfortunately, this combination leads to reducing reduction in the hormones that effect the menstrual cycle. This could reach the point to completely stop the menstrual cycle. If the menstrual cycle discontinues for more than three months it is then labeled as **amenorrhea**. If continued, then there is a risk of premature osteoporosis. It is not uncommon for young women in their 20s and 30s who develop this complication to look like their bones are 40–50 years older than their age. It is believed that this may be more common than people realized and since they are not informed they do not worry about the loss of their menstruation cycle and what it could mean. However, if it is allowed to continue, it has been known to lead to risking death by shutting down organs in the body. Intervening early tends to be the solution, but the longer it goes on, the more damage that may occur with no way to recover from it. It is worth noting that sports or activities that focus on extreme endurance activities or may have a emphasis on weight control tend to be more likely to have these risks (track, cross-country, rowing, figure skating, gymnastics, cheerleading, etc.) Many of the notable signs and symptoms are those found in general eating disorders:

- Swelling around hands and ankles
- Low blood pressure
- Weakened bones and stress fractures (hairline cracks appearing in the bone)
- Brittle fingernails
- Cold hands and feet
- Dry skin and hair loss
- Extreme weight loss

HOW I SEE ME ...

At the end of the day, we may talk a lot about health, but most individuals are also concerned about how they are perceived by themselves and by others. Most of us look in the mirror and wish there were things we could change, especially if there is extra weight in locations on our body. This is where the advantage of frequent physical activity and exercise can help in many ways. Research in **self-efficacy** continues to show that those engaging in regular physical activity typically improve their emotions, moods, and issues with anxiety. This is only partially because they begin looking better over time, but also because as people engage in regular exercise they begin to feel a sense of accomplishment and control. Many people are more satisfied and comfortable with their bodies even when only small changes have been obtained. Several studies showed that as there was a healthy increase in physical activity or exercise behavior, there was an increase in positive feelings of self-worth.

However, some individuals become obsessed with flaws in their body and cannot become satisfied with the way they see themselves, regardless of the time they put into exercise or even plastic surgery. This is called **Body Dysmorphic Disorder**, which is when a fixation occurs on the flaws or flaw in appearance until it becomes obsessive, and considered a chronic mental illness.[7] Besides surgery, individuals suffering from this disorder may begin to take exercise to unhealthy levels, and usually go well above the recommended levels of exercise. Oftentimes, the thought process is, "why run for 30 minutes when you can run for three hours, and isn't it more healthy to do more exercise?" However, researchers point out that individuals with exercise addictions are different than those who exercise for general health due to the fact that they begin building the rest of their lives around their exercise habits. They consistently keep changing plans to fit their need for exercise, and eventually this begins to have an effect on their personal and social lives and behaviors. Long-term effects can lead to injuries, depression, exhaustion, and even suicidal tendencies.[8]

FIGURING OUT YOUR BODY MASS V. PERCENT BODY FAT

The most common way that most people measure their "fat" is by stepping onto the scale. Why this may be helpful in determining if you lost "weight" or are gaining it, it does not tell you if that weight is fat or potentially muscles mass. Due to this we have created ways for us to assess the amount of fat that people may have on their bodies, and if it is a serious health risk.

BODY MASS INDEX

We use the term **Body Mass Index (BMI)** as a way to categorize what health risks you may have based on the number you receive. Research has shown that BMI can be a reliable measure for average human beings. However, extreme or heavily athletic individuals may often not fit well into the categories, and other methods of assessment should be used. This is because BMI cannot tell if you are looking at fat or fat-free mass, and it is not very useful in tracking changes in the mass (muscle or fat). Oftentimes, when used for research, it is in conjunction with waist circumference and it is recommended that highly athletic people use a different form of measurement.

It is worth noting that normal BMI is categorized as 18.5–24.9, and although 25–29.9 is considered overweight, more and more people are falling into the categories above 30. As before, it is worth noting that women typically will have a higher BMI than men due to fat storage differences. Although happening less often in American society, a score that is low enough to fall below the 17.5 marker into mild thinness often is flagged as a potential eating disorder consideration. Low scores can also happen due to other health concerns and are associated with specific diseases or unhealthy habits like smoking. The bottom line is that there are several things that designate if you have a good category for BMI or not. Note that the way to calculate Body Mass Index is located in Lab 4.

WEIGHT CATEGORIES

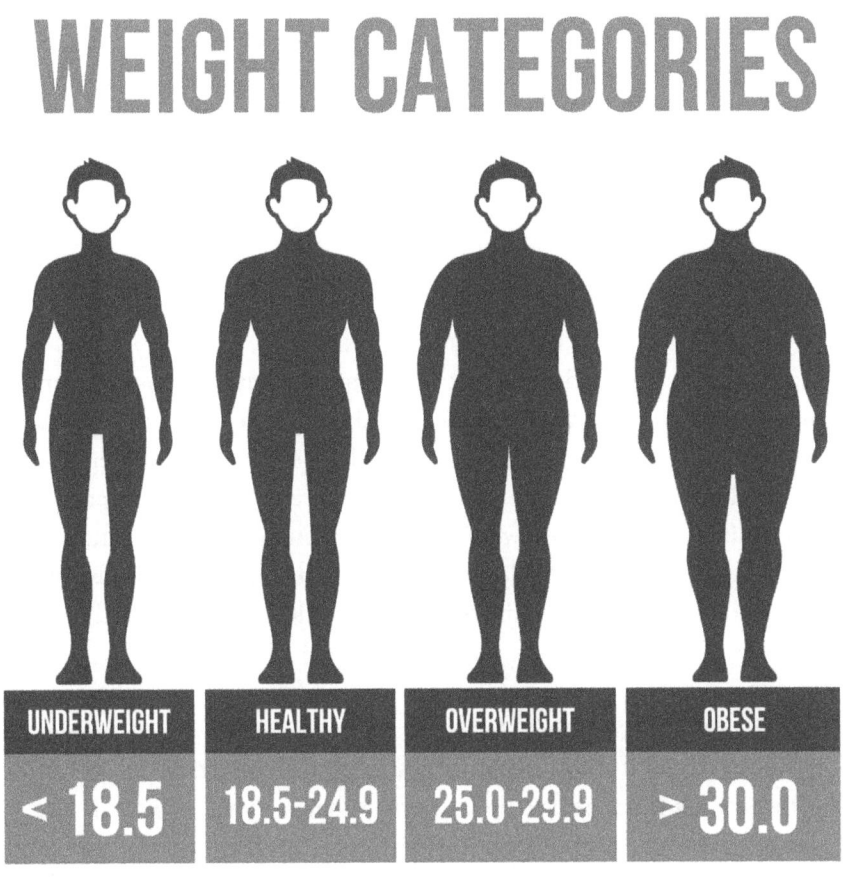

UNDERWEIGHT	HEALTHY	OVERWEIGHT	OBESE
< 18.5	18.5-24.9	25.0-29.9	> 30.0

Figure 3.1: Body Mass Index.

PERCENT BODY FAT

More accurate, especially in unique cases for athletes, is the concept of measuring the percentage of body fat that makes up a person. There are many ways to perform this, ranging from easy to complex, as well as cheap to expensive. Although none of these methods is 100% perfect and contain some degree of error, they are considered acceptable methods for research.

SKINFOLD CALIPERS

Probably one of the cheapest and easiest methods for measuring the percent body fat is the use of skinfold calipers. The calipers are typically better if made of a high quality material, like metal, and have a spring to make them "pinch." However, cheaper ones made of plastic can be purchased, but usually are not as trusted for producing accurate results. Measuring requires multiple different sites. Therefore, this combination is considered an indirect method for measuring. It is worth noting that the skinfold calipers methods has an error of 4% and that is only with a person who has proper training

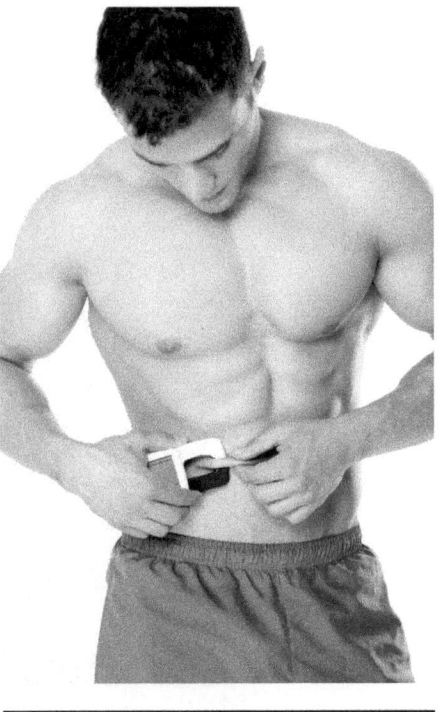

Figure 3.2: Skinfold Calipers.

and experience in using the calipers. The key for this is to follow the protocols to accurately know where to pinch the skinfolds, and it is also worth noting that skinfold thickness can be altered by how hydrated an individual being measured is. This means that this may change not only day-by-day, but even differ inside the same day. A recommendation is to track this often and around the same time of day for every scheduled evaluation, to keep the test accurate.

HYDROSTATIC WEIGHING (UNDERWATER WEIGHING)

In hydrostatic weighing, a person is placed on a seat and then submerged into water and weighed. The body density is then measured and percentage of body fat and the fat-free mass are estimated. This works due to fat having a lower density than water, and on the flip side, muscle has more density then water. Yes, technically a person dumped out of a canoe into a river floats more with more fat mass, however, less fat may make you more streamlined and less tired when swimming…which is important when that alligator decides to come your way. For decades, the gold standard in measuring percent body fat was hydrostatic weighing, so it is very common to find one in university exercise science labs across the country.

BIOELECTRICAL IMPEDANCE ANALYSIS (BIA)

A BIA measurement is unique in that it uses a machine to send a small electrical current through the body and then measures how much the tissue resists the current. What makes this work is that water is more heavily located in the fat-free areas of the body, making them excellent conductors. Fat, on the other hand, is not a good conductor. Basically, the least resistance the current encounters, the less fat there is. The error potential for BIA is pretty high at 4- to 5%. It can also be affected by the quality of product being used; a

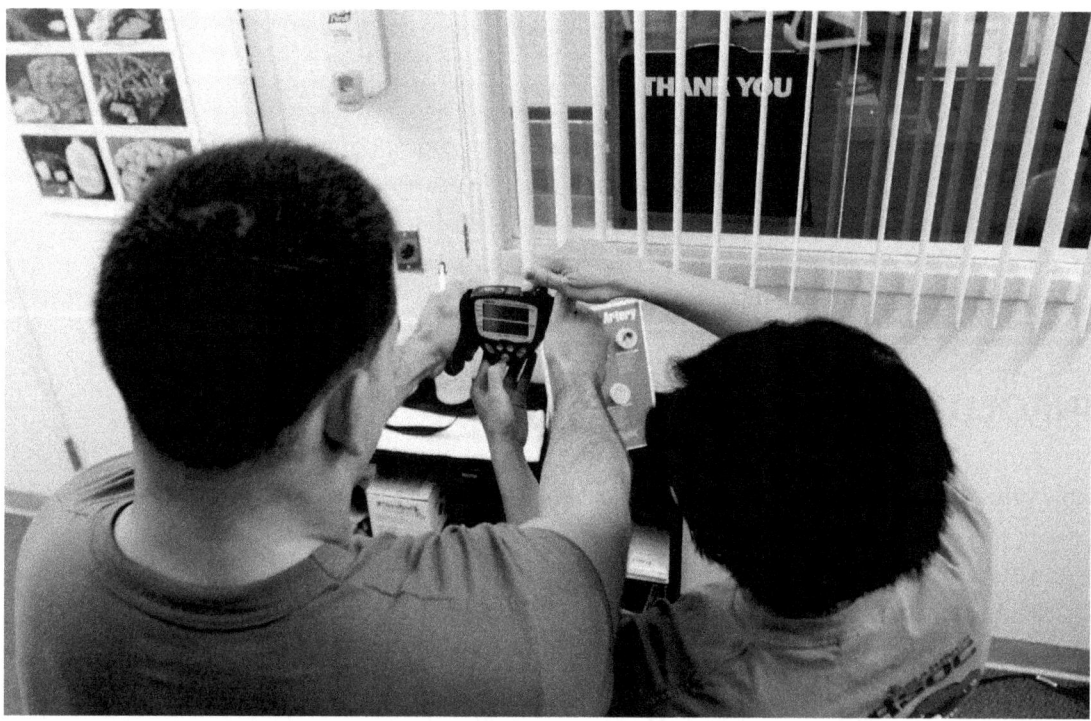

Figure 3.3: Bioelectrical Impedance Analysis (BIA) in Use.

cheap, hand-held machine could be bought online easily, but would not be nearly as accurate as a larger, more expensive machine found in the lab. Even if using a cheaper one (many are now combined with a weight scale so you can check when you stand on it for your weight), consistent use would allow for a solid baseline for your percent of body fat and can track alterations over time. It is highly recommended that you follow the instructions that come with the machine for an accurate reading. Since the amount of water in the body plays a role of conducting the electrical charge, it is recommended to be well hydrated, and to not test if dehydrated or overhydrated to keep it accurate.

BOD POD

The Bod Pod is a small egg-shaped chamber that measures a person's body composition by air displacement. It notes how much it is displaced or altered when a person sits in the chamber. The scientific name is called plethysmography, and has an error percentage of 2–4%.

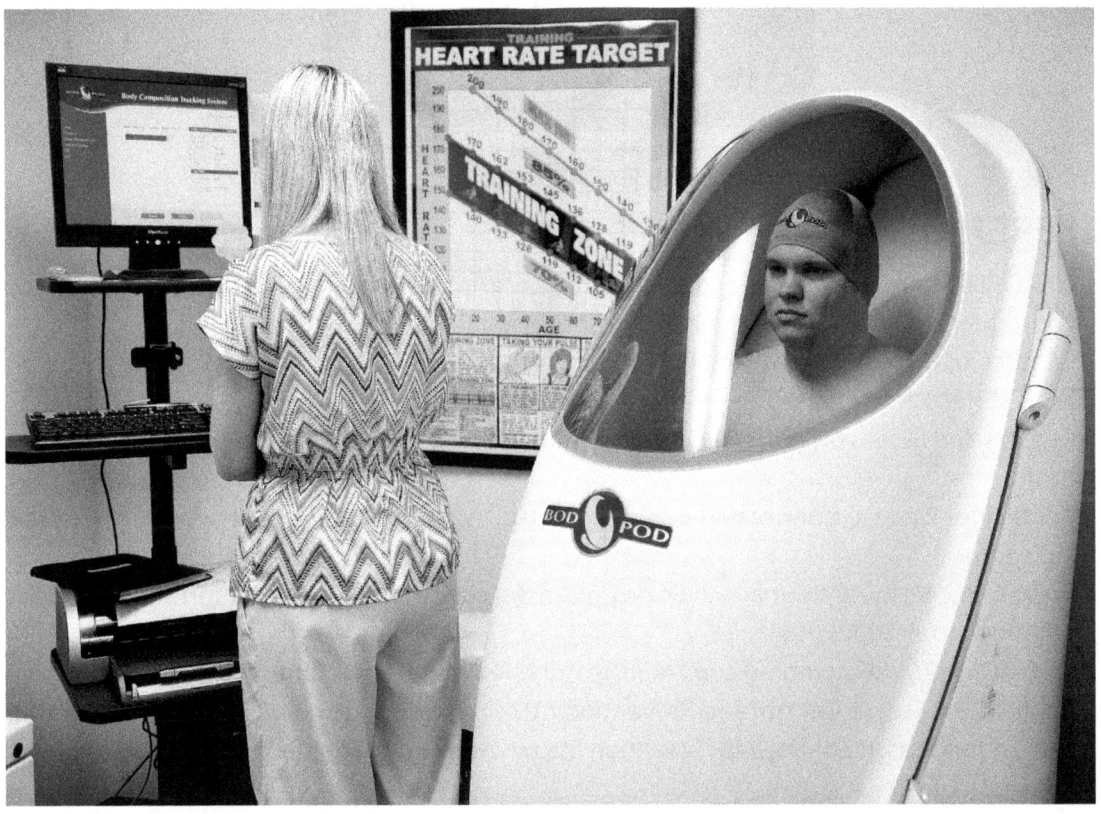

Figure 3.4: Using a Bod Pod to Assess Body Composition.

DEXA (DUAL-ENERGY X-RAY ABSORPTIOMETRY)

DEXA uses high and low energy beams to X-ray into tissue. This has an error rate around 2%.

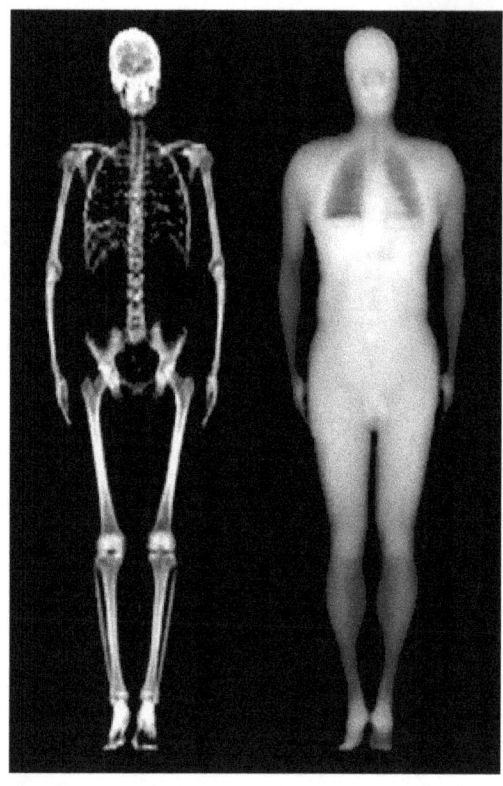

Figure 3.5: Results from a DEXA Scan.

REFERENCES

1. Food Research & Action Center. http://frac.org/initiatives/hunger-and-obesity/what-are-the-consequences-of-adult-overweight-and-obesity/.
2. Centers for Disease Control and Prevention. http://nccd.cdc.gov/NPAO_DTM/LocationSummary.aspx?statecode=94.
3. Centers for Disease Control and Prevention http://www.cdc.gov/healthyyouth/obesity/facts.htm.
4. Centers for Disease Control and Prevention http://www.cdc.gov/healthyyouth/physicalactivity/facts.htm.
5. Mayo Clinic http://www.mayoclinic.org/diseases-conditions/body-dysmorphic-disorder/basics/definition/con-20029953.
6. WebMDhttp://www.webmd.com/men/features/exercise-addiction.
7. Centers for Disease Control and Prevention http://www.cdc.gov/obesity/data/adult.html.
8. Centers for Disease Control and Prevention http://www.cdc.gov/minorityhealth/CHDIReport.html.

IMAGE CREDITS

4 CARDIORESPIRATORY ENDURANCE

Cardiorespiratory endurance is the body performing prolonged, large-muscle, dynamic movements. This is usually performed at a moderately vigorous intensity, and is considered a building block towards healthy living. It is also the most popular form of exercise that people perform, specifically walking.[1] This leads to the massive benefits that are gained in preventing both acute and chronic illnesses, as well as managing chronic illness that a person may already have.

HOW DOES THE CARDIORESPIRATORY SYSTEM WORK?

The cardiorespiratory system is essential for your life and bodily function. It does several amazing things like moving blood throughout your body, carrying oxygen and other nutrients to muscles and organs, while removing waste and toxins out of those same areas. It is made up of three parts:

- Your heart
- Your blood vessels
- Your respiratory system

YOUR HEART

Your heart is about the size of your closed fist, and is made up of four important chambers. While in specific settings, like when the American National Anthem is played, we reference the heart as on the left side of the chest; however, it is actually located predominately under your sternum. The heart's major purpose is to be the pump that sends blood into the lungs to be oxygenated (i.e., adding oxygen to the blood stream) and then pump it out to the rest of the body where it is needed, and the oxygen is removed. The design of the heart works through a process called **pulmonary circulation,** where the right side of the heart takes in the deoxygenated blood, and the left side sends out the oxygenated blood. When the body is circulating the oxygen-rich blood throughout the body and removing waste products, this is called **systemic circulation.**

What occurs is that oxygen-deprived blood returns from the rest of the body with waste, and enters the upper right chamber of the heart, known as the **right atrium** (also called the venae cavae). After the chamber is filled with blood, it contracts and pumps the blood into the **right ventricle**. After the ventricle becomes full, it also contracts and sends the blood through the **pulmonary artery** and into the lungs. In the lungs, blood removes waste products (i.e. carbon dioxide) that we **exhale,** and then picks up and adds oxygen from when we **inhale**. Now fresh oxygen-rich blood leaves the lungs through the **pulmonary veins** into the **left atrium** of the heart. After filling up, the atrium contracts and pushes the blood into the **left ventricle.** When the left ventricle becomes full, it pumps through the **aorta**, and out into the body. The aorta is the largest artery in the body, which is understandable since it's job is to push the oxygenated blood to other arteries throughout the body.

CIRCULATION OF BLOOD THROUGH THE HEART

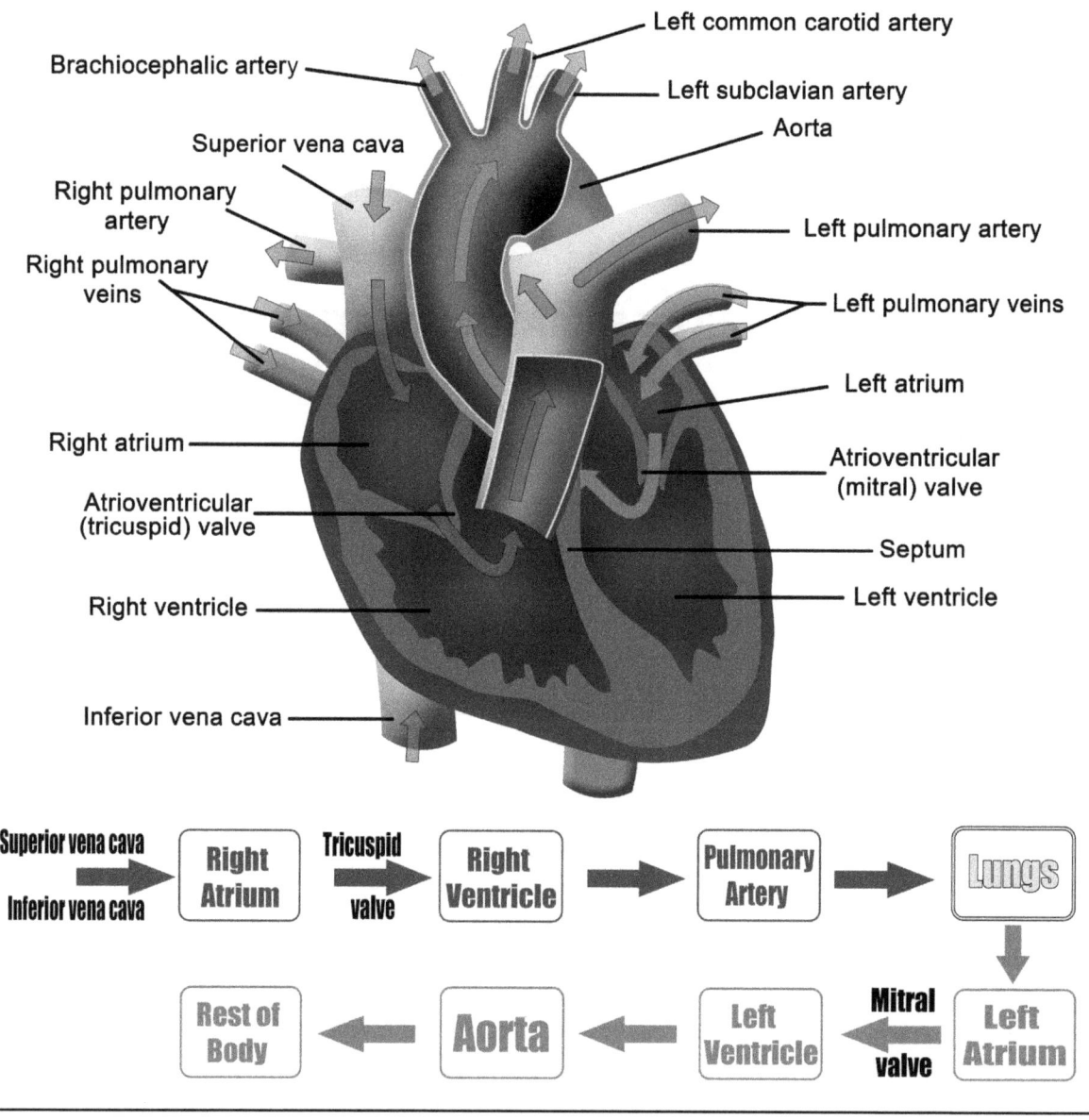

Figure 4.1: Anatomy and Circulation of the Heart.

YOUR BLOOD VESSELS

Blood vessels are divided into different categories by their function. As stated earlier, **arteries** carry oxygen-ated blood away from the heart and have thick, very elastic walls that can flex and relax as needed. When blood leaves the aorta, it branches into smaller vessels and correspondingly smaller arteries. Eventually it ends in **capillaries**, which are still considered blood vessels that are tiny to the point of being about a single cell in thickness. At this level, the blood coming in with oxygen and other nutrients will be exchanged with the depleted blood and waste. This depleted blood will then make its way back towards the heart through continuously larger vessels. First, going into **venules**, which then lead to the **veins**. Interestingly, the heart doesn't naturally "replenish" itself just by having blood pumped through its chambers; it has quite a few of its own arteries and veins that wrap around it after branching from the aorta.

Circulatory System Capilary Blood Flow

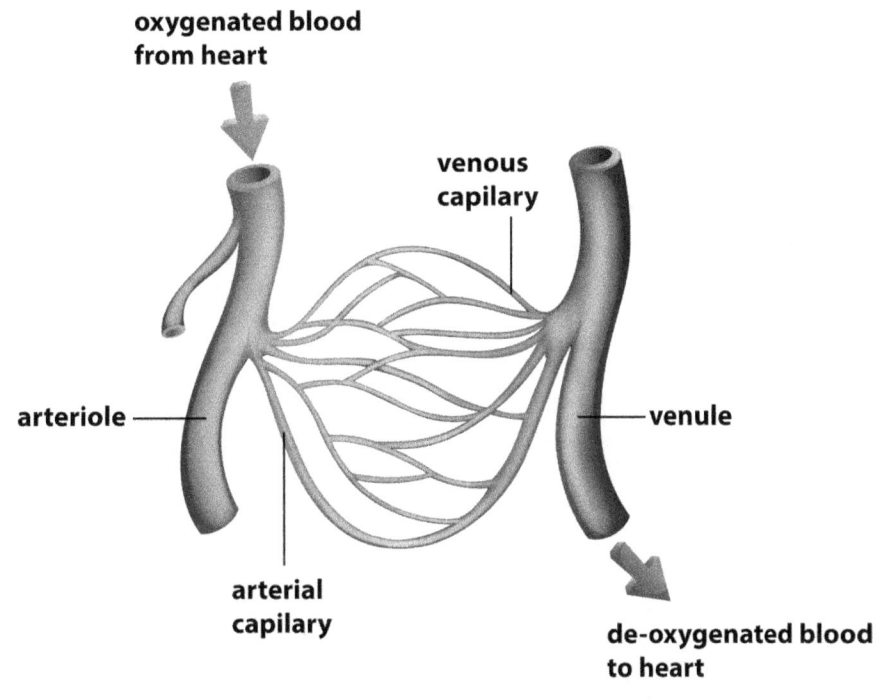

Figure 4.2: Capillary Function.

YOUR RESPIRATORY SYSTEM

The main job of the respiratory system is to provide oxygen through the lungs and remove waste. This helps us balance out the acid in our bodies as we activate our metabolism during increasing activities. How this works is that there is a change in pressure when you take a breath and fill your lungs with air. As you inhale and inflate your lungs, the air passes through **aveoli**. At this point, the oxygen molecules will pass from the aveoli, through the capillaries, and into the blood. Happening in reverse is how waste like carbon dioxide exits the blood stream. The now oxygenated blood returns to the heart, while the waste is then exhaled out of the body. Since oxygen intake and waste removal is essential to the body's functionality, this process must also be able to speed up to handle the intense demands placed on it when we increase our activity levels.

CONCEPTS OF THE RESPIRATORY SYSTEM

Normally when we are going about our day, or if we are resting, our hearts beat steadily. Our normal heart beat range tends to be between 50 and 80 beats per minute, with 60 being considered average. This results in around 12–18 breaths per minute to oxygenate the body. When the heart contracts during a heart beat, the phase is called **systole**. With systole, the heart pumps the blood from the atria and into the ventricles (i.e., the "lub" sound). Immediately a "dub" sound follows as the ventricles contract and push blood into lungs and body to circulate. When it goes into the brief period of rest after a heartbeat, the phase is called **diastole.** These components lead up to the concept of **blood pressure,** which is the amount of force placed on the walls of the blood vessel by the blood flowing through them. This force is created by the contraction of the heart, and you circulate all of your blood usually once per hour.[2] A typical blood pressure is considered a systolic of 120 and a diastolic of 80, commonly written as 120/80. There are various reasons for an increase in blood pressure, a common issue in the U.S. One could be constricting blood vessels, and an increase in heart rate, essentially forcing more blood through tighter tunnels. This issue also happens when blood vessels and arteries become blocked or harden, so that they cannot flex with the increased blood flow.

Our cardiorespiratory system alters when we place stress on it through vigorous physical activity. To handle this, our heart rate increases into the range of 170–210 beats per minute. Often this is accompanied by an increase in **stroke volume**, how much blood is pumped with each contraction. A continuation of this leads to an increase in the amount of total blood being processed through the body per minute, also known as the **cardiac output**. This can lead to an increase in higher blood pressure, like 180/90. It also creates a need for more oxygen and causes an increase in respiration rates, breathing as many as 40–60 breaths per minute. When we are operating normally, about 20% of blood goes to the muscles that control the skeleton. However, when we start intense exercise that can increase to as high as 90%.[3]

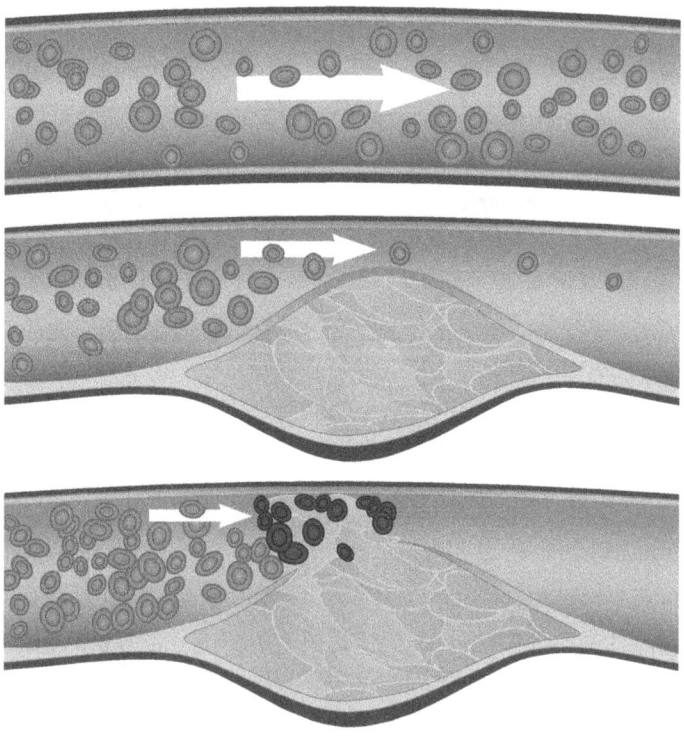

Figure 4.3: Blood Vessels Blocked.

BENEFITS OF CARDIORESPIRATORY ENDURANCE

PHYSIOLOGICAL BENEFITS

One of the best benefits of consistent and regular moderate exercise is that it can boost our immune functions. When combined with a healthy diet and plenty of rest, exercise places minor stress on the body, which causes an increase in the immune system due to repair work. This helps fight off colds and infections, and is also believed to help curb other issues like cancer.[4]

We also gain benefits from the continued increase of our heart rate, respiration rate, blood pressure, and cardiac output as we exercise over time. While this helps us improve our overall physical performance capability, it also helps us with the function of our everyday lives. Our left ventricle adapts by increasing in size and allowing it to push out more blood to the rest of the body with every contraction. This ends up allowing for a lower resting heart rate, as well as a decrease in blood pressure. Our blood's ability to transport oxygen also increases, meaning that we are able to transport more oxygen than before. This is good for also handling acute health, like preventing heart attacks, or handling the stress of a heart attack if one occurs, and increasing the chances of survival.

Our body also becomes more efficient in operating our metabolism. This leads to better control of energy use in our cells. This can be seen in the adaptation of the body using lactic acid and fat as fuel more efficiently, gaining better control of glycogen function, And increasing the number, as well as size, of mitochondria in your skeletal muscles cells. Your total number of capillaries increases, allowing an increase in oxygen and waste transfer. This also leads to an increase in general recovery from exercise, as well as injuries.

SELF-ESTEEM AND BODY COMPOSITION

When we eat excess calories that we do not use for fuel, our body is designed to store them for later. This made a lot of sense in the hunter and gatherer society that we had thousands of years ago when we didn't know where our next meal was coming from. Now though, usually some kind of restaurant is merely

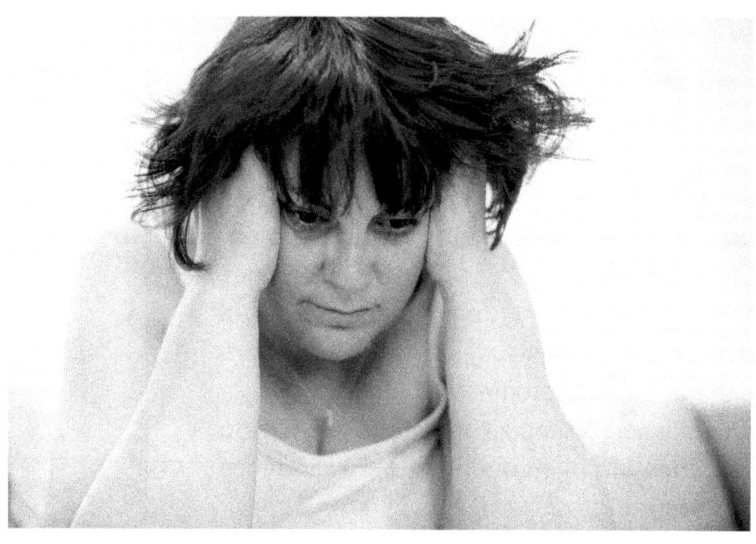

Figure 4.4: Depressed Overweight Woman.

a few blocks away from us, or within a decent reach. We also don't tend to have to spend a lot of calories trying to "catch" or find our own food sources. Combine this with the fact that we have more salt, sugars, and fats in our diets, as well as a continued decrease in physical activity (especially since more and more jobs are at desks and on the computer), then it isn't surprising that this built-in storage design has led to bigger waistlines. For most people, a major reason to exercise is to look better. As we use fat for fuel, it reduces that side of our body's composition and shows more of the muscular development that we may have. Cardiorespiratory endurance also releases dopamine, a feel good drug for the brain. Continued exercise leads to improved moods, and decreases in stress, anxiety, and depression. Research also shows that it leads to better sleep, and that as your body improves delivery of oxygen through the bloodstream, it also improves mental functionality.[5]

CHRONIC ILLNESS

As we engage in continued cardiorespiratory endurance exercise, we reduce the risk and are able to regress many chronic illnesses, especially for a beginning exerciser. The overall benefits of exercise on chronic illness are discussed in chapter 8, but we will briefly cover some of the benefits of endurance exercise here. Research has shown that various forms of cancer (colon, breast, lung, prostate, etc.) can be prevented through the continued use of endurance training. Since endurance training is considered a "weight bearing" exercise using your own body weight, it has some benefits for your bones. This form of exercise can prevent osteoporosis by placing stress on your bones in the early years (20–40s) and having them adapt and strengthen in response to the training. By strengthening and thickening the bones, it keeps the effects of osteoporosis, which reduces the bone density, at a minimum. This helps in preventing future bone fractures. Endurance exercise also causes glycogen (sugar) to be burned as fuel, and this prevents the need for the body to regulate your blood sugar levels and store the excess as fats. Sugar that isn't burned causes the body to become resistant to the insulin hormone and develop type 2 diabetes. As stated before, the heart also adapts to exercise and becomes stronger, putting it at less risk for various heart diseases and an acute heart attack. It will also make you have a stronger chance for survival if a heart attack does occur.

The benefits can also be lost relatively quickly if not maintained. Many people can reach their health-related goals in 4–6 months, and then enter a minimum 3-day a week maintenance phase to keep the benefits. Yet, if exercise stops, then the benefits can begin to drop in a matter of a few weeks. The recommendation is to start over from a lower level then you previous reached and work your way back up.

CREATING AN ENDURANCE PLAN WITH FITT

When you develop a program for cardiorespiratory endurance, what is accomplished depends on how you plan your goals. Part of all designs need to include a warm up and cool down (see below), a gradual start, and an increase of your FITT as you begin to adapt to the training, based on your endurance goals.

The *frequency* of training that is recommended by American College of Sport Medicine (ACSM) is 3–5 days a week. Some rest days must be included since repairs need to occur. That being said, we are referring to training, so it is okay to walk pretty much every day within distances that are your normal routine. While having some physical activity is better than engaging in no physical activity, it is stressed that usually a minimum of three days is required for performance improvement and activating fat loss. The total recommendation is 160 minutes of moderate activity, or 75 minutes of vigorous activity a week.

Intensity plays a huge role since typically our bodies are used to moving on a regular bases. The body must be forced to adapt by placing appropriate stress via training on it. Intensity can be measured in several different ways. The first of which is the **rating of perceived exertion (RPE)**, which is where a person states how much they feel like they are placing effort into the activity. This is usually on a scale of 1–20, ranging from no exertion to maximum exertion level. After exercising a few times, people will have a feel for how much effort and intensity various activities take. This is pretty subjective to each person though, and can vary and be quite inaccurate. The recommendation is that individuals begin to associate the perceived exertions with specific heart rate ranges. This is done by associating it to your target heart rate zone. A quick and easy way to see your intensity level is called the **talk test**. Along with the heart rate increasing, the respiration rate will also increase. Moderate intensity tends to make speech somewhat complicated, but a conversation is still possible. In vigorous physical activity, speech becomes reduced to very brief phrases.

The **target heart rate zone** is basing your endurance training around ranges that correspond to your maximum heart rate. The ACSM states that people should tend to use an equation to find their maximum heart rate, and then operate around 65%–90% for proper benefits. The closer to 90%, the more immediate benefits, like fat burning will be gained. However, if you are beginning an endurance program for the first time, then it is recommended to begin closer to the 65% part of the range and work your way up. The calculation for your Target Heart Rate is:

Maximum Heart Rate (MHR) = 220 − age
Target Heart Rate Zone (65% to 90%) = MHR × .65 and MHR × .90

Another short calculation that is sometimes used is the **heart rate reserve**, and it is considered the difference between the maximum heart rate minus the resting heart rate. The amount of reserve should be about 45–85% of your maximum heart rate, depending on how low your resting heart rate is. If the reserve is 40% or lower, then there is great concern.

Time is also an important consideration when discussing endurance training. The ACSM typically recommends that an average session for working cardiorespiratory endurance be 20–60 minutes for health benefits. Training longer can occur for those who are training for specific fitness goals. This can be broken up over multiple sessions so long as there is a minimum of 30 minutes. So instead of a 30-minute brisk walk, you may do a brisk walk of 10 minutes three times during the day. It is worth noting that the lower the intensity, the longer the exercise is recommended for equitable benefits. So a walk with a lower intensity rating (usually based on your heart rate) may be 40–60 minutes, compared to an intense job that might be 20–30 minutes. Some people use time to train at varied intensities. There is research support for pushing your body hard for a short amount of time, and then backing off to a slower pace for a while. For those trying to run for the first time, this is also a method to improve. It might be that

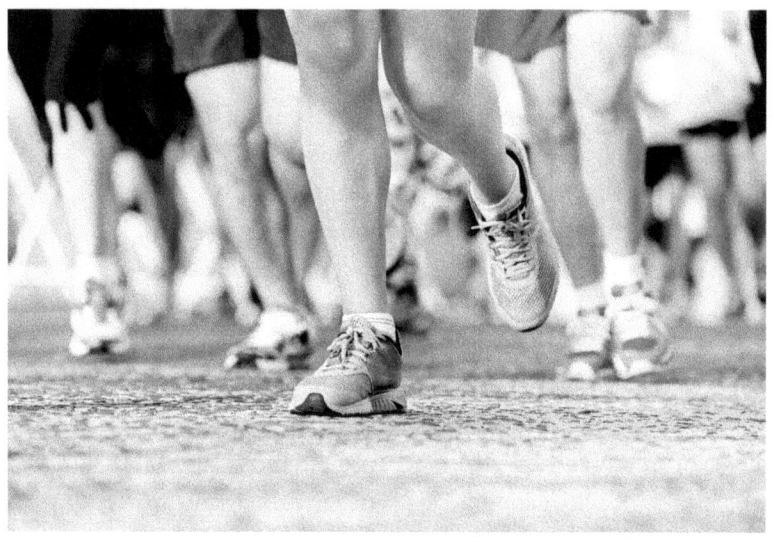

Figure 4.5: People Running Marathon.

the individual walks for four minutes and then begins to run for a full minute. Over time, they start to alter it so more of the 5-minute time is dedicated to running.

Different *Types* of endurance training are very common to see. This can be seen in triathlons, where a person does swimming, running, and bicycling. All of which are considered excellent, but the benefits from measuring distance vary heavily with these different activities. The recommendation is to use your heart rate to know your intensity level, and the amount of time that you hold it at certain levels to determine your training benefits. Individuals who have been injured can benefit greatly from exercises that have removed even weight-bearing capability like swimming.

WHY HAVE A WARM-UP AND COOL DOWN?

The importance of a warm up and cool down cannot be stressed enough for cardiorespiratory endurance. There is the benefit of injury prevention by warming up the muscles and through using them slowly, and increasing blood flow into those areas and their corresponding joints. The heart also has time to gradually ease into the required demands placed on it. As far as a warm up goes, it usually only needs to be 5–10 minutes. A beginning exerciser may need more time to warm up then someone who has been doing endurance exercises for a while. As pointed out in the other chapters, stretching is considered important, but isn't the same as a warm up and so cannot be counted in the time of the warm up. While further explained in Chapter 6, stretching has proven to have little to do with injury prevention and may reduce your performance capability.

A cool down is equally important, and in some ways potentially more so. As you slow your body's physical activity down over a 5–10 minute period, it allows the blood to quit being directly sent to your active muscles and back into the rest of the body to make it back its resting phase. If for some reasons a person just completely stops moving after a strenuous run, then there is a risk of plummeting blood pressure and **syncope** (passing out). This occurs due to the heart pushing blood out quickly and **vasodilation** of the blood vessels. When resting, the body tends to move the blood back to the heart easily, but when exercising this is more complicated since there is no form of arterial push for blood return. Our muscles squeeze our veins, pushing the blood back to the heart when it is operating at rapid speed. However, when we just stop after running for a long time, our heart will continue to pump out blood at a rapid rate, but our muscles are not returning the blood flow. This tends to lead to a lack of oxygen and a risk of dizziness or the potential to pass out. This is a perfect response, since if you pass out and fall to the ground then gravity will allow blood to flow into the heart. Yet, if for some reason you do not end up on the floor, and say collapse against a wall, without gravity's aid to return the blood flow at the rate of your increased heart rate, then this can lead to sudden cardiac arrest (not the same as a heart attack and is completely unrelated to heart disease).[6] A recommendation is to decrease you speed by half repeatedly every minute until you are in a normal restful walk.

ASSESSING CARDIORESPIRATORY ENDURANCE

The most common way we look at measuring an individual's cardiorespiratory endurance in a lab is through assessing his or her VO_{2max}. VO_{2max} refers to your body's maximum oxygen consumption and its efficient utilization of oxygen. The more this increases, the better our body becomes at handling endurance-related activities. Our body can adapt towards increasing VO_{2max} with a range of 10–30%. However, this is based on several of the following factors:

- Fitness level
- Health level
- Genetics
- Age

The largest benefits will be for those who are just starting programs and they can usually start seeing the effects in a few weeks. Yet, when someone has been operating for years, the increase may occur from minor alterations in training, but those alterations will be tiny and hard to notice unless precise assessment is occurring. Also, continued use of endurance training will cause your heart rate to lower at a resting state. This may occur as early as four weeks after training, and a heart rate can lower as much as 10–15 beats per minute. These are all observable changes a person beginning training can see without much formal assessment, but there are also more commonly used assessments.

COMMON ASSESSMENTS

One of the most popular tests for young adults is the *1.5 mile run/walk test*. The concept behind this test is that we consume more oxygen when we increase our speed while running. So scoring a faster time on this test tends to indicate a high VO_{2max}. Another popular test is the *1 mile walk test*, which measures your VO_{2max} based on how long it takes to quickly walk a mile. The measurement is based on the time it takes to finish the mile and how fast your heart rate is on a chart. The last common type of assessment is the

3-minute step test. An individual will step up and down onto a step and cause an increase in heart rate. After the three minutes has ended, the measurement is how long it takes for the heart rate to return to normal.

HEART RATES

As mentioned previously, your heart rate will adapt to endurance exercise over time so that it is lower when at rest. Beyond this, we can monitor it to reflect our intensity (discussed above) while we are actually exercising. This is typically done by placing two fingers (index and middle fingers) on your neck, called the carotid artery, and on the inside of your wrist, known as the radial pulse. Do remember to avoid using your thumb since it contains its own pulse. Light pressure is usually enough to detect your heartbeat; press too hard and it can cut off the blood flow. Often, we count the beats detected per minute. However, holding your pulse while running for a full minute could be complicated. Yet, only counting beats for ten seconds and then multiplying by six will let you check it quickly. With the advent of new technology, we are seeing heart rate monitors outside of the lab and medical settings. They also now integrate with smart phone software to provide it as one variable to the overall assessment of your digital health profile.

METS

Another way we tend to assess endurance exercise is through monitoring how our metabolism increases with exercise. It baselines at one MET, which represents the body's metabolic point while at rest. As people begin to exercise and use twice as much energy than when they are at rest, then they are considered using two METs. Exercises tend to be reflected on a scale of one to twelve. With low intensity, having MET ratings of three to four could be walking. Moderate intensity exercises, like heavy hiking, can be up to seven METs. High intensity exercises like jogging can be as high as ten or twelve METs. Again, this means more energy requirements, which in turn means more calories burned. Using METs shows us that upping the intensity allows us to burn more fat as fuel, and begin to alter our body composition. Factors that affect the METs increasing and decreasing beyond intensity are:

- The environment exercise is performed in
- Body composition
- Body weight
- Skill level for the exercise performed

COMMON SAFETY CONCERNS

Being that cardiorespiratory endurance is the most common form of fitness and exercise that people engage in, there is always some form of risk that can occur.

COMMON INJURIES

Although it usually isn't considered an injury, **blisters** happen often enough that they need to be dealt with. This occurs when friction has rubbed the skin enough to cause fluid to accumulate under the skin. Avoid draining or tearing it unless it is absolutely necessary. They make small covers that cushion around them to decrease the pressure being placed on it. If it does tear, try to keep the skin intact and clean with antiseptic

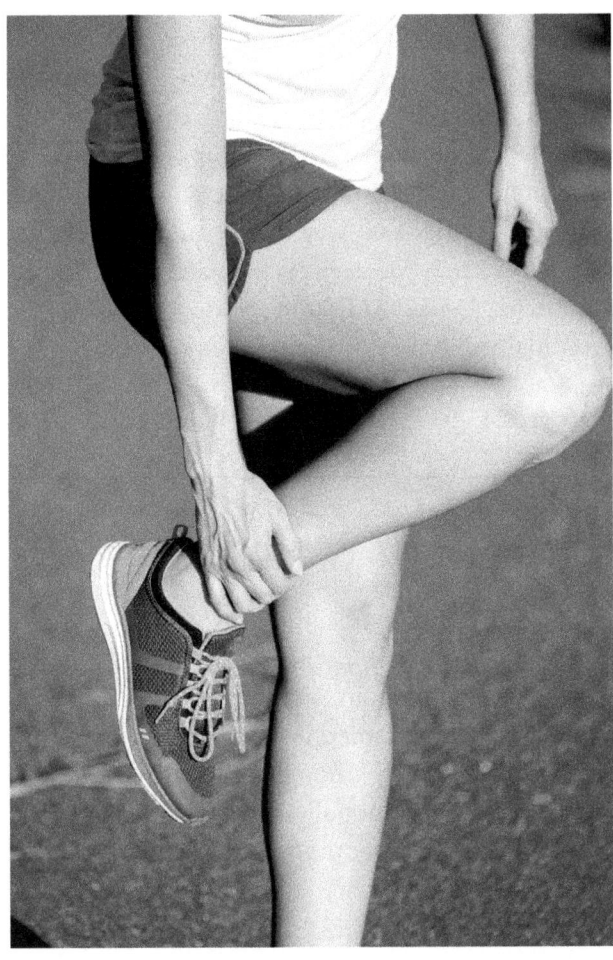

Figure 4.6: Injuries can easily occur if prevention isn't planned.

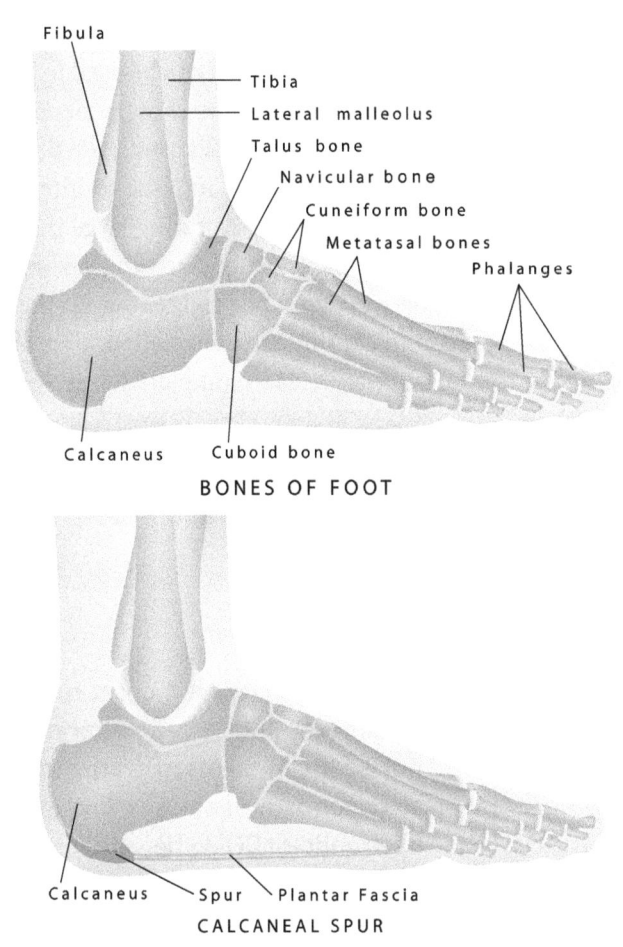

Fibula
Tibia
Lateral malleolus
Talus bone
Navicular bone
Cuneiform bone
Metatasal bones
Phalanges

Calcaneus   Cuboid bone
BONES OF FOOT

Calcaneus   Spur   Plantar Fascia
CALCANEAL SPUR

Figure 4.7: Heel Spur.

before bandaging, as this avoids infections. Some people purchase a product called moleskin that is thin and can be placed on the skin so rubbing doesn't bother your skin.

A **sprain** is when there is an over-stretched or torn ligament, and typically this happens around joints. A **strain** is when there is a stretch or tear that occurs in the muscles or tendons.[7] This could be felt at different points in the muscle, and therefore may not hurt at the biggest part of the muscle. Typically, this is associated with the local area of injury having pain, tenderness to touch, swelling, some discoloration, and minor loss of function. The primary recommendation is to apply Rest, Ice, Compression, and Elevation (RICE). After the swelling goes down, switch to warm cloths to help circulation in the area, and then carefully work on stretching and strengthening the injured location.

Sometimes you will hear people complain of **shin splints**, which is a pain usually located in the front of the lower leg, opposite of the calves. This can be common in people changing their routines or intensities, and is not abnormal since it is usually an indication that the muscles are being overworked in some way. Major recommendations are to rest, and use ice to mitigate swelling before and after exercising. When performance is required, then adding support by tapping the area may be required. Making sure to strengthen and stretch the area is vital, as well as using excellent footwear and support.

Plantar fasciitis is a common heel pain for runners. It is inflammation over a band of tissue the goes along the bottom of your foot to your heel. It often feels like a stabbing pain in the foot. The recommendation is to apply ice, and use flexibility training to help flex the area out. There are a number of footwear products that can be used to help support through compression, which often reduces the pain.

Side stitch is a term that many people are familiar with, which is a sharp, stabbing pain in the side. However, knowing what causes it is a little more complicated. There are a variety of things that might be related, most involving an issue of intense exercise and pulling on internal organs in some way. There have been some links to eating large meals or high sugar intakes, but no way to determine if there is a cause and effect relationship. The recommendations are to stretch the arm on the pain side, then try bending forward while tightening up the abdominal muscles. Usually side stitch passes and allows the person to continue to exercise, but they are so painful initially that they can cause even the best-trained endurance athletes to completely stop where they are at.

FAQS CHECK!

What is DOMS?

This refers to delayed onset muscle soreness. It refers to the pain and muscle soreness occurring 24 hours or so after exercising. In the past people blamed lactic acid build up, but it actually seems to relate more with the repair work the body is doing. It can also show some tenderness and swelling in the areas being effected. Traditionally, there is not really treatment for DOMS beyond rest. Prevention is possible by using equipment properly, and to progress gradually with increasing intensity or time in an exercise.

ENVIRONMENTAL CONCERNS

HEAT

While operating in warm and hot weather is common, there are always risks associated with endurance training in this type of weather. **Dehydration** can easily occur if the individual is not taking in or replacing proper fluids during exercise. It should be noted that this can technically happen in any form of weather, but is more typical in hot weather due to the amount of sweat removing fluid from the body. You begin to feel dehydration early on, and will notice the first signs of feeling thirsty, which you shouldn't ignore. The recommendation is to drink enough to match fluid loss about every 30 minutes, and if the temperature increases (or your intensity) then the time might need to be more every 10–20 minutes. It isn't enough to just drink while you're exercising, but also plan ahead by drinking a cup or two of water a few hours before hand, depending on your hydration habits. This will also prevent a decrease in performance capability.

Heat exhaustion happens when not enough blood is returning to the heart since it is going to the active muscles, as well as the skin to cause you to cool down. Symptoms begin to show in the form of a weak but quick pulse, headaches, feeling weak and dizzy, becoming pale, sweating heavily, and potentially being confused. The most common way to handle this is to sit in a shaded or cool area, use cool clothes to help lower body temperature, and drink plenty of fluids. Typically this person should avoid more training or exercise for the day so that their body can rest and recover. **Heatstroke** usually occurs if heat exhaustion is not addressed, and is a serious medical issue that can result in death if not treated. The body temperature has risen to the point that sweating has shut down, which in turn causes the temperature to increase further and rapidly. It results in very severe symptoms such as a hot, flushed and dry face, chills or shivering, confusion and odd or irregular behavior, and may lead to a person collapsing or convulsing. The body temperature is so high and even survival can risk brain damage, so it is recommended to cool them as quickly as possible, and to seek medical attention at a hospital.

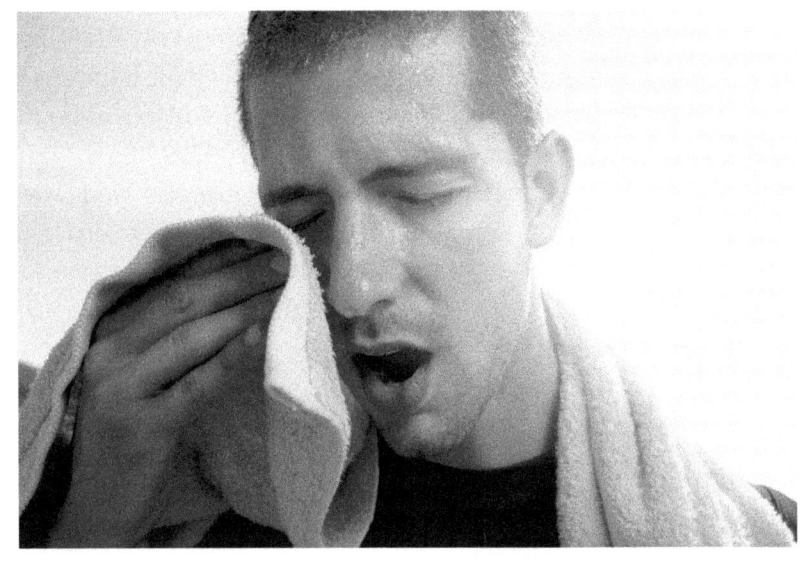

Figure 4.8: Drinking fluids during exercise is essential when temperatures increase.

COLD

Cold weather issues arise from a person's core body temperature dropping too low to the point that he or she is no longer able to regain heat at the rate they are losing it, which is also known as **hypothermia**. The end result is the nervous system decreasing until a person feels sleepy, and their energy consumption decreases. During hypothermia, it isn't uncommon for individuals to go so far as to slip into a coma and risk death.

Frostbite also can occur in extremely cold temperatures, and it is when the body's tissue begins to freeze. Oftentimes, it is the small parts that tend to stick out, like ears, noses, and fingers, that are affected the most. The cold temperature causes poor circulation to the area to the point the tissue doesn't circulate blood and freezes. Keep in mind that cold is not just based on the actual temperature outside, but the amount of wind and the temperature change that can occur. Meaning that it is worth looking at the *wind chill* reported by the news for this information since it is a better reflection of that combination. Dressing for the temperature change, and in layers of clothing go a long way to preventing this. While you may dress light to run and decrease sweating in the cooler temperature, you need to be prepared to risk stopping while on your run and have clothes to add layers to keep you warm, since moderately cold temperatures can still cause frostbite in 20–30 minutes.

REFERENCES

1. Bureau of Labor Statistics. Sports and Exercise. http://www.bls.gov/spotlight/2008/sports/.
2. "How Long Does it Take Your Heart to Circulate the Total Amount of Blood in Your Body?" *Lansing State Journal*. http://www.pa.msu.edu/sciencet/ask_st/120193.html.
3. Boone, T. *Introduction to Exercise Physiology*. Burlington, MA: Jones & Bartlett, 2014.
4. National Cancer Institute. "Physical Activity and Cancer." http://www.cancer.gov/about-cancer/causes-prevention/risk/obesity/physical-activity-fact-sheet.

5. WebMD. "Shocking Heart Deaths: Why They Happen." http://www.webmd.com/heart-disease/features/sudden-cardiac-arrest-why-it-happens?page=4.
6. Mayo Clinic."Sprains and strains." http://www.mayoclinic.org/diseases-conditions/sprains-and-strains/basics/definition/con-20020958.
7. Mental Health Foundation. "Exercise and Mental Health." http://www.mentalhealth.org.uk/help-information/mental-health-a-z/e/exercise-mental-health/.

FIGURE CREDITS

5 DEVELOPING MUSCULAR STRENGTH AND ENDURANCE

WHY IS IT IMPORTANT?

Muscles are essential for movement and function. Not only could we not move or grab things we might need, muscles also protect us from injury and help us with calorie expenditure and weight loss. When we discuss **muscular strength**, we are referring to the amount of force we can produce on a single maximum effort. Depending on the muscle movement, this often is measured by how much weight we can use while doing the movement just once. If we can do the movement more than once, or not at all, then we are not looking at our optimal muscular strength for that movement. By developing **muscular endurance**, we are working on how many times a muscle can contract and repeat a movement, or how long the muscle can hold the contraction or action. A great example of muscular endurance can be seen in push-ups, which are common in exercise assessment. The strength portion is being able to lift your body; however, we usually see how many a participant can do, which is measuring muscular endurance. Both muscular strength and endurance play a major role in not only our physical performance, but also our short and long-term health. To fully understand their roles, it needs to be understood how they work.

FAQs CHECK!

So when we quit working out, does muscle transform into fat?

For some reason, younger people seem to believe that these two types of body tissue are similar, but they are in fact very different types. While one tissue may shrink thereby making the other one seem larger, it is not one tissue becoming another. Stopping working out just results in the muscle shrinking due to inactivity. Unfortunately, if physical activities decrease and calorie consumption continues, then usually an increase in body fat occurs.

PHYSIOLOGY OF MUSCLES AND TRAINING

Muscles are designed to move the skeleton from point A to point B, and they also allow us to generate and exert force on objects. This works due to a muscle contracting, shortening it, and pulling on the tendons that attach the muscle to the bone. In a simple example, when we contract the bicep muscle, the tendons are located at the shoulder and below the elbow on the inside of the arm. Even though the muscle is visible in the upper arm, the lower tendons connect to the inside forearm and as the bicep contracts, it pulls the skeletal muscles in the forearms closer. The muscle that is focused on being worked during a contraction is called the **agonist**. The muscle that is opposite to the agonist, which is contracting, relaxes in response and is known as the **antagonist.** In the case of a bicep curl, a bicep is the agonist during contraction, and the triceps relax and are the antagonist.[1]

MUSCLE FIBERS

Like the rest of your body, muscles are made up of cells. These cells are actually quite unique and are called **muscle fibers.** Muscle fibers are not the normal rounded-looking cells we usually discuss in biology class, but instead are elongated so that they can work like a bungee cord that can stretch, and then tighten and contract, pulling on both ends. Inside the muscle fibers are bundles of similar and tiny protein structures called **myofibrils.** These myofibrils are the actual containers for the **sarcomeres,** which contract the muscles through a hook and pull motion by the actin and myosin molecules (which is fascinating, but far more detailed then needed for this book). It is often stated that we "grow" muscle, but in reality, after we become adults we really stop growing new muscle fibers as we adapt. Increasing the number of muscle fibers is called **hyperplasia.** We do, however, cause fibers to increase in their size, effectively making bigger muscles. This increasing in muscle fiber size is called **hypertrophy.** There is a reverse to this process; with inactivity there can be shrinkage of muscle fiber size, called **atrophy.** Many people who have had to place an arm or leg in a cast will be familiar with the casted limb being much smaller than its counterpart when the cast is removed.

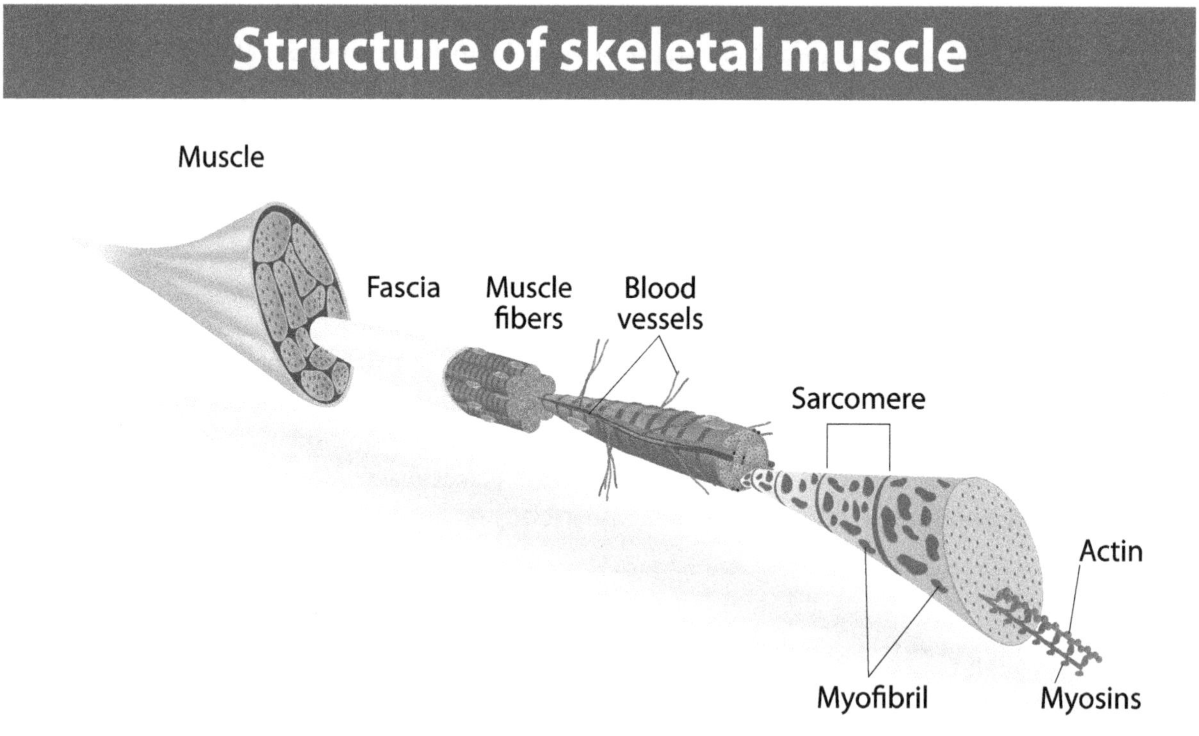

Structure of skeletal muscle

Muscle

Fascia Muscle fibers Blood vessels

Sarcomere

Actin

Myofibril Myosins

Figure 5.1: The human muscle is deeply complex, and involves layer of working components.

TYPES OF FIBERS

While we have talked about fibers in general, there are two types of fibers and they play very essential but different roles in our movement ability. **Slow-twitch fibers** typically are not able to contract quickly or as strong as their counterpart. However, they are not at a complete disadvantage because they are extremely resistant to fatigue and tend to not tire as quickly. They are considered oxidative in nature, and work better with that energy system more efficiently (as seen in Chapter 2). **Fast-twitch muscles** contract very quickly and are far more powerful, operating on the anaerobic system (not requiring oxygen). They tend to tire quickly though. They are also whitish in color.

While human beings are made up of a mixture of these types in all of our muscles, we do have a variance percentage from person to person. Which means some people may be well balanced, others may lean more towards having fast-twitch or slow-twitch fibers. Most of this is determined by genetics, which is why it is common to see athletes who become parents tend to have children who seem physically gifted in a similar sport or activity. Meaning those who have slow-twitch fibers tend to excel at endurance activities like cross-country running, and the fast-twitch fibers tend to benefit those who are engaged in sports for speed, strength, and power. This can be seen in power lifting and sprinting. The only real way to test and know which predominate muscle fiber type you might have requires a muscle biopsy (most people don't jump at the chance to have a small incision and piece of muscle snipped out). Before you worry that you may never be able to complete a marathon because you may lean the other direction, you need to understand that you also have a few indeterminate types of muscle fibers that tend to be neutral. These specific types are amazing in the fact that they can be trained over time to fit more in line with the goal of your training; meaning if you are training for a marathon, than these neutral fibers will begin to act like slow-twitch fibers. So why we may have a tendency to be better at some activities, it does not mean we cannot be adequate in our performance goals.[2]

FAQs CHECK!

Do you prefer dark or light meat on the Turkey on Thanksgiving?

An interesting fact is that when we place slow-twitch fibers under a microscope they appear reddish in color. On the other hand, if we place fast-twitch muscles under the same microscope, they would appear whiter looking. This appearance can be seen clearly in some species even upon visual inspection. Turkeys are not well known for their ability to fly very far. Even though their wings are extremely powerful, they tend to tire extremely quickly and are usually used to moving around complex obstacles, or moving quickly away from a threat. However, a turkey's legs are built to be in constant motion and can run around all day. This is why when you inspect a turkey (Thanksgiving being a perfect time!), it can be seen that the wing and breast meat is typically white looking from the amount of fast-twitch muscle fibers, and the legs and corresponding areas are red due to being slow-twitch muscle fibers.[3]

MOTOR UNITS

While the physical makeup of a muscle and its performance has been discussed, the actual trigger called a **motor unit** has not. The motor unit is the **motor neuron** (the nerve) and it's connected to the muscle fibers. This relays the message from the brain through the nervous system, to the specific nerve that recruits the required muscle fibers. The more strength that's required, the more the motor units will be activated. A single motor unit could be connected to a few muscle fibers, or several hundred. The more complex and precise movements need many fibers connected to the motor unit. An example could be seen in the eye and the precision movements needed to direct and focus one's vision. Interestingly, motor units adapt as they go through training, especially strength training. Usually the first eight weeks of strength training does not have much muscle growth, but individuals feel like they are making gains and are often are able to increase the load of weight on their chosen exercises. However, the actual term for this is **muscle learning,** where physical performance and strength increase before increased muscle size occurs.[4]

MOTOR NEURON

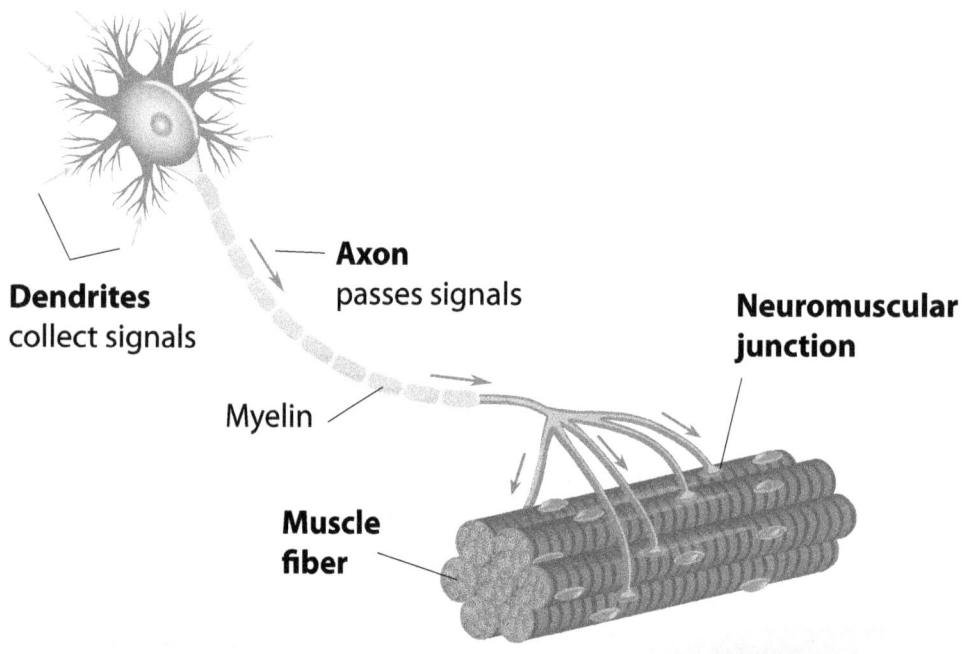

Dendrites
collect signals

Axon
passes signals

Myelin

Muscle fiber

Neuromuscular junction

Figure 5.2: Motor Neuron.

BENEFITS OF MUSCULAR STRENGTH AND ENDURANCE

PERFORMANCE AND INJURY

Muscular development can help prevent injury for numerous reasons, most importantly in supporting your posture and also strengthening the body's ability to perform everyday lifting. With the major complaint of back pain by many adults, correcting both those issues is a priority that can be solved through muscular strength and endurance training. This can help prevent acute and chronic injuries. Besides general everyday movements, improving muscular development can also make performance in sport or recreational activities far more enjoyable by mastering advance techniques in those activities.

AGING AND HEALTH

Unfortunately, as we age and pass 30-years old, we no longer retain muscle mass as easily. This doesn't mean we can't build muscle mass as we get older, just that as every year goes by it takes more work to maintain the mass we currently have. Muscle soreness and injury tend to take longer to recover from as we age as well. Individuals need to learn to adjust for their body's aging process. Other issues are not just the muscle mass reduction, but also the motor units do not adequately connect as we age. Also chronic diseases can be managed and avoided by training, by effecting glucose control, oxygen consumption, blood pressure, and cholesterol.

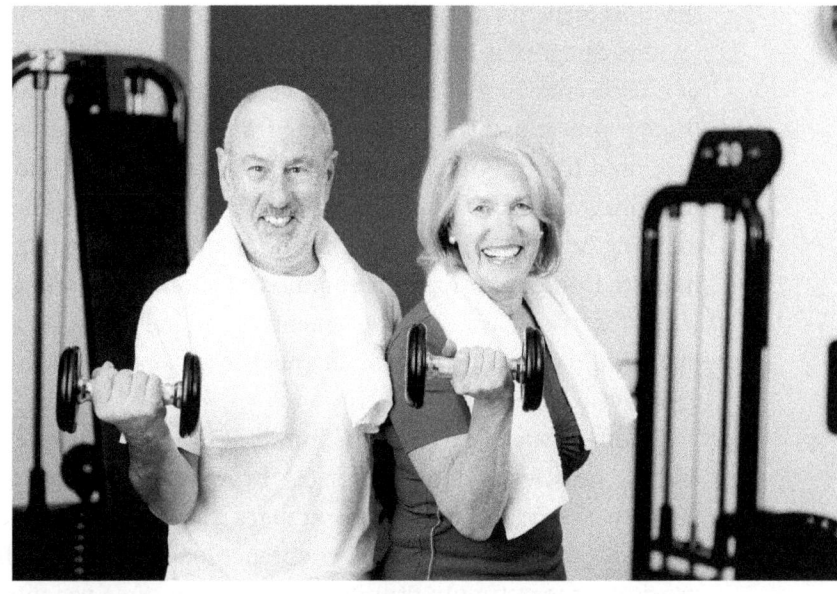

Figure 5.3: Strength training doesn't have to end just because we age.

QUALITY OF LIFE AND BODY COMPOSITION

Training muscular strength and endurance helps in balancing body composition (as seen in chapter 3). This occurs by increasing the muscle mass, raising that side of the proportion. Also, increased muscle mass uses more calories per day for function. Meaning the more muscle mass on your body, the more calories you burn by increasing your metabolism, the more reduction of fat can occur. There is also the afterburning effect that occurs after a strength training session, which can last for several hours by burning additional calories for that day. For most people, a major goal of strength training is to look better, and feel more comfortable in their clothes and how they look. This tends to lead to more self-confidence and a better quality of life.

FAQs CHECK!

So increasing my protein intake will help me lift more?

This is sort of a half yes and no. Protein does not make you stronger; no matter how much you take in, it doesn't make bigger muscles. Being in the gym and forcing your body to make adaptations is how you get bigger muscles. That being said, protein is a building block in muscle repair, especially for recovery after heavy workouts. Meaning that if you engage in a heavy strength training routine and ingest a recommended protein amount pretty quickly after, then it helps repair the muscles, leading to increased muscle growth as a response.[5]

TYPES OF STRENGTH TRAINING

There are three categories that we place strength training movements in. These categories have to deal with the movement, if any at all, that the muscle is making while it is contracting.

One category is **isometric exercise**, which means that the muscle is contracting, without the length of muscle changing. Placing your hands on a wall or table and pressing hard can demonstrate this. Even though your muscles are contracting from the exertion, they are not actually changing length. Although they used to be popular with door-to-door salesmen at the beginning of the 20th century, and they do improve muscular strength, there are limits. They are not commonly used much by athletes and those focusing beyond health, since they do not operate a strength movement through a joint's full range of motion. Isometric training is common in some situations. It often can be seen in calisthenics and body weight exercises, as well as movements found in Pilates. Besides being excellent exercises to start with for people who do not exercise often, they are also useful for those who have had injuries or chronic illness. This is also called static exercise.

Another type of exercise is **isotonic**, also called dynamic exercise. This is where the muscle contracts and the muscle length also changes. By far, isotonic exercises are the most popular form of muscular strength exercise performed by athletes and the general populace. This is because isotonic exercises gradually increase strength and endurance loads, and move them through the joint's full range of motion, providing the optimum training in most cases. Free weights help provide the most benefit by engaging not only the muscles needed for the movement, but also the muscles that support the body during that movement. These can also be performed on weight machines for specific muscle targeting, or if the person is recovering from injury or aging.

The last type of muscular exercise category is **isokinetic.** Isokinetic workouts are unique. They involve moving a muscle at a constant speed, at a set level of force, through a specialized machine. The strongest part of our lift during a movement is around the halfway point, often when joints are at a 90 degree angle. We can see this by using a weight that does not alter the resistance throughout the activity, which is called **constant resistance.** Typically, we only lift weights that are easy to move at our weakest points, meaning that our strongest parts are not being

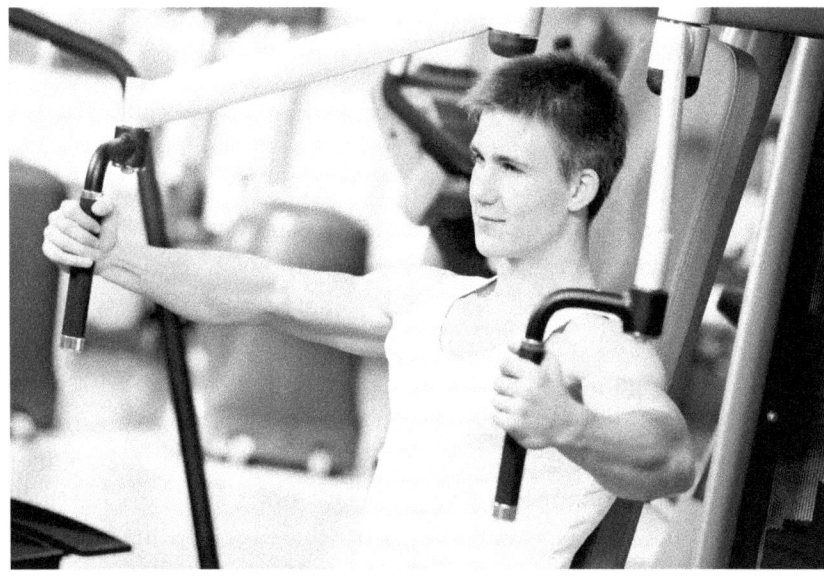

Figure 5.4: Using machines is beneficial if injured or targeting specific muscles.

stressed enough, or we are lifting weights for the strongest parts, and then skimping on the full range of motion (which makes the lift look more like a throwing motion). A specialized machine for isokinetic workouts adjusts the weight load to stay equal throughout the movement, reducing the load on weak points and increasing it on the stronger points of the lift. This altering of the resistance is commonly called **variable resistance.**

ASSESSMENT OF STRENGTH TRAINING AND ENDURANCE

Assessment of strength and endurance commonly focuses around one major concept: the one repetition maximum (usually referred to as 1RM). The largest amount of force that can be generated in one activity movement (i.e. amount of weight that can be benched pressed), in ONE lift. If you are able to do more than one repetition with the weight load, then wait, rest awhile, and gradually add a little more weight, and then try again. Endurance usually looks at how many times a movement can be done, or how long a position could be held. Many well-known governmental tests assess this by having participants engage in as many push-ups as they can perform.

USING FITT PRINCIPLES

As learned in chapter 1, the FITT principle is how we look into the requirements for building comprehensive and health-related exercise programming for maximum benefits. Unlike cardiorespiratory endurance training, it takes a lot more activity and a variety of them to reach the majority of the body's muscles, about 8–12 exercises. With the *frequency*, the recommendation is a minimum of two days per week and that workouts on the same muscle do not happen on back-to-back days. However, just because you might be training different muscles on different days doesn't mean that you won't suffer overall fatigue, and going too many days a week also will keep muscles from having time to repair. By having split routines, cutting it so that some days are for specific muscles, like arms and back, while other days cover the other muscles.

Intensity tends to alter depending on your goals. This is usually considered the amount of resistance (in most cases weight), and this forces the body to adapt to that resistance. You should base your resistance on your goals, by choosing resistance that forces your body to adapt. For those interested in strength and building muscle mass, then you should set your resistance to 80% of what your one repetition maximum (1RM) is, and do less repetitions. If muscular endurance is the goal, then the ACSM recommends 40–60% of your one repetition maximum, with more repetitions. This means that those who max their bench press at 200 pounds would use about 160 pounds, and if they were going for endurance then the weight would be closer to 80–120 pounds.

Time would be different than the way we view cardiorespiratory endurance and flexibility. Instead of an actual time, we look at repetitions and sets. The point of repetitions is to cause muscle fatigue, usually to the point that proper form is not continual. Due to the heavy weights in a strength-oriented plan, the lifting capability is usually low for repetitions, about 1–5. With an endurance-oriented plan, a high volume of repetitions, about 15–20 is commonly used. Oftentimes, people just want to improve their general health. With that in mind, about 8–12 repetitions are recommended. With specific exercises that are focused on body weight, stomach crunches and occasionally push-ups, more than the recommended number may be necessary since you will be adapting the weight. This can easily be seen in the gym with people doing 50, 70, even 200 of them in a row. Sets are the collection of repetitions that are usually separated by a rest period. So, if a strength-oriented plan has repetitions of 8, one group of 8 is considered a set. While we may have muscle fatigue at the end of one set, the rest period before the next set begins often provides adequate recovery of ATP (discussed in chapter 2) to continue without reducing further repetitions. Research shows that multiple sets tend to increase the development of strength. So, how long do you rest between sets? The recommendation for those who have a strength-oriented plan is to have more than three minutes of rest between sets.[6] Those focusing on endurance need to use shorter rest periods since handling fatigue is part of the goal, and about 1–3 minutes is considered typical. There are high intensity training regimens that use less than a minute, and they are highly effective. However, it is recommended that beginners work their way up to this type of training. People also use **circuit training**, where similar exercises can be alternated using different muscle groups. This would mean doing bicep curls to target your biceps, and then 30 seconds later doing bent-over dumbbell flyes for your back, and then 30 seconds after that doing the bicep curls again. This massively cuts down gym time, trains your cardiorespiratory endurance, and still gives the targeted muscles a minute or more to recover.

There are various options for *types* of training and many are listed in the section below. The complete body should be worked, targeting all the muscles.. Usually people have no problem exercising the arms, legs, chest and back, but often they leave out the neck, calves, and other more precise areas. The recommendation when setting up an exercise program is that large muscles and their movements must be worked before moving onto smaller muscles. This is due to fatigue occurring far more quickly with smaller muscles, and they are needed for the larger muscle movements. If starting with small muscles, then they often are too exhausted to properly perform the larger exercises. The way most people write out their exercises is by focusing on the three major components. Imagine that a person is going to do a bench press using 2 sets of 6 repetitions with 140 pounds of weight

Sets × Reps. × lbs.
  2 × 6 × 140

TYPES OF TRAINING AND EQUIPMENT

CONCENTRIC AND ECCENTRIC MOVEMENT

The foundation for training muscular strength and endurance is found in **concentric** and **eccentric** movement. Concentric movement is when force is exerted by the muscle to the point that it contracts and can manipulate the resistance placed on it. Eccentric movement is when the force produced by the muscle is less than the resistance placed on it and the contraction occurs as the muscle lengthens; in many weight rooms this is called doing "negatives." To illustrate this, imagine a leg curl that is designed to contract the hamstring. As we bend the leg against the resistance of weights, that would be a concentric action. Yet, when we slowly move the leg back into a straightened position, it is still applying force against the resistance, and this is the eccentric action. To have the full benefits to the motion, it is recommended to move muscles through the full range of motion, with both actions slow and controlled.

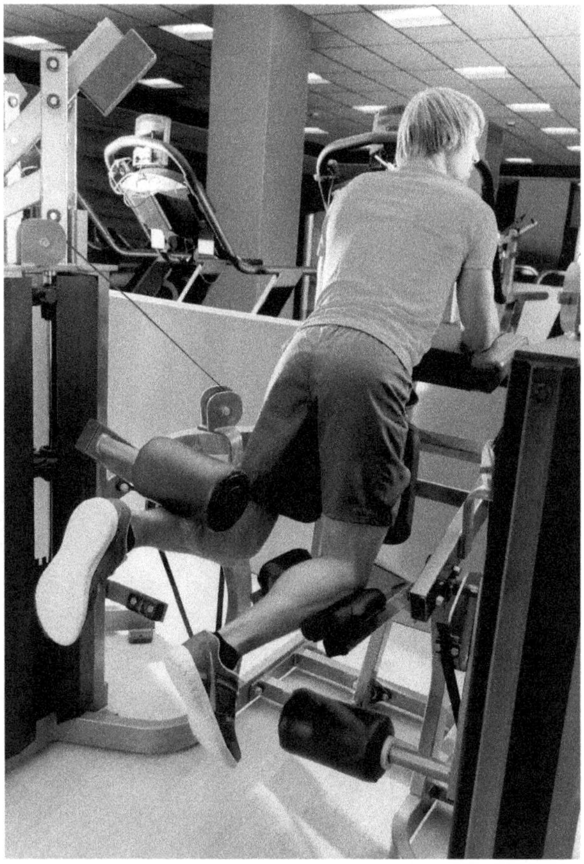

Figure 5.5: Leg Curls.

FREE WEIGHTS

The uses of barbells and weights with the body moving freely are the most commonly looked at form of strength training. The major benefit is the ability to control and manipulate the weights for movements you need to properly reach your goals. From a health perspective, it is immensely helpful since it allows you to also use your support muscles during lifts, and mimic real life movements. There is risk though, especially if you are not using proper techniques. Every year individuals seek emergency care for not using weights correctly or with a spotter to assist when a weight becomes too hard to use. This can result in a weight crashing down on the lifter.

MACHINES

The advantages of machines are that they allow you to lift without much concern for safety, and they are highly convenient. Usually it takes just a few seconds to adjust the seating for a proper fit and the peg or handle that changes the weight, and that is all that is needed to start. This works well when crunched for time, if you're a beginner, or recovering from an injury. The safety built into the machine also eliminates the need for a spotter on lifts. The major drawback tends to be that they target the specific muscle to be worked, but do not help with the support muscles. This means they do not really mimic movement in the realistic setting, and can lead to injury if care is not taken when using those support muscles in heavy lifting and moving.

RESISTANCE BANDS

Resistance bands, also called exercise bands, are stretchable elastic strips or tubing that provide increasing resistance as they are stretched. They come in a variety of resistance tensions and lengths so that different movements and muscles can be worked. Almost all major muscle movements can be achieved with resistance bands, and they are relatively cheap and easy to transport.

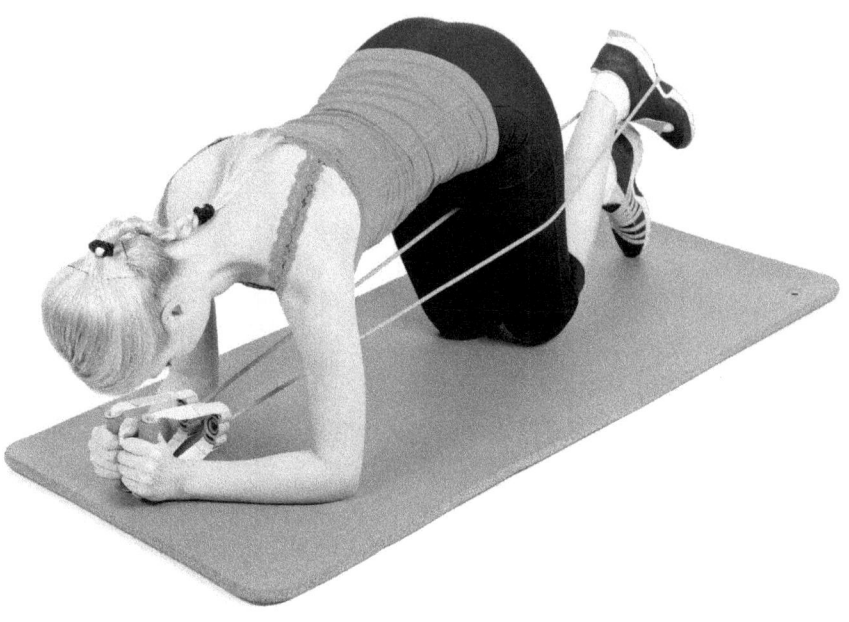

Figure 5.6: Resistence Bands are Versatile.

SPEED LOADING

With speed loading, an individual will move the resistance through an activity at the speed of the actual activity. Oftentimes, the resistance is low so that there is not a risk of injury. An example of this can be seen with batters taking multiple swings at full speed with a heavily weighted bat to develop power.

KETTLEBELLS

Over the past few decades, the popularity of kettlebells has exploded, even though they are not really new to weight training in other countries. The history of kettlebells is that they were designed by Russian soldiers to work on fitness when around camp. Cannon balls had handles welded onto them and then provided instant weights. They are most commonly use in isotonic movements since the handle allows for them to be swung and easily gripped. Oftentimes, the concentric and eccentric actions of muscles are used as they explode the movement and then quickly slow the movement phase down as part of the training.

STABILITY BALLS

While originally used for therapy and injury recovery, they have become pretty standard in many gyms. The primary function of the ball is to work the core area, however, it is able to support a full body workout. Stability balls are excellent for using support muscles and developing realistic movement abilities. Different weighted balls and ball sizes can be used to alter the resistance and muscle engagement.

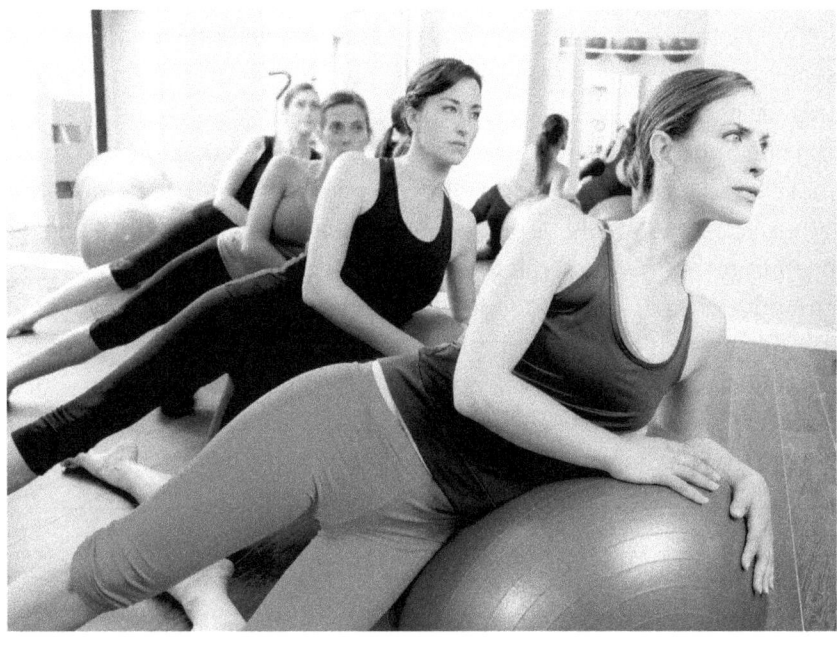

Figure 5.7: Stability balls for your body to support itself.

PLYOMETRICS

Another exercise that has gained traction over the past few decades is plyometrics. Its core philosophy is developing ballistic and explosive movements by developing muscular power. This is done by focusing on the eccentric actions of the muscle, and then the concentric motion. It can be seen in the popular box jumping used by many athletes. The performer crouches on the box and explode his or her legs into a straight position off the box and onto the floor. Landing into a crouch position, they would immediately explode them into eccentric action again, and jump onto the box.

PILATES

Pilates has been around for almost a century and is named after a former soldier, boxer, and gymnast enthusiast, Joseph Pilates. Many times people immediately assume this is similar to yoga, and while there are some movements that are similar, the strength-training component is vastly more intensified. While there are some specialized machines (Joe Pilates was famed for tinkering with new equipment ideas), most of the work can be done on the floor with a mat. Pilates tends to focus on the core: the stomach, back, and buttocks. Then it moves on to working the whole body. Due to its often rigorous strength component, it is recommended to take a day off in between the muscle groups being worked.

STRENGTH TRAINING SAFE PRACTICES

- If just beginning, try to find qualified instruction or hire a personal trainer to help design a program and show proper lifting techniques.
- Make sure to use good posture and be stable before attempting a lift, especially for your back/spine area.
- If a piece of equipment looks wrong or damaged, do not use it, and report it to the staff.
- If you're sick, already training heavily, or injured, it is recommended to wait until you're recovered. Otherwise, compromised immune systems pushed harder will continue to fail and you will get more ill and fatigued.
- If you feel pain, stop, as chances are there is a risk for serious injury.
- Do not twist your body using heavy weights.
- Always lift with your legs.
- Always load a weight bar evenly, placing equal weight on each side before adding more weight (Yes, people have tipped bars with too much weight on one side.) Remember to always use collars to keep plates from falling off.
- Lift smoothly, and do not jerk the weight around or bounce it off you. This creates a high risk for your body, and potentially harmful to those in your environment.
- Always use a spotter(s) for exercises that compromise your spine, head, or involve moving things from the front to overhead.
- Typically, people only have one spotter who should stand behind an individual to grip the bar in an emergency. If there are two spotters, then they each take an end of a bar to stand next to, so that they are able to grab it and lift it with ease if needed.
- The best recommendation for spotters is to have clear communication and signals worked out between the spotters and the lifter. This includes for situations where long answers may not be possible.

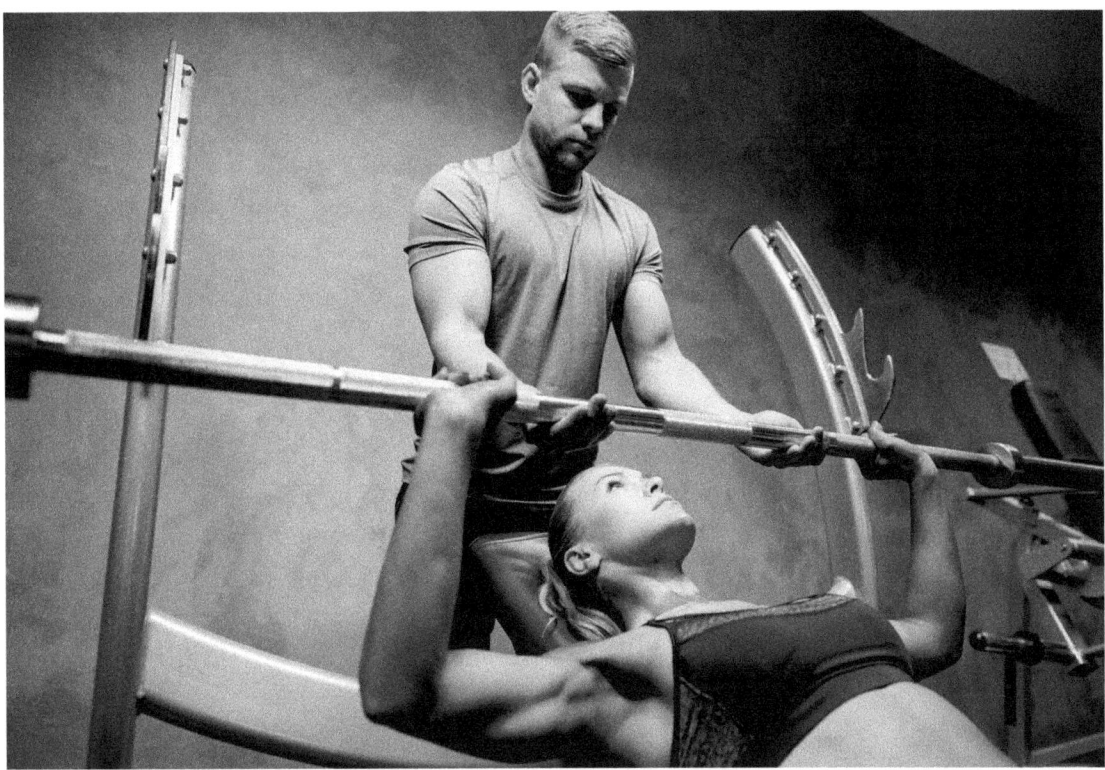

Figure 5.8: Spotter are the safest way to lift.

REFERENCES

1. Tsatalas, T., Spyropoulos, G., Sileloglou, P., Sideris, V., & Giakas, G. "The Role of Co-Activation of Agonist and Antagonist Muscles in Neural Adaptations of Strength Training." *Inquiries In Sport & Physical Education*,7 no. 2 (2009): 232–243.
2. Hopker, J. G., Coleman, D. A., Gregson, H. C., Jobson, S. A., Von der Haar, T., Wiles, J., & Passfield, L. "The Influence of Training Status, Age, and Muscle Fiber Type on Cycling Efficiency and Endurance Performance." *Journal Of Applied Physiology* 115 no. 3 (2013): 723–729.
3. Library of Congress. https://www.loc.gov/rr/scitech/mysteries/turkeymeat.html
4. McComas, A. "Human Neuromuscular Adaptations that Accompany Changes in Activity. *Medicine & Science In Sports & Exercise* 26 no. 12 (1994): 1498–1509.
5. Haraguchi, F., Silva, M., Neves, L., Santos, R., & Pedrosa, M. "Whey Protein Precludes Lipid and Protein Oxidation and Improves Body Weight Gain in Resistance-Exercised Rats." *European Journal Of Nutrition* 50 no. 5 (2011): 331–339.
6. de Salles, B. F., Simão, R., Miranda, H., Bottaro, M., Fontana, F., & Willardson, J. M. "Strength Increases in Upper and Lower Body are Larger with Longer Inter-Set Rest Intervals in Trained Men." *Journal Of Science & Medicine In Sport*, 13 no. 4 (2010): 429–433.

IMAGE CREDITS

6 FLEXIBILITY

WHAT IS FLEXIBILITY AND DOES IT MATTER?

When discussing the term flexibility, we are referring to the movement of a joint through its *full* range of motion. As discussed in this chapter, flexibility plays a vital role in our health. From increasing our physical performance to decreasing risk of injury, it helps in our everyday lives. However, of all the components of health discussed, it is probably the most skipped over by individuals who are working on their health. Oftentimes, the direct benefits are not as obvious as the bigger muscles of strength training, or the weight loss associated with cardiovascular exercise, but that doesn't make it less important. Compared to the other health components, flexibility really can be done anywhere, without special equipment, taking little time, and if using no resistance, can be done every day.[1]

FAQs CHECK!

Stretching? Isn't that the same as warming-up for other exercises?

They are not the same thing, even if stretching is sometimes added to warm-ups. Typically a warm-up involves moving the joints that are going to be used through their full range of motion. This allows the temperature in the muscle to become warm and function better for exercise. It also jump starts your metabolism so that it is ready to function well as you transition to increased exercise intensity.

TYPES OF FLEXIBILITY/STRETCHING

Flexibility has three different types when considering its context in health and physical performance. Typically we refer to this as stretching in general society.

STATIC STRETCHING

The most common type of stretching is **static stretching**. In a static stretch, an individual will extend a joint to the end of its range of motion and then, when in minor discomfort, hold that position for a set amount of time before relaxing the muscle. This is the most commonly used form of stretching and is one of the safest. Usually your ability to perform stretches is dependent on your joint structure, frequency of stretching, and how loose you can make your muscles in preparation for a stretch.

DYNAMIC STRETCHING

Another type is **dynamic stretching**, which involves moving a joint through the full range of motion possible with no, or little, resistance. This can be seen when athletes are warming up for sport performances. An example could be a baseball player slowly swinging a weighted bat, or a kicker practicing a slow warm-up kick through the full range of motion. The slow, but constant motion is what separates this from the static stretching discussed before. It is commonly seen in many warm-ups for sport or performance requirements, and encouraged if an individual has already reached the level of performance required for the activity they are engaging in.

BALLISTIC STRETCHING

The third type is **ballistic stretching**, and this is where the stretch is moving, similar to dynamic, but at a much faster rate through the joint's full range of motion. As stated with dynamic, and as will be pointed out in nervous system regulation later in the chapter, the person must be in proper shape to engage in moving stretches. However, ballistic stretching moves at the actual speed of a performance requirement, and this creates a risk of over-stretching in the form of a strain or sprain. Due to this, it is recommended that individuals do not engage in ballistic stretching, and typically it is still only seen in dancing and martial arts. Research also tends to support more benefits found static stretching.[2]

WHAT ARE FACTORS IN FLEXIBILITY?

MUSCLE LENGTH AND ELASTICITY

There are limits to your physical capability in flexibility. What this means is that the muscles, tendons and ligaments, as well as the skin around the joint that is being moved, can limit how far a person may stretch. The joint's tendons and ligaments play an extremely important role in allowing stretching, since it allows the range of motion and is joined to the muscles themselves. Since 1/3rd of a muscle is made of this connective tissue, it can be improved for optimum lengthening if used regularly in a flexibility program. There are two types of connective tissue: collagen and elastin. **Elastin** are elastic and flexible yellow fibers that create the stretchability in the connective tissue. **Collagen** are the fibers in connective tissue that provide support and structure and appear white. Muscles tend to be made up of both forms of connective tissue and they tend to overlap. When we choose to stretch our muscles, the elastin fibers tend to straighten out. As we relax our muscle stretching, they then snap back to normal shape (think a bit like a rubber band). This short-term stretching off and on is known as **elastin elongation**. Doing this often enough can cause an increase in the flexibility of the muscles being used, and oddly, this long-term process is called **plastic**

elongation. Unfortunately, if we do not stretch enough, the connective tissue can actually work in in reverse and begin to shorten and decrease flexibility.

FAQs CHECK!

Overstretching

Unfortunately, like most forms of exercising there can be too much of a "good" thing. There is a risk of stretching too much and too far, and this causes stretching (damaging elasticity) and/or tears in the muscle tissue. If this goes too far you can rip or rupture the muscle, causing severe damage. Some people naturally are able to over-stretch for numerous reasons, and should take care that this doesn't happen even though they feel used to it. Outside items used in stretching, like weights and partners, must also take care not to push or pull too far, causing overstretching.

JOINT STRUCTURE

How the joint is designed is probably the most obvious factor in a joint's flexibility. The most notable examples are hinge joints and ball-and-socket joints. A hinge joint can be seen in the fingers, toes, and knees. These joints can flex, but when they extend they also lock, moving only back and forth. Compare this to ball-and-socket joints, as seen in the hip and shoulder, which allow for a large range of motion and move in multiple directions. Although the general structure of a joint doesn't really change from person to person, there are some minor alterations that can occur due to gender and heredity. Some studies have noted that females are more likely to have more flexibility in specific joints than males. Some people also have a biological tendency to be more flexible than others since their parents tend to be more flexible. Additional flexibility in joints seems to pass down from parent to child.

The inside of a joint has several components. The bones that make up a joint are covered with cartilage and a **joint capsule** sits between the bones. The joint capsule is mostly connective tissue that is semi-elastic and contains synovial fluid that keeps the bone ends from touching and grinding on each other.

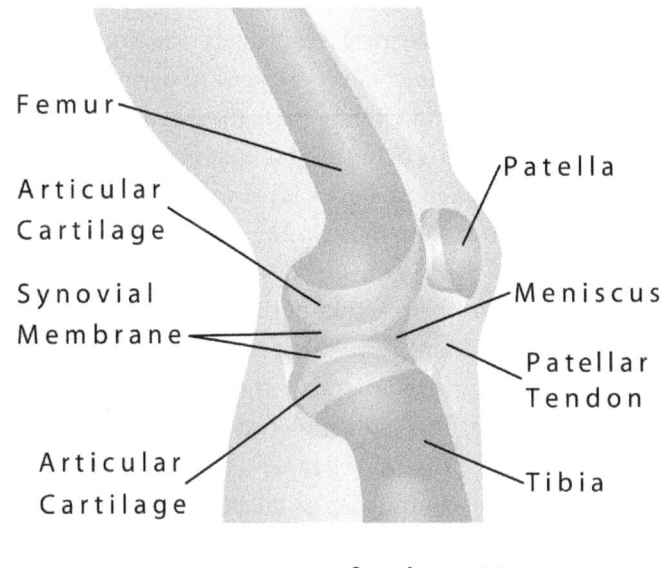

Anatomy of the Knee

Figure 6.1: Anatomy of the Knee Joint.

FAQs CHECK!

Cracking Your Knuckles

While many of us absolutely hate the sound of cracking knuckles, a few of us also feel like it is a necessity. Will this be a problem for your hand joints in the long term? Due to a recent MRI study on the topic this past year, we have learned that when a joint separates during cracking, a gas bubble forms in the synovial fluid. As the joints separate further, the gap created releases this bubble from the fluid, and makes the cracking sound. While the amount of force placed on the joints being cracked is enough to risk damage, research so far has not led to any beliefs that it will cause long-term harm or arthritis.

NERVOUS SYSTEM REGULATION

Nerves that send information about the function and movement of the skeletal and muscular systems to the nervous system are called **proprioceptors**. The proprioceptors note any movement or alteration in pressure and directionality of your muscles, joints, and tendons. There are two different types located in skeletal muscles: **muscles spindles** and the **Golgi tendon organ**. Spindles are located in the bulkiest part of the muscle (usually called the "belly" of the muscle) and they note changes in the length of the muscle. The Golgi tendon organ is found where the muscle joins the muscle tendon, and is designed to force a contraction if the muscle feels overstretched. This information is then used by the brain to determine the next movement, reaction, or alteration needed by the body. This is beneficial for more than health since it has a direct effect on physical performance. The feedback from the proprioceptors allows for adjustments in an individual's strength, speed, power, and balance. It also informs the body when too much strain or torque is being used so that you can adjust and avoid injury.

The way injury is prevented by proprioceptors is by noting the length and speed of alteration occurring in the muscle. This allows the brain to cause the muscle to contract and resist the change occurring in the muscle's extension and length. Typically, if a lengthening or stretching of the muscle is small, then the reaction of the proprioceptor is small. This has little to no risk and is only a minor protection function. However, if the individual stretches in a very quick, bouncy, and dynamic movement, then the proprioceptors may trigger a very direct and extremely strong response in terms of muscular contraction. This has a high risk of injury in and of itself, since the strong reactive contraction may occur at the same time as the rapid stretch, and then it can cause a strain or tear in the muscle. This is why stretching is also a training of the nervous system. As you practice slow stretching and holding positions with the muscle lengthening, you are also training the proprioceptors to accept, and not react to the stretch. This keeps them from hindering a deeper stretch with a muscle contraction at the same time.

BENEFITS OF FLEXIBILITY

Several of the most notable benefits of practicing regular flexibility training are that it can help create and maintain great posture, balance, and strength. Our society tends to have us engage in more jobs that involve sitting, which gives us the bad habit of hunching over. This hunching oftentimes causes the back and spine muscles to be overstretched and the chest muscles to be constantly brought together, and then they shorten. There is a common rounding hump that used to be seen in older people, but now is becoming common with younger age groups in the current technological-age generation. This humped look is called **kyphosis**, and is easily prevented and can be corrected by practicing good posture and engaging in regular flexibility training. Strength is also a benefit of regular flexibility training by allowing an individual who is more flexible to exert more power and force throughout their full range of motion, instead of just the optimal angle. This is extremely helpful if a physical performance involves large movements, and an example can be seen with a rower performing a strong pulling motion through the majority of the range in the shoulder joint.

Other benefits of flexibility training are that the tension that builds up from not using muscles and joints can be painful. Flexibility helps keep the muscles loose and reduces acute and chronic pain. In the reverse issue, the constant use of muscles can cause them to tense up and can cause muscle cramps; consistent flexibility training, especially static stretching, can reduce both of these issues. This also allows them to improve their mobility, especially as aging plays a toll. Flexibility has shown to reduce aging's effects on mobility, and even reverse it to a point. It also can be seen to help with recovery from major surgery or traumatic injuries. Research also shows that stretching and activities that associate flexibility (examples can be seen in Tai Chi and Yoga) can help reduce mental fatigue and tension. It allows people to help control their breathing and has been known to reduce blood pressure.[3]

FAQs CHECK!

Can my other health component training affect flexibility?

Very much so, and it's one of the reasons we encourage adding it to an overall training program for health. Exercises tend to use and tighten muscles when engaged in exercise, and then cause a decrease in flexibility. Typically, if muscular strength and endurance training are done correctly, they will use the full range of motion during a lift or movement, and do not limit the flexibility too much. However, cardiorespiratory exercises often times just move through a limited range of motion and start to tighten the muscle to the point of limiting their flexibility if not addressed.

AGE

Like other health components, namely muscular strength, flexibility training is invaluable over the course of one's life, becoming more important with age. As we age, we naturally begin to lose flexibility, which causes us to be less mobile and decreases our range of motion in joints. If an individual does not try to develop a program for increasing and maintaining flexibility, then it is common to see restriction in the trunk and neck area. This stands out especially when elderly people try to drive and are unable to turn their necks to take in the view along the side, and behind the vehicle. Most of the issues with the elderly and mobility become a combination of inactivity that leads to muscle tightness, and limited range of motion, due to these issues and the related pain they cause with age, so they continue to be even more inactive. This circular problem can be easily avoided by implementing a regular flexibility training program.

LOWER BACK AND JOINT ISSUES

Lower back pain is one of the most common complaints in the US. It currently ranks as the third most burdensome condition in terms of poor health, only behind ischemic heart disease and chronic obstructive pulmonary disease.[4] Oftentimes, this is caused by lack of the spine being stable. Over-stretching your back by sitting hunched in a chair leaves the back with a lack of protection. This is a two-part problem: the first is the lack of muscular strength and that the muscles surrounding the spine have not been strengthened with training, and therefore cannot support the movement and motions of the spine as it is used (solutions to this are covered in Chapter 5). The second is that the muscles may be weak, but they are typically tense, and place strain on the spine, which does not allow it to move as smoothly as needed.. Beginning and maintaining a regular flexibility program will prevent this from happening, and protect against injury and pain. Besides the risk of being inactive, certain activities can have extreme risks as well. An example could be in any job or sport when a quick change of direction may cause the spine to rapidly snap or twist in a specific direction. This is often seen in sports like basketball, where players have to twist their upper bodies to catch a ball, and even more so if contact is involved while the twist is occurring, as seen in football. Jobs that involve carrying heavy objects, as seen in many construction roles, also can be a concern if people try to lift more than they are capable of, or if they are trying to lift improperly, with their backs instead of their legs (Figure 6.2).

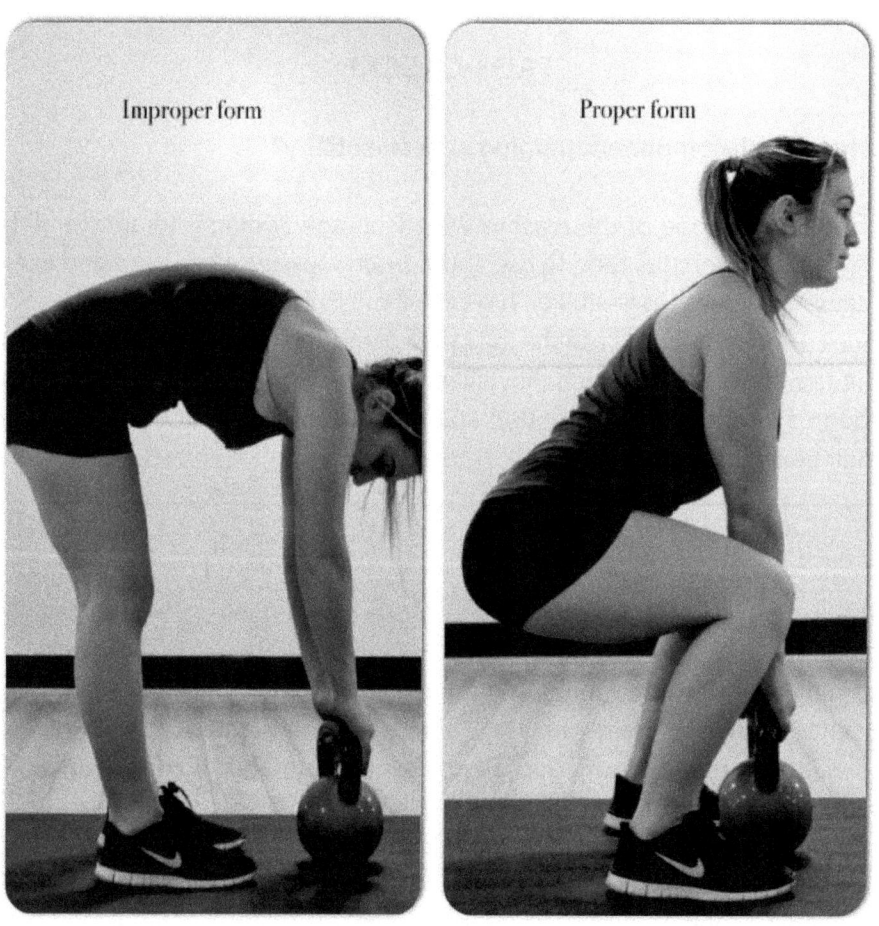

Figure 6.2: Improper lifting can cause major harm or pain to areas like the lower back.

Joints are often a problem for people as they move into middle age, since many people do not focus on what is needed to take care of them, even if they are engaging in training for health and fitness. The issues that arise with joints are similar to those with the spine. Developing the muscles around the joint increases stability and protection, and allows it to move easier through its range of motion. However, lack of use can also cause the muscles and tendons to be taut, and place unnecessary pressure on the joint. This can directly cause joint pain, as well as have the joint itself react in damaging ways as it matures and ages. Examples of this can be seen in damaged cartilage and improper joint lubrication. Lack of use causes a decrease in the mobility and elasticity of the connective tissue around a joint. **Arthritis** is another issue that can plague joints, especially with age. Commonly known as osteoarthritis, damage is caused by constant wear and tear on the on the cartridge, and if continued, it can result in bone grinding on bone.[5] This tends to lead to pain, and then people reduce their range of motion due to the pain. Besides age, common causes in the U.S. tend to be from obesity and the lack of physical activity, which as stated earlier, can protect the joint if done before damage occurs. Usually if damage and pain are extensive, the pain will be controlled with prescription drugs, and if it inhibits quality of life, many people opt for joint replacement via surgery.

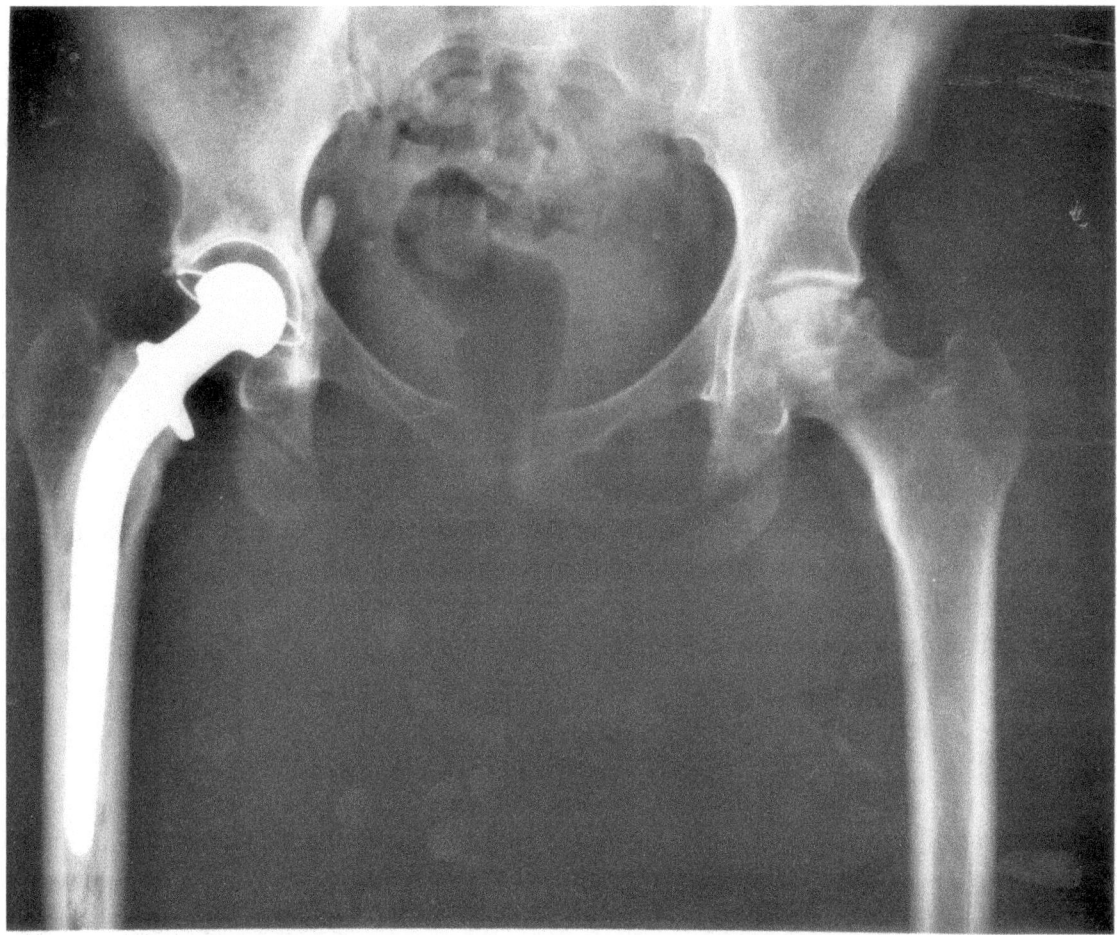

Figure 6.3: Example of a Hip Replacement.

ASSESSMENT AND GUIDELINES

The key to understanding flexibility assessment and developing a training program is that there are a variety of joints in the body, and their mere structure forces more individuality in developing a program then one might expect. While the ideal is to be more flexible, the idea is to obtain average flexibility, not to have more than average flexibility. As much as having low, or next to no flexibility is a problem, research indicates that having too much flexibility can also be problematic and detrimental to your health. Even people who have worked hard on having excellent fitness levels risk causing damage to their bodies by overextending their joints. The body is not made to stabilize motions that move beyond its range of motion and this could lead to **subluxation**, a partial dislocation of the joint.

WHEN SHOULD I STRETCH?

Many people associate stretching with the warm-up to their exercise. While they can be done before a major exercise, they are not the same. For improved stretching, it is recommended to do the warm-up before the stretch. When your exercises involve high intensity or a lot of changes in direction, as seen in many sports, then the stretching component becomes even more encouraged after the warm-up. That being said, stretching is always the most effective after an exercise session. With your muscles extremely warm from the activity, they are easier to stretch out without worry about straining them. After intense exercise, your muscles tend to also shorten and tighten in response to the heavy use. Stretching them can reduce the potential spasms and soreness that can occur due to this shortening.

USING FITT

According to ACSM guidelines, a general flexibility program should be 2–3 days a week; however, if there isn't a strength or fatigue component, then the program can go 5, or even all 7 days a week. While this meets the *Frequency* portion of the FITT principle, what about the others? In *Intensity*, we usually recommend that a person engage in static stretching. With this in mind, stretch a muscle until slight tension is felt, and then hold it for 15–30 seconds. Use deep breaths and remain relaxed so not to cause muscle contractions during the stretch. Then relax the stretch for about 30–60 seconds before engaging in another stretch. Usually this is recommended to do for 2–4 repetitions. For *Time*, a flexibility session can be done around 10–30 minutes, and if a strength component or additional exercise considerations are combined, then 45 to

60 minutes tends to often happen. In regards to *Type*, there are a variety of types mentioned in this chapter to follow in general. There is also the need to recognize that joints require specific care and movements, and there are recommendations on how to stretch specific joints and muscles.

Although you see a reduction in aches in pains within days of starting a flexibility program, increased flexibility does not often become noticeable until 2–3 weeks later. However, it usually takes 2–3 months to reach major improvements, and often joint flexibility can be increased by 10–20% after that time.

FAQs Check!

Can flexibility training limit my muscular strength?

Overall, doing flexibility training or stretching can help benefit muscular strength. However, research has noted that if you engage in stretching right before muscular strength training, then there is a chance to reduce the amount of power or strength that can be used during the strength training. This is due to the lengthening the muscles before they are used, and it is recommended that you make stretching part of your cool-down, not your warm-up. This doesn't mean you shouldn't have a warm-up, since blood going into the muscles helps prevent injury and improves muscle use. Taking a walk or light jog 5–12 minutes before engaging in muscular strength exercises can achieve this goal.

UNIQUE TECHNIQUES

PROPRIOCEPTIVE NEUROMUSCULAR FACILITATION

One popular technique in physical performance is **PNF (Proprioceptive Neuromuscular Facilitation)**. PNF stretching techniques involve contracting and then relaxing a muscle before stretching it (Figure 6.4). This allows the proprioceptors, previously discussed, to activate and then allows for a deeper stretch, since it will relax the muscle being used. It also allows some additional blood flow into the muscles to help warm them for improved stretching. An example can be the front of the thigh, your quadriceps, with your leg in front of you; you can contract the muscle for about 6 seconds and then briefly let it relax. Then you can move into a step stretch, by stepping forward with the opposite leg and leaning forward with it, letting the leg you are stretching drag out behind you, and stretching the now relaxed quadriceps. You hold this stretched for 15–30 seconds and then repeat the whole process from contraction to stretch with the other leg.

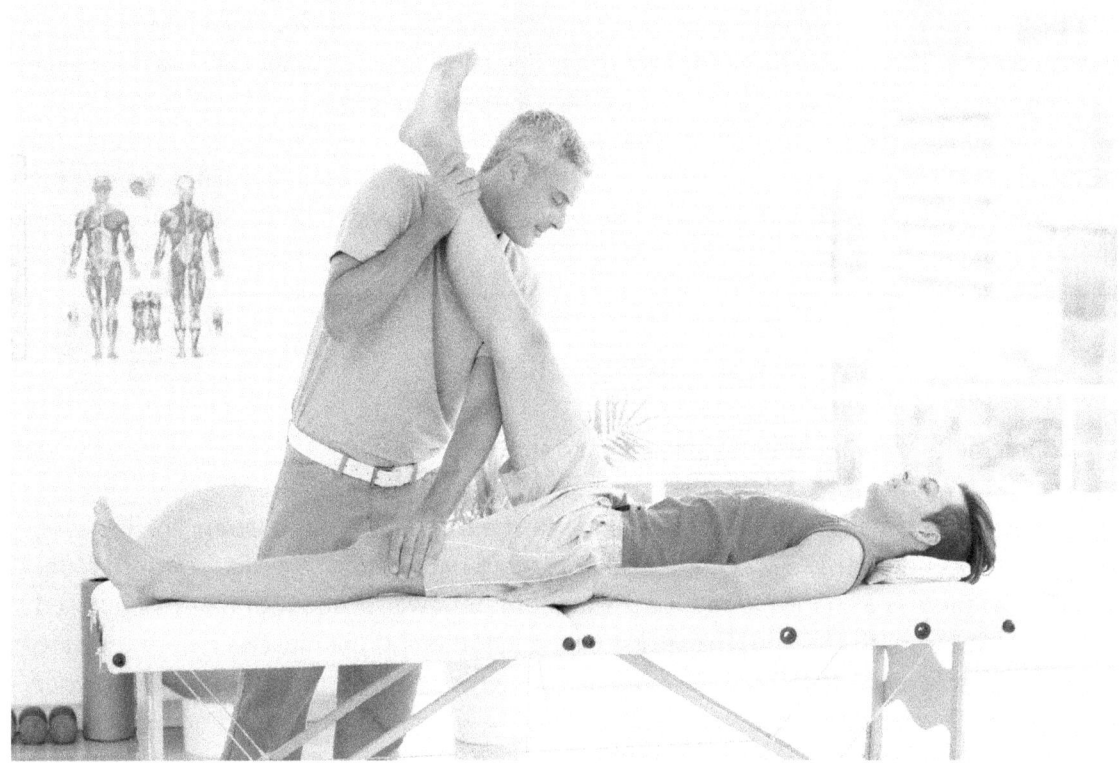

Figure 6.4: Using PNF Techniques.

Another method of PNF used, although very similar, is to engage the muscle with contract-relax-contract. However, it is important to note that the first contraction and relaxation occur as mentioned in the previous stretch, with the last contraction being the antagonist muscle (opposite muscle) of the stretch. In the case of the above example, you would contract the quadriceps for around 6 seconds, then relax it, then contract the hamstring for about 6 seconds before moving into the step stretch as stated above. The benefit of using a contracted antagonist muscle is that it engages the proprioceptors and they typically will not try to create contractions during the stretch, allowing for a deeper stretch and more flexibility. However, it must be noted that this is one of the few stretches to cause more soreness the next day instead of relieving it, due to the contraction portions. For some of the stretch movements and muscles this can be difficult, and the use of a partner may make it easier.

ACTIVE AND PASSIVE STRETCHING

Active Stretching

Active stretching is a unique technique that causes a stretch of the target muscle by contracting the antagonist muscle. By contracting the muscle, it pulls the target muscle into a stretched position via a reflex action. This typically is a low-risk way to engage in a stretch, and is often recommended to beginners. The issue becomes that it doesn't take too long maximize the flexibility with this method. While this may be great for beginners, usually after a few weeks to months, deeper stretches might be needed and a stronger, more specific flexibility program might be needed.

Passive Stretching

With Passive Stretching, you use a person or outside object to provide resistance for a joint to move through its full range of motion. This is often seen when athletes stretch posterior hip muscles with a trainer or partner. The athlete will lie on his back and place his leg at a 90 degree angle. The partner will then bend down on one knee and place the leg on his shoulder; they will then bend forward, forcing the leg closer to their trunk. Examples of outside forces that can be used are a partner, gravity, weight, or ropes/bands. While this is an excellent way to move into a deep stretch, there is a very serious risk since the stretch isn't controlled by the individual and there is no way to stop the stretch if it goes too far.

FAQs CHECK!

How much pain should a stretch cause?

None … while a stretch should be pressing your comfort level, it should not cause pain in anyway. Typically, pain is indicative of overstretching and is a precursor to injury. It is your body's way of informing you to stop what you are doing before an injury occurs.

LIFE TIPS AND RECOMMENDATIONS FOR HEALTHY MUSCLES AND FLEXIBILITY

- If it is "hard" to lift, then don't do it alone.
- Do not use overly soft or plush chairs, as they tend to weaken muscles due to lack of support.
- Do not lift heavy objects above your waist.
- To relax your back muscles while sitting, cross your legs.
- Your body is more optimal with heavy objects being carried in front of you.
- Placing foot rests under desks at workstations helps with back strain.
- Do not bend at the waist; always bend from the hips and knees.
- Hold your head up so it stays straight with the spine to reduce back strain.
- For parents, do not lean over to change a diaper; try placing the baby on a safe, elevated surface or to your side.
- If possible, consider buying a rocking chair, as the rocking motion helps your back muscles rest by changing muscles being used as you rock back and forth.

REFERENCES

1. Mayo Clinic http://www.mayoclinic.org/healthy-lifestyle/fitness/in-depth/stretching/art-20047931
2. Covert, C., Alexander, M., Petronis, J., and Davis, D. "Comparison of Ballistic and Static Stretching on Hamstring Muscle Length Using an Equal Stretching does." *Journal of Strength and Conditioning Research*, 24 no. 11 (2010): 3008–3015.

3. Lacaze, D., Sacco, I. Roche, L., Pereira, C., and Casarotto, R. "Stretching and Joint Mobilization Exercises Reduce Call-Center Operators' Musculoskeletal Discomfort and Fatigue. http://www.ncbi.nlm.nih.gov/pubmed/20668622.
4. National Institute of Neurological Disorders and Stroke. http://www.ninds.nih.gov/disorders/backpain/detail_backpain.htm.
5. Mayo Clinic. http://www.mayoclinic.org/diseases-conditions/arthritis/basics/causes/con-20034095.

FIGURE CREDITS

7 ASSESSING AND COPING WITH STRESS

BY ASHLEE BURT

ADAPTATION TO STRESS

Our body goes through changes, or adaptations, in order to cope with stress. Hans Selye identified this protective stress response system as the general adaptation syndrome (GAS). Many variables can affect how well this system works, including nutrition and the sleep status of an individual. Keep in mind that each of us handles stress differently. What may drastically stress one person negatively, might only mildly negatively stress another with the same situation or event. Other factors that play a role are personality types, which will be talked about later, locus of control, and self-esteem. **Locus of control** is what we believe has control over the events in our lives. Those with an internal locus of control (meaning they believe that a person has an effect on his or her own outcomes), self-motivation, and optimistic personality types are believed to have faster healing and better immune system responses. However, individuals who rely mainly on an external locus of control (those who believe that things outside themselves are responsible for all outcomes in their lives), and have low self-esteem with a pessimistic viewpoint are believed to heal more slowly, get sick more often, and have a higher risk of certain diseases, etc. We are all going to have stress in our lives; there is no way around it, you will have some positive and some negative. The goal is to have more positive than negative, however keep in mind even too much positive stress is still too much stress.

Stress is the body's response to any situation. This includes mental, emotional, and physiological, and can be caused by a threatening or exciting situation. A **stressor** is the item, event, or person that upsets or excites us and causes the stress. The term **eustress** refers to positive stress. This stress challenges a person to grow, adapt, and solve problems. Compare this to **distress**, which is considered negative stress. It can cause health deterioration and harm to the body.

There are three stages to the GAS system: alarm, resistance, and exhaustion/recovery. The body's first reaction is to go into the **alarm stage**; think of this stage as the body's quick response, like an alarm going off on your phone to alert you, or wake you up to a fire alarm. It's meant to startle your body. During this stage, the body's sympathetic nervous system kicks in and initiates the fight-or-flight response. Physiological adaptations

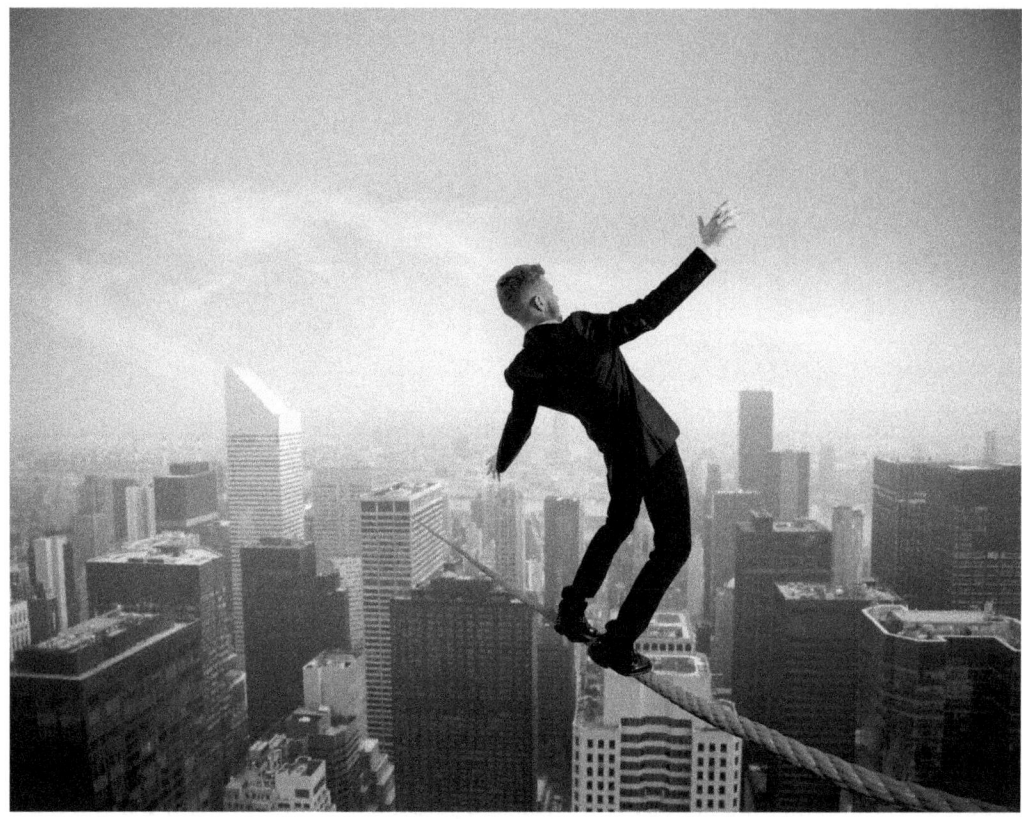

Figure 7.1: Everyone has stress.

someone might experience during this stage include an increased heart rate, sweating, shaking, diarrhea, etc. Let's look at an example of a situation. The alarm stage is a short-term solution to the stress. If someone is called in for an important meeting, but not told what the meeting is about, his body could begin responding to that stress while he is sitting in the waiting area. Physically, he may experience clammy hands, a fast pulse, sweating, and flushed skin. These continue even when he is called into the meeting and even during the meeting. Once the body acknowledges that there isn't a threat (he finds out he is not getting fired, maybe he's getting promoted!) then the body gradually returns to homeostasis (the heart rate goes back to normal, and trembling subsides).

The second stage, **resistance**, no longer has the initial high stress (fight-or-flight) response that the alarm stage had. During this stage, the body will continue to adapt as necessary to desensitize itself from the stressor. This still utilizes internal resources (blood pressure now might run a little higher for example). Let's continue the situational example given during the alarm stage. Instead, during the meeting the individual is fired. Now the fight-or-flight response begins to decline because he has an answer, but his body will move on to the resistance stage as he starts to work out plans for new employment, financial concerns, family concerns, and so forth.

The last stage incorporates two parts, **exhaustion** and **recovery**. During exhaustion, physiological responses may become opposite of the alarm phase, to reserve energy such as a decreased heart rate. Once in this stage, the individual continues to exhaust himself, and energy levels drop. Continuing in this stage may lead to complications such as heart disease, kidney failure, and even death. If the situation is resolved too slowly and the individual begins the recovery stage, the body heads back towards homeostasis. If the aforementioned individual is unable to find employment before his savings run out, then his body may be in the exhaustion phase and slowly tire itself out. If he finds a good job and feels confident that he will be financially secure, then he may enter the recovery phase, as the body attempts to go back to homeostasis.[1]

Depending on where an individual is in his stage of life affects what types of stressors he encounters. For example, college students have different stressors than older working adults. A study was conducted that categorized stressors by interpersonal, intrapersonal, academic, and environmental. The highest stressors reported from the college students for each category were changes in social activities, change in sleeping habits, increased class workload, and vacation/breaks, respectively.[2] You will be able to identify your own sources of stress when you complete lab 12. You will then be able to see how vulnerable you are to stress by completing lab 13.

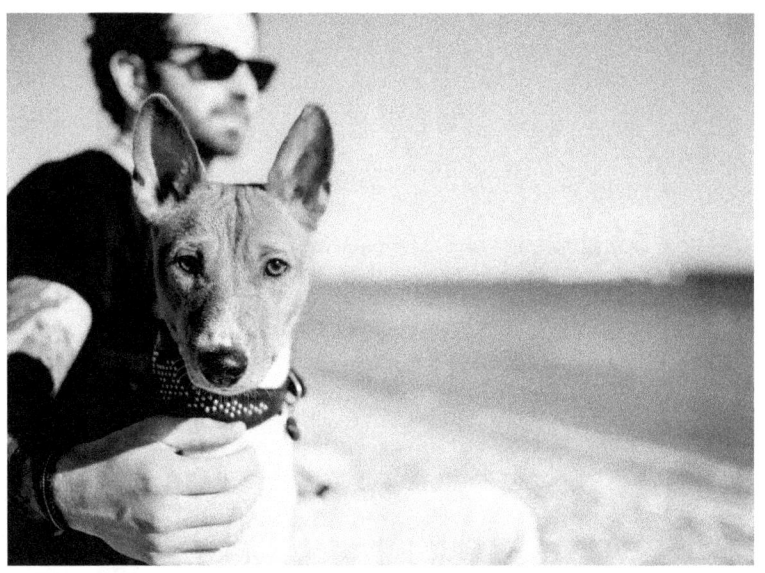

Figure 7.2: Breaks are needed in life.

FAQs CHECK!

When stress is too normal

When you wake up in the morning, it's the start of a new day. No one has cut you off in traffic yet, or hurt your feelings. The homework hasn't piled up yet, and you were able to accomplish all of yesterday's deadlines. You should wake up feeling fresh and rejuvenated, not stressed. Sounds nice, doesn't it? Do you wake up feeling that way? Probably not, and you might find yourself dealing with stress most the time. It isn't uncommon that if you have been stressed for so long, that your body sees that as your emotional norm. High stress can turn dangerous if it goes unchecked, and it can increase your risk for health problems, such as depression, sleep problems, memory impairment, obesity, digestive problems and more.

PERSONALITY TYPES

There are three main personality types: Type A, Type B and Type C. Among these types, individuals may be a mix of more than one, in which researchers will classify as A-1, A-2, etc., or X as a mix of A and B. We are going to discuss the basic components of each type.

Type A personalities are generally goal-minded individuals, which include personality traits that show as aggressive, ambitious, competitive and sometimes hostile behavior. In the extreme part of this spectrum, Type A individuals may seem easily angered and overly stressed, which puts them at a higher risk for heart disease, high blood pressure, and other conditions. They may struggle to get along with

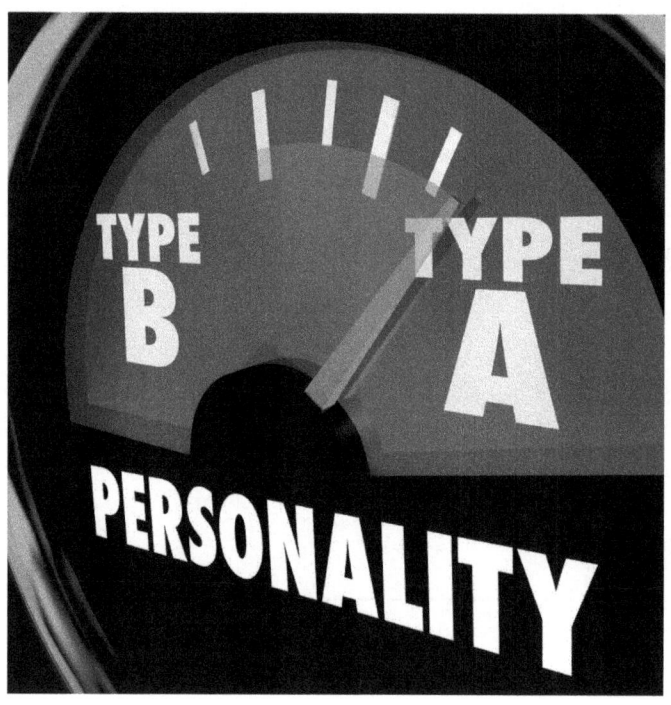

Figure 7.3: Type A Personality Words.

others that they work with, since often they may only like things accomplished their way. They are often in a hurry to accomplish their goals as they consistently feel behind.

Type B individuals have the opposite behavior to Type A. Extreme Type B personalities are generally calm, relaxed and easygoing. The majority of the time they do not feel rushed or pressured. While this may seem ideal, in extreme cases, many may not even set their own goals or deadlines, leading to not accomplishing things. This lack of accomplishment or completing objectives, over time, may lead to similar stress that Type A's feel, including issues with depression, as nothing around them gets done, and leads to additional issues with relationships when others feel they cannot count on them.

As researchers further look into personality types in relation to workload and stress, a third type has been categorized. Type C is considered to be often just as stressed as extreme Type A individuals, however, they are at a decreased risk for disease. They tend to be hard working, polite, responsible, and ambitious, but unlike Type As, they attempt to control their emotions and avoid conflict. They are better at controlling a situation to meet the needs of everyone, and not just themselves. Type C individuals accomplish this by utilizing what has been described as the three Cs: confidence, commitment, and control. This means that these individuals focus on being confident, and they can work on a project and meet deadlines so that they do not feel overwhelmed. They can commit to the projects they are engaged on, and avoid taking on too much additional work. They also focus on control, and the ability to work within a project and also control their own lives, allowing individuals to focus and accomplish goals.

Research has been strongly linked to emotional stress and chronic conditions such as heart disease and high blood pressure, specifically in relation to anger and depression. Stress especially affects college students. A survey was conducted by the American College Health Association (ACHA) in 2015 that showed almost half, 49.6%, of the undergraduate students surveyed (16,760) reported that things were hopeless within the last 12 months. The survey also showed that within the last 12 months, 32.2% of students identified stress as a factor that affected their academic performance.[3] There are a variety of factors that play into college student's stress, and they can stem from a history of psychological disorders, previous childhood issues such as self-cutting, sexual abuse, and eating disorders. Whereas some become depressed in college due to work overload and burnout, parental pressure, financial pressure, romantic involvement and/or breakups and therefore may turn to substance abuse. The American College Health Association has a program called Healthy Campus 2020 where any student or faculty member can join the coalition. Their objectives are listed on their website, and there is a pledge each person can take. They also provide information on how to transform your campus into a healthy one.[4]

COPING WITH STRESS THROUGH EXERCISE AND COMPLEMENTARY ALTERNATIVE MEDICINES (CAM)

For young adults leaving their parents' homes for the first time for college, living on their own and having to make their own decisions, pressure from parents, friends, partners, school, and finally the stress felt when graduation is around the corner and they now having to find a job and actually make it on their own is stressful! Each of us will handle these stressors differently, and that's what makes us unique. We each also have different levels of support from friends and family, whereas other individuals may not have efficient family support. There are many ways we can cope with stress and these can be positive or negative. Some individuals may express anger and irritability when they become stressed; this is not conducive to relieving the stress or to solving problems, but it is the easiest way to react. For some, coping with stress means listening to music, watching TV, playing a video game, etc., but for the purpose of this textbook, we are going to focus on specific methods that have been shown in research to help cope and/or reduce stress in individuals and are not recreationally based. We will also look at some well-used strategies that may lack or need further research support, but are popular regardless in handling stress. These are also known as Complementary Alternative Medicines (CAM).

PHYSICAL ACTIVITY

Exercise is the easiest and often the cheapest method for people to reduce their stress levels. It does not require a gym membership; walking or jogging outside is free! You can get roommates or friends involved, and if you have access to a student recreation center on campus, then you have the choice to participate in activity classes, lift weights, use the track or pool if they have one, get involved in intramurals—the list goes on. By that point, you have the resources available, it's getting yourself to go (although many of us feel we don't have time between (homework, classes, relationships, families, jobs, etc.) and you HAVE to make time. It will give you more energy and help manage all these things going on in your life. We will discuss motivation later in this chapter.

YOGA

As the Mayo Clinic describes, "Your mobile phone is ringing, your boss wants to talk to you, and your partner wants to know what's for dinner." This is a typical way that stress builds. Not each individual item is necessarily stressful, but they build up, and technology allows us to have faster access to one another, and thus creates the stack of stress. Yoga is an exercise technique that incorporates physical poses, utilizes the mind and controlled breathing. It has been shown to help reduce stress, lower blood pressure, lower the heart rate, and provide an overall increase in health.[5]

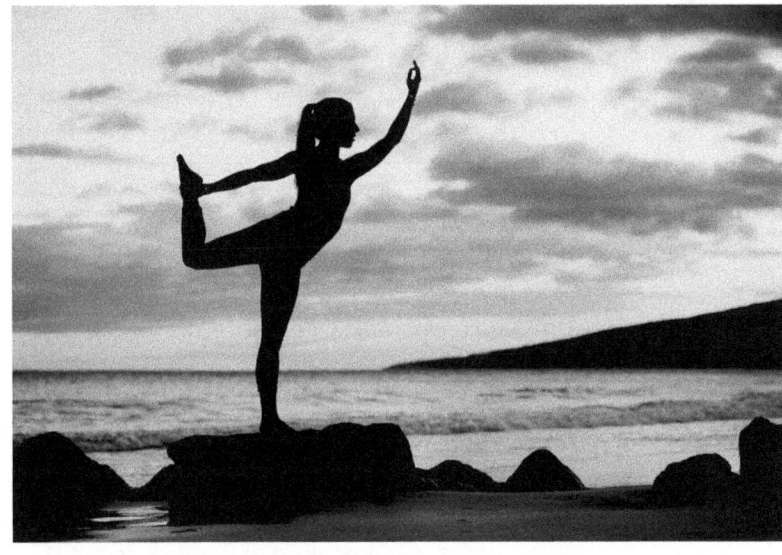

Figure 7.4: Yoga can be done daily.

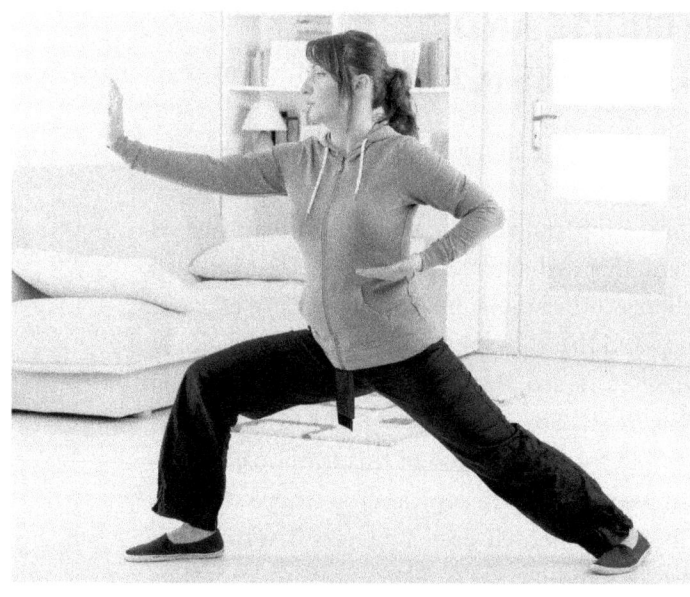

Figure 7.5: Woman Doing Qi Gong Tai Chi.

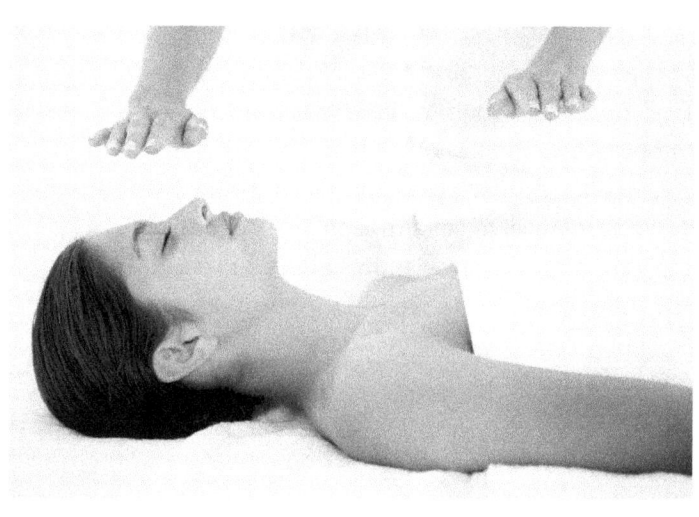

Figure 7.6: Reiki.

TAI CHI

Tai Chi is originally a Chinese form of self-defense, however, today it has been implemented to help reduce stress and anxiety, and increase flexibility and balance. It's similar to yoga in that it involves meditation and deep breathing, however Tai Chi is not in poses, but instead involves slow, flowing, and gentle movements. Anyone can perform Tai Chi as it requires no equipment, or no specific environment. It is a low impact exercise and therefore safe for muscles and joints, which is why this method is a great choice for elderly.[6]

REIKI

Reiki is considered a CAM method that originated in Japan. It involves specific hand placement by the practitioner either lightly on, or just above the client. It is believed that energy (chi) helps the body to naturally heal itself (there is no research that has proven this). When the practitioners use their hands on or above the client, they are able to transfer their energy as well as move the client's energy around to help bring them back to balance (reducing stress, pain, and illnesses). There is no science that supports the effectiveness of Reiki, however it is generally safe to do.[7]

PROGRESSIVE MUSCLE RELAXATION

Progressive Muscle Relaxation is another free and easy stress reducing method. Again, you should be in a quiet environment where you can focus. All you need to do is focus on which muscle group you want to tighten, then relax that muscle group and repeat the process. You should tense the muscle groups for about five seconds, and relax for up to 30 seconds. The goal is to do a variety of muscle groups and to focus on the blood warming your muscle as you tighten and then relax it. Many times this method is combined with others, such as guided imagery and breathing exercises.[8]

BREATHING EXERCISES (LIKE LAMAZE CLASSES)

This stress reducing technique is straightforward. It does not require any equipment, is free, and can be done anywhere, anytime. To perform this method, you must breathe from your diaphragm and establish a slow, deep, and efficient breathing technique. You can use it if you find yourself in an acutely stressful situation: before a big game as an athlete, before you have to present for a class, among many other situations. Controlling your breathing helps your body to take control and calm down,[9] which is why it is used by women who are in labor and preparing for birth (e.g., Lamaze).

MEDITATION

Another simple and free method to help reduce stress and anxiety is meditation. It is a mind-body treatment that is considered a complementary alternative medicine (CAM). In doing this, an individual is to focus his attention and work on removing all the other items bouncing around in his mind, and the goal is to produce a deep state of relaxation and to have a tranquil mind. Meditation can provide multiple physical and emotional benefits as well as help manage certain conditions such as asthma and depression, although more research needs to be done on these.[10]

MASSAGE THERAPY

Another form of CAM, massage therapy, involves a certified professional to manipulate the tissues throughout your body (e.g., muscle and tendons) with various amounts of pressure and specific movements. Many studies have shown massage to help reduce stress as well as pain and tension in the muscles. Specifically, the Mayo Clinic oftentimes recommends massage therapy for those who need to cope with pain and stress due to cancer, heart disease, and other conditions.[11]

ACUPRESSURE/ACUPUNCTURE

Acupuncture and acupressure are both forms of CAM, and are similar to one another. With acupuncture, very fine, thin needles are inserted into the skin at specific points in the body. In acupressure, the same specific points are tended to, but instead of fine needles, therapists use their hands and fingers and to apply pressure. Like Tai Chi, these methods are also based on traditional Chinese practices. These methods are most often used to help treat pain. The Chinese belief is that puncturing specific locations on the body helps balance the flow of energy/life force (i.e., chi), whereas the Western use believes the punctured points stimulate nerves, muscles, and connective tissue, and thus in turn will boost the body's natural painkiller as well as increase blood flow.[12]

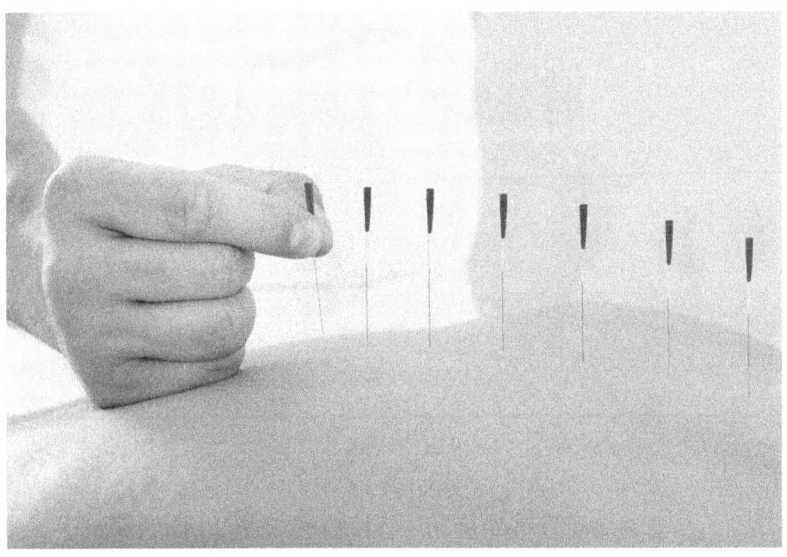

Figure 7.7: Acupuncture.

VISUAL/GUIDED IMAGERY

To use imagery as a method to reduce stress, the individual must focus on pleasant images or environments to replace the negative or stressful feelings she may be having. It can be done anywhere, however, it is recommended it be somewhere quiet that you can sit and focus. Individuals may choose to direct themselves, use a practitioner, or a recording. The goal is to place yourself wherever you are imagining, not to just close your eyes and see a picture. Include all of your senses; see the pleasant image/environment you created, imagine what the area smells like, feels like (sun on your face, etc.)[13,14]

BIOFEEDBACK

This method of stress reduction requires equipment that has electrical sensors connected to you to obtain information about your body such as temperature, heart rate, respiration rate, brainwaves, muscles and sweat glands. The purpose of gathering this information is to allow an individual to understand her body and her body's reactions to stress, and to then be able to focus on making changes, such as relaxing certain muscles to help reduce pain. Biofeedback provides individuals the information so that they may have the ability and power to use their thoughts in controlling their bodies, and thus improve their health. One biofeedback device has been approved by the FDA to help reduce stress and lower blood pressure; it is a portable device that individuals can carry around that helps promote slow, deep breathing.[15,16]

AROMATHERAPY (ESSENTIAL OILS & DIFFUSERS)

Aromatherapy is another alternative medicine technique with not enough research to fully support it. This industry has grown tremendously with the use of essential oils (i.e., extracted from plants), which can be used topically, ingested, or diffused. Keep in mind that just because something is "natural" it can

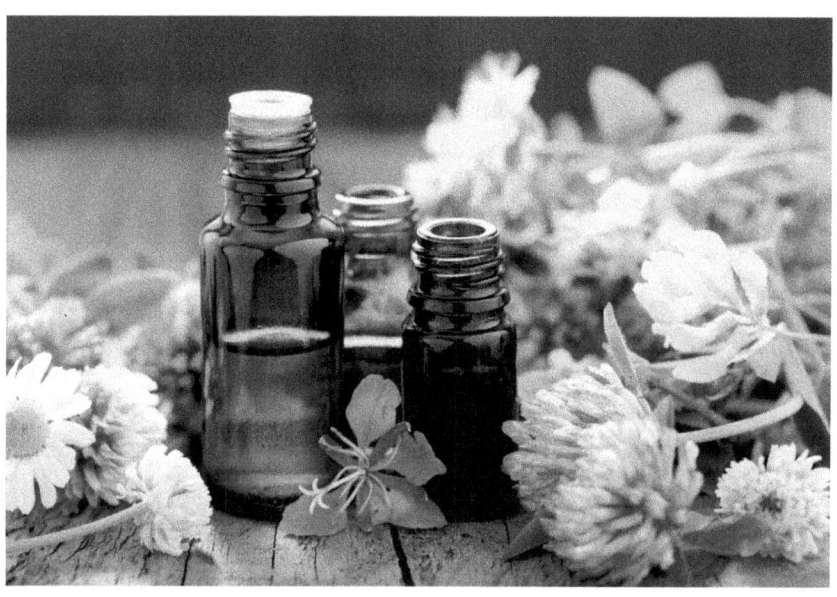

still have side effects (e.g., an allergic skin reaction) or interact with other medications you may be taking. These items are also not regulated by the Food and Drug Administration. You must always inform your health care provider(s) of any alternative medicines you may be using. The concept behind aromatherapy is that certain herbs, when inhaled, help reduce stress, depression, and anxiety, and may also help with sleep and even increase happiness. This occurs by the aroma stimulating the olfactory receptors in your nose, and in return, sending a message through your central nervous system to your limbic system, the part of the brain that controls your emotions. One meta-analysis concluded that aromatherapy is effective as an intervention to reduce

Figure 7.8: Essential Oils and Medical Flowers.

stress,[17] however in another research article, they concluded that although aromatherapy has been reported to reduce stress and anxiety, that it does not necessarily work for individuals who are having an acute mental stress situation.[18,19]

HERBAL THERAPY

Herbal treatments for conditions such as migraines, stress, heart disease, joint inflammation, etc., have slowly become more researched as their popularity grows. Many herbs have a variety of uses, some of which help with stress reduction including chamomile, lavender, valerian, and kava. However, some of these have been shown to have serious side effects, including liver damage. Remember, not all herbs are monitored by the FDA, therefore, as a consumer you must utilize what resources you can to understand herbs before using them. A great site that has a list of herbs with what they can be used for and how, as well as research that has been conducted on them can be found on the National Center for Complementary and Integrative Health website https://nccih.nih.gov/.[20]

OTHER WAYS TO HELP REDUCE STRESS

- *Time Management*: Prioritize and use your time well, and don't feel like you "wasted" time doing something. You may keep a daily log for a few days of what you are doing each day and then sit down and point out where you had free time or wasted time.
- *Delegating*: It's okay to ask for help! If you have group work, delegate who has to do what, and if you live with roommates, cleanup needs to be evenly delegated.
- *Saying "no"*: Don't be overly involved. You do not have to volunteer every week for church, your fraternity, or attend every get together you're invited to. All these things may seem fantastic, but again you do not want to max out your stress level.
- *Remove distractions*: Turn off the TV, take out your headphones, and go to the library when you have to focus on assignments.
- *Goal setting*: Make a list and be specific so you know what you are trying to achieve and when.
- *Planner/Calendar use*: Stick to the plan, as this will help keep you organized and on task, and therefore hopefully less stressed.
- *Include time for yourself and reward yourself for accomplishments*: If you cannot have "me" time and do not positively reward yourself for any accomplishments, you may become depressed which in turn leads to stress—so take care of yourself!
- *Be able to adapt*: Situations change and things happen, but don't get stuck in a rut because something didn't go the way it was supposed to; be able to adapt, analyze, solve, and move forward!

HOW TO GET (AND STAY) MOTIVATED!

First, let's distinguish the difference between **ambition** and **motivation**. Ambition is the *desire* to want to be active and/or achieve a goal. Motivation is the *force of influence* that gives you a reason for doing something (being active/obtaining goal). Without motivation, you more than likely will not reach your ambition. Someone can have all the ambition in the world: "I'm going to open up a flower shop," or "I'm going to start running every day." However, if the individual does not have a strong internal locus of control, and does not have any other reason to drive him, then the likeliness of obtaining his ambition decreases. Part of this is understanding that believing in you is a start to accomplishing goals. **Self-efficacy**, according to the American Psychological Association, is a person's belief in his ability to have the skill or behavior to produce specific attainments/goals.[21]

To start, you should figure out which locus of control you are more like. Those with a strong internal locus of control tend to believe they control themselves as well as influence the environment around them. They generally have a strong self-efficacy that they can accomplish anything they need to in order to succeed. individuals with an external locus of control do not believe they have control over events or what other people do. These people are generally more resigned in thinking things happen to them because of luck or fate, and that there is nothing they can do about it. This makes them passive and willing to accept the things occurring around them. Oftentimes, those with a stronger external locus of control tend to be those of younger or older age groups, whereas middle-aged individuals tend to have higher internal locus of control.

TIPS FOR STAYING MOTIVATED

- Set goals: This is a must! Without goals, you have nothing you are looking forward to achieve, and therefore no ambition or motivation! Remember they should be SMART goals!
- Make it fun: Whether your goal is to become more physically active or more focused for studying and homework, make it fun. Exercise does not have to be lifting weights and running—take a dance class. Take breaks when you're studying, and allow a small amount of time (e.g., 20 minutes) to do something fun during those breaks (e.g., play a game, go for a short walk). You will come back with a clearer and refreshed mind.
- Make it consistent: If it's exercise, make a plan, daily or however many times a week you set your goal. If it's for assignments, follow the same routine, and give yourself the same amount of time for breaks, etc.
- Incorporate friends: Social support can be extremely helpful with motivation. You can hold each other accountable. In some cases, it may have a negative effect. For example, roommates or a couple where one may beg the other to "stay in and watch a movie instead," consistently interrupting the other one's goal(s).
- Use behavior change models: Using a behavior change model lets you visually see where you are on reaching your ambition. The stages of a change model also provide processes for you to utilize to help you stay motivated!
- Put it on paper: Write it down or use sticky notes for you to read every morning to help motivate you to reach your goal(s).
- Rewards: Always reward yourself somehow when you have met a short-term goal, as this will help with your commitment to continue.
- Join a gym or pay for a trainer: Maybe paying money will help you stay motivated! Knowing you are in a contract with a monthly fee, or having a personal trainer waiting on you to show up will help motivate you to get to the gym.
- Journal: Keeping a daily log of your day's events can also help "write out your stress," and some people find this to be very helpful in allowing them to let their thoughts run free and de-stress.
- And of course, eating a healthy, well-balanced diet and getting enough sleep will help your motivation to remain consistent![22,23]

SLEEP CONSISTENCY MATTERS

According to a 2015 survey by ACHA, 21.7% of undergraduate students reported sleep difficulties as effecting their academic performance.[24] Sleep deprivation has been linked to multiple negative outcomes, such as increasing the risk of obesity and stress levels, and decreasing the immune system and academic performance, among many other chronic conditions. With lack of sleep comes napping for too long, over-sleeping, and chronic fatigue or exhaustion. Our body's like a consistent sleep schedule. Our internal sleep pattern does not like to go to bed early one night and stay up late the next, and even if you sleep in, your body does not recognize those hours as "catching up" on sleep, hence why many of you may have had the experience of feeling MORE exhausted after sleeping in. Research has proven that efficient sleep is linked to better learning and memory, and has a positive effect on our metabolism.

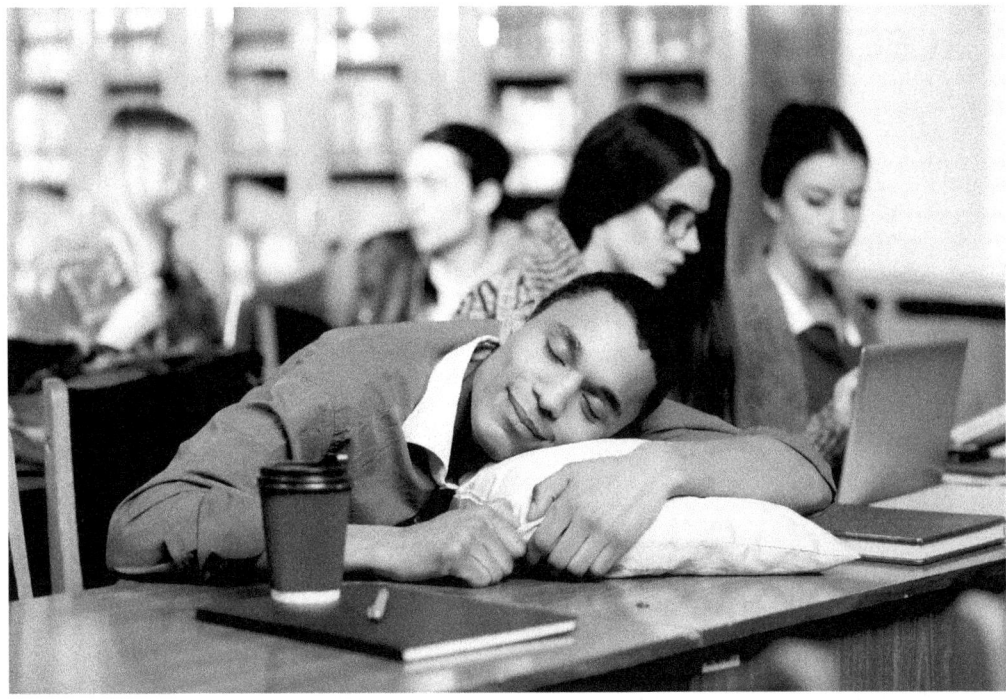

Figure 7.9: Man Sleeping During Class.

Our body needs a certain amount of rest and though there is no formula to figure out exactly how many hours you need, the average person requires about seven and one-half hours every night. One way you can try to pinpoint exactly how many hours you personally need would be to wake up at the exact same time every day and keep a log of how you feel. If you went to bed late the night before and woke up groggy, try to go to bed earlier the next night and wake up at the same time, then write down how you feel. Repeat this until you find the correct amount of time sleeping you require, and keep it consistent.

The reason we need a consistent sleep schedule with a consistent amount of hours each night is due to our body going through **stages of sleep**. When we are awake, our brain waves are small and rapid because we are constantly thinking and moving around. When we lie down to sleep, our body first goes into stage one, where the waves are still small and rapid but our muscles begin to relax, and our breathing starts to slow down. During stage one, you may be sleepy with your eyes half open, between wake and sleep. In stage two, the waves become larger and slightly less rapid, compared to stage one. During stage two, our eyes are no longer responding to light, and our breathing slows as more and more muscles become more relaxed. In stage three, the waves are even longer compared to one and two, and there may be a spike in brain activity. Stage four is when we start producing delta waves, and this stage is also known as the deep sleep stage where our brain waves are very long and far apart. Respirations and heart rate decrease tremendously as the body goes into an almost comatose state while it is in its full rest period. Approximately an hour into the four stages of sleep, an individual will then move into the active dream sleep, known as rapid eye movement (REM). Brain waves now change to look similar to that of being awake; however your body is still fully asleep.

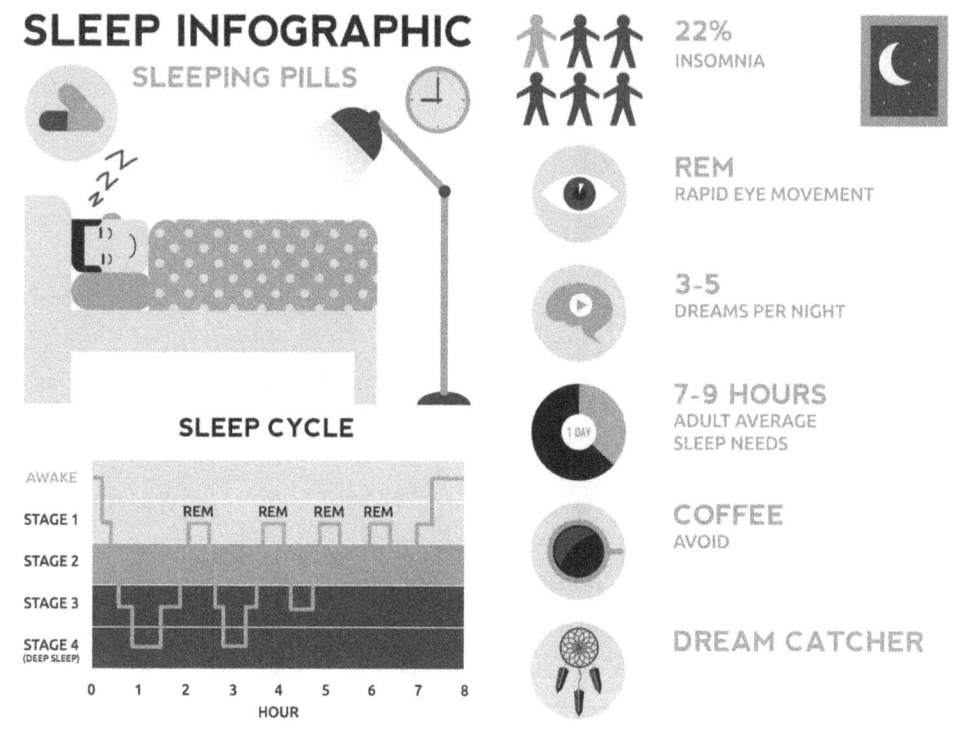

Figure 7.10: REM and the Sleep Cycle.

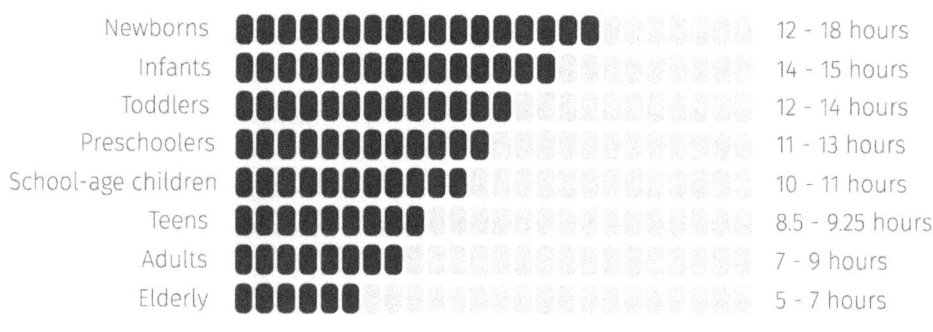

Figure 7.11: How much sleep do we need?

TIPS FOR BETTER, MORE CONSISTENT, SLEEP

- Avoid eating late at night (this keeps your body from working on digesting)
- Don't exercise just before bed (it will take a while for your body to calm down back to homeostasis)
- Limit distractions (phone, TV, etc.)
- Foods with magnesium and tryptophan (walnuts, almonds, bananas) have been shown to help induce sleep
- Have a consistent sleep schedule with the same amount of hours each night
- Avoid coffee and other caffeinated items later in the day
- Avoid relying on alcohol and other sleep medications
- Avoid long naps, as research has shown short naps 15–30 minutes in duration can refresh individuals and lower stress, but a long nap could do the opposite.

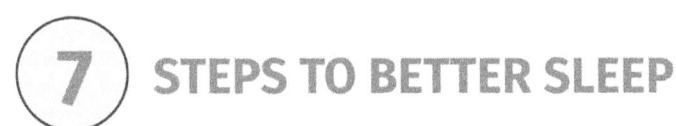

STEPS TO BETTER SLEEP

SLEEP HYGIENE

1. Allow enough time for sleep

2. Make your bedroom a peaceful, tidy environment

3. Get a regular schedule

4. Avoid heavy meals, alcohol, caffeine before sleep

5. Avoid exercising 3 hours before sleep

6. Avoid TV beds and other media-furniture

7. Avoid bright light for two hours before bed

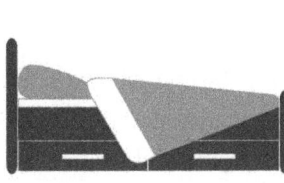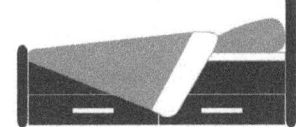

Figure 7.12: Sleeping Well.

REFERENCES

1. Story, L.. *Pathophysiology: A practical Approach*. Sudbary, MA: Jones & Bartlett Learning, 2012.

2. Ross, S. E., Niebling, B. C., & Heckert, T. M. Sources of Stress Among College Students. *College Student Journal,* 33 no. 2 (1999): 312. http://www.rosehulman.edu/StudentAffairs/ra/files/CLSK/PDF/Section%20Two%20Instructor%20Resources/Sources%20of%20Stress%20Among%20College%20Students.pdf.

3. American College Health Association. National College Health Assessment Publications and Reports. Retrieved from http://www.acha-ncha.org/reports_ACHA-NCHAIIc.html.

4. American College Health Association. "Health Campus 2020." Retrieved from http://www.acha.org/HealthyCampus

5. Mayo Clinic. "Yoga: Fight Stress and Find Serenity.http://www.mayoclinic.org/healthy-lifestyle/stress-management/in-depth/yoga/art-20044733.

6. Mayo Clinic. "Tai Chi: A Gentle Way to Fight Stress. http://www.mayoclinic.org/healthy-lifestyle/stress-management/in-depth/tai-chi/art-20045184.

7. National Institute of Health. Reiki Information. https://nccih.nih.gov/health/reiki.

8. Mayo Clinic. "Reduce Tension Through Muscle Relaxation. http://www.mayoclinic.org/healthy-lifestyle/stress-management/in-depth/health-tip/art-20048705.

9. Mayo Clinic. "Tests and Procedures: Stress." http://www.mayoclinic.org/tests-procedures/stress-management/basics/definition/prc-20021046.

10. Mayo Clinic. "Meditation: A Simple, Fast Way to Reduce Stress." Retrieved from http://www.mayoclinic.org/tests-procedures/meditation/in-depth/meditation/art-20045858.

11. Mayo Clinic."MassageTherapyOverview."http://www.mayoclinic.org/tests-procedures/massage-therapy/home/ovc-20170282.

12. Mayo Clinic. "Tests and Procedures: Acupuncture." http://www.mayoclinic.org/tests-procedures/acupuncture/basics/definition/prc-20020778.

13. National Center for Complementary and Integrative Health. "Relaxation Techniques for Health." https://nccih.nih.gov/health/stress/relaxation.htm.

14. Michigan Comprehensive Cancer Center. "Guided Imagery." http://www.mcancer.org/support/managing-emotions/complementary-therapies/guided-imagery.

15. Mayo Clinic. "Tests and Procedures: Biofeedback." http://www.mayoclinic.org/tests-procedures/biofeedback/home/ovc-20169724.

16. National Center for Complementary and Integrative Health. "Relaxation Techniques for Health." https://nccih.nih.gov/health/stress/relaxation.htm.

17. Kim, G. & Suh, S. "Meta-Analysis About Effect of Aromatherapy on Stress." *The Korean Journal of Hospice and Palliative Care* 11 no. 4 (2008): 188–195.http://www.koreascience.or.kr/article/ArticleFullRecord.jsp?cn=OHORBM_2008_v11n4_188.

18. Sgoutas-Emch, S., Fox T., Preston, M., Brooks, C. & Serber, E. "Stress Management: Aromatherapy as an Alternative." *The Scientific Review of Alternative Medicine,* 5 no. 2 (2001): 90–95. http://www.sram.org/media/documents/uploads/article_pdfs/5-2-03.Sgoutas-Emch.pdf.

19. Mayo Clinic. "What are the Benefits of Aromatherapy?" http://www.mayoclinic.org/healthy-lifestyle/consumer-health/expert-answers/aromatherapy/faq-20058566.

20. Mayo Clinic. "Is There an Effective Herbal Treatment for Anxiety?" Retrieved from http://www.mayoclinic.org/diseases-conditions/generalized-anxiety-disorder/expert-answers/herbal-treatment-for-anxiety/faq-20057945.

21. American Psychological Association. "Teaching Tip Sheet: Self-Efficacy." http://www.apa.org/pi/aids/resources/education/self-efficacy.aspx.
22. Mayo Clinic. "Fitness: Tips for Staying Motivated." http://www.mayoclinic.org/healthy-lifestyle/fitness/in-depth/fitness/art-20047624?pg=2.
23. American Psychological Association. "Five Tips to Help Manage Stress." http://www.apa.org/helpcenter/manage-stress.aspx.
24. American College Health Association. "ACHA-NCHA IIc Report" (Fall 2015-present). http://www.acha-ncha.org/reports_ACHA-NCHAIIc.html.

IMAGE CREDITS

Fig. 7.1: Copyright © Depositphotos/alphaspirit.

Fig. 7.2: Copyright © Depositphotos/avemario.

Fig. 7.4: Copyright © Depositphotos/EpicStockMedia.

Fig. 7.3: Copyright © Depositphotos/iqoncept.

Fig. 7.5: Copyright © Depositphotos/Amaviael.

Fig. 7.6: Copyright © Depositphotos/Wavebreakmedia.

Fig. 7.7: Copyright © Depositphotos/AndreyPopov.

Fig. 7.8: Copyright © Depositphotos/duskbabe.

Fig. 7.9: Copyright © Depositphotos/svyatoslavlipik.

Fig. 7.10: Copyright © Depositphotos/nongpimmy.

Fig. 7.11: Copyright © Depositphotos/Volha.Belausava.

Fig. 7.12: Copyright © Depositphotos/Volha.Belausava.

8 SEXUAL HEALTH

BY ASHLEE BURT

WHAT IS SEXUALITY?

Before we dive into sexual health, let's take a moment and discuss some key terminology that may come up. **Sexuality** incorporates more than just the act; it includes behaviors, attitudes, and instincts associated with being sexual. Organizations, such as the World Health Organization (WHO) and the American School Health Association (ASHA), define **sexual health** in different ways. According to the WHO, sexual health is a state of physical, emotional, mental and social well being in relation to sexuality, so you see here many of the dimensions of wellness are incorporated into sexual health. The WHO states that sexual health does not just indicate the absence of a disease or dysfunction, but requires individuals to have a positive and respectful approach to sexuality and their corresponding relationships. This means both parties have safe and pleasurable experiences that include mutual consent, free from discrimination and violence. Overall, sexual health is achieved when the sexual rights of all persons involved receive respect, trust one another, and that all parties have their sexuality fulfilled.[1]

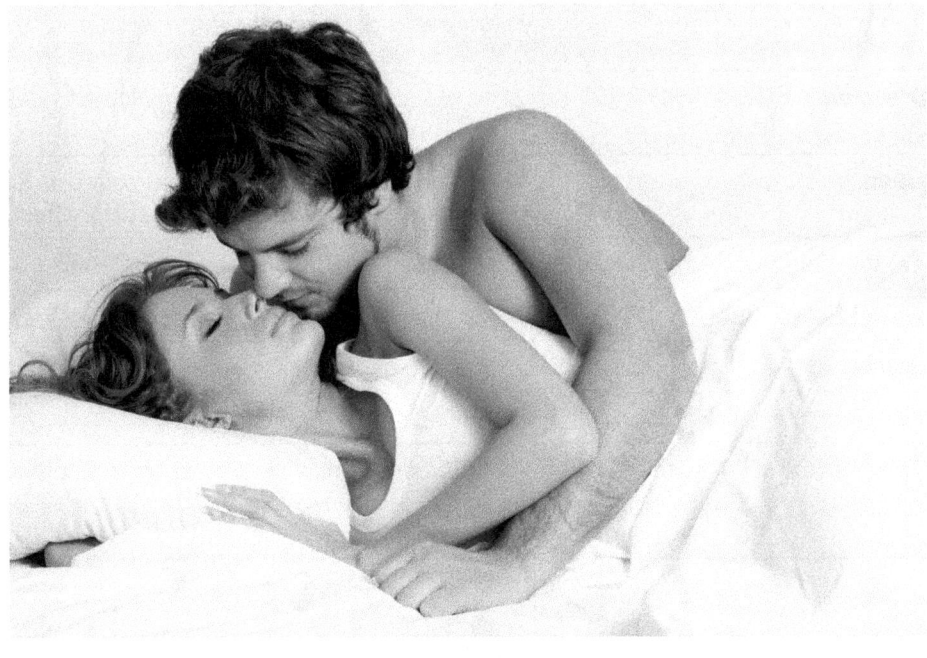

Figure 8.1: Sexual Health.

SEXUAL HEALTH

Sexual health, as described by ASHA, is being able to accept and enjoy individual sexuality throughout a lifetime. ASHA also discusses the importance of physical and emotional health in regards to sexuality. Specifically, they make a list of what being sexually healthy means:

- Understanding that sexuality is a natural part of life
- Recognizing and respecting the sexual rights of others
- Having access to sexual health information, education, and care
- Preventing unintended pregnancies as well as STI/D's, and to seek care and treatment when needed
- Ability to experience sexual pleasure, satisfaction, and intimacy when desired
- Ability to communicate about sexual health with others including partners and healthcare providers[2]

We have discussed sexual health, and within that we mentioned **sexual rights.** Before we move on let's discuss how ASHA describes sexual rights. We already recognize basic human rights that are found in our national laws as well as in international documents that state that all persons have the right to be free of coercion, discrimination and violence. In regards to sexual rights, it specifically means the aforementioned items should be met to the highest standard of sexual health, including access to sexual reproductive health care services, to be able to seek and receive information related to sexuality, education on sexuality, to have respect for bodily integrity, the ability to choose their partner and to decide to be sexually active or not, consensual sexual relationships and marriage, ability to decide whether or not, and when, to have children and to be able to pursue a satisfying, safe and enjoyable sexual life.

Please refer to the table below for other key terms that you may want to be aware of:[3,4]

Term	Definition
Cross-Dressing	Act or practice of wearing clothes made for the opposite sex.
Drag-queen	A male homosexual who dresses as a woman, especially for comic or theatrical effect.
Heterosexual Relationship	Those of opposite sex (male-female).
Homosexual Relationship	Those of the same sex (male-male, female-female).
Monogamy	One partner.
Polygamy	Multiple partners.
Sexually Transmitted Disease (STD)	A communicable disease that is spread through sexual contact (vaginal, anal, or oral sex) that is a symptomatic disease.

(Continued)

Term	Definition
Sexually Transmitted Infection (STI)	A communicable infection that is spread through sexual contact (vaginal, anal, or oral sex, that is not yet classified as a disease as there are none to mild symptoms.
Transgender	Relating to or being a person who identifies with a gender identity that differs from the one that corresponds to the person's sex at birth.
Transsexual	A person who strongly identifies with the opposite sex and may seek to live as a member of this sex especially by undergoing surgery and hormone therapy to obtain the necessary physical appearance (as by changing the external sex organs).
Transvestite	A person and especially a male who adopts the dress and often the behavior typical of the opposite sex especially for purposes of emotional or sexual gratification[44].

PERSONAL SAFETY AND HEALTHY RELATIONSHIPS

How do you keep yourself sexually safe and what are the components of a healthy relationship? Many may say that good relationships are common sense; however, the majority of kids, parents, and schools, do not receive education on these topics, including how to keep yourself safe sexually, or how to create and manage a healthy relationship. Let's break down basic concepts that will help create a safe and healthy relationship. Many of you can agree that individuals should avoid risky behaviors. This can include going for a run in the middle of the night without telling a friend or family member, with headphones in, and not on a well-lit path. This is increasing the risk to your personal safety. To give a sexual scenario, going to a party without a friend, trusting strangers, not observing your surroundings—again this increases risk to your personal safety. In regards to a relationship between partners, while it's not necessarily avoiding risky behaviors the same way you would if you were going to a party or on a late run, but it's communicating and taking preventative action to avoid any unhealthy outcomes.

A healthy relationship must have clear and open communication; this is the only way each of you will know what the other's expectations are, and to work on compromises to meet each other's needs. If you do not have communication in the relationship, then trust will not develop between the partners, and it will most likely fail, or one partner will be left unsatisfied. Partners must agree on boundaries with their intimate life, both must agree their needs are being met, and discussion on how to protect against STI's and unintended pregnancies needs to take place. If the relationship is an open relationship, then the partners must agree on how often to get screened for STI's and HIV as well as whether or not protection will be used and what that will be. Risky behavior may also include using birth control methods that do not have a high success rate, such as the calendar method or pull out method, which are discussed later in the chapter.

WHAT ARE STI'S/STD'S?

CHLAMYDIA

Chlamydia is a bacterial infection, known as a "silent" infection that can be spread through vaginal, anal, or oral sex (i.e., contact with mucous membranes). According to the Centers for Disease Control and Prevention (CDC), as of 2014, there were a total of 1,441,789 cases of the infection. This puts the rate of 456.1 cases per 100,000 people. Overall, this infection showed a 2.8% increase in cases and is still the most frequently reported bacterial STI. The age group most affected by this infection is 14–24 year olds. Researchers believe the bacteria can incubate in an individual for seven to fourteen days. If a pregnant woman gives birth while infected, the infant will contract the infection as they pass through the birth canal and can have complications such as conjunctivitis (eye infection) and pneumonia. With a chlamydia infection, both males and females may be asymptomatic, or without symptoms. However, when there are symptoms present it usually includes discharge from the penis or vagina, swelling of the testes in men, or painful urination for women. Specifically in women it can cause a more serious infection called pelvic inflammatory disease (PID), which we will discuss later in this chapter. Also, if this infection goes untreated over the long term, it can cause infertility in both men and women. Other symptoms that can occur depending on the sexual activity, but are less common, are in the rectum and throat. If the rectum is infected, it can cause proctitis (i.e., rectal pain, discharge, and or bleeding), and if the throat becomes infected through oral sex, the infection can be found in the back of the throat, however this is usually asymptomatic. To treat this infection, an individual needs to see a health care provider to be tested and diagnosed, and then they will receive antibiotics[6,9].

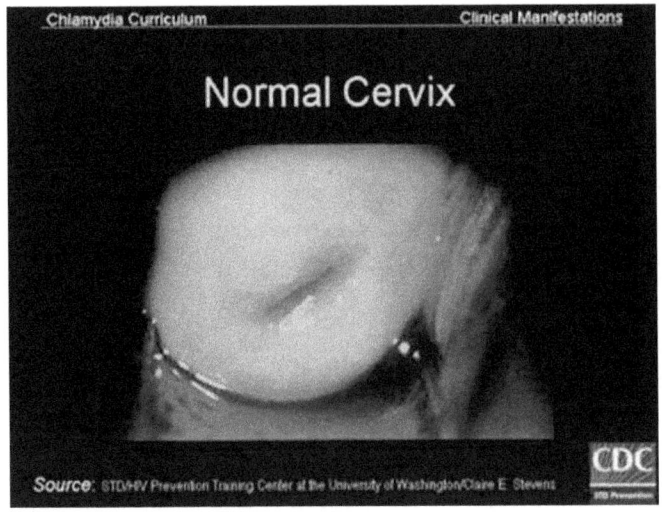

Figure 8.2: Normal Cervix.

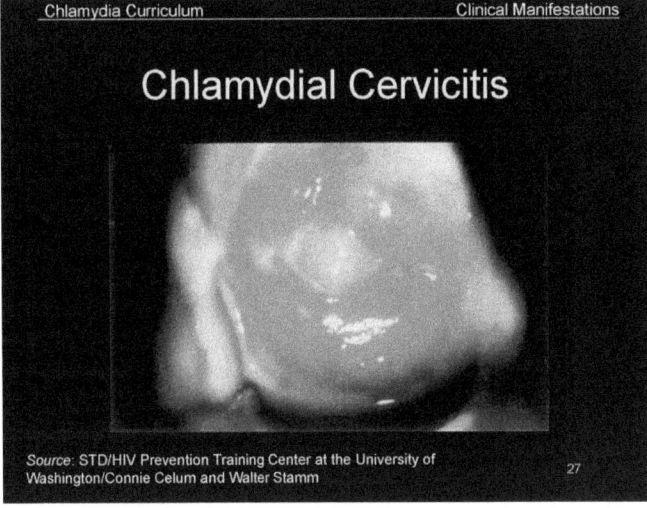

Figure 8.3: Cervix with Chlamydia.

GONORRHEA

Gonorrhea has been around for a very long time, and there are references to this disease by the Chinese, the Egyptians, and even in the Bible. It is widely known as "the clap," and years ago it was the most common STI, but today it is second to chlamydia. This infection is bacterial and incubates two to seven days in its host. Similar to chlamydia, it is spread through sexual contact (e.g., vaginal, anal, or oral sex). Since 2013, the rate of gonorrhea cases has increased by 5.1% in the United States. Again, many men and women are asymptomatic. Symptoms can consist of urethral infection in men with pain upon urinating, and white, yellow, or green discharge from the penis. This generally occurs approximately fourteen days after the infection. Men may also experience testicular or scrotal pain. Many women will go without symptoms until the infection reaches the fallopian tubes. Women with symptoms may experience vaginal discharge or burning upon urination, which many times is mistaken for a bladder or vaginal infection. Women may also experience redness, swelling, and itching of the vulva. If an individual contracts an infection through anal sex, he may have symptoms of discharge, itching, soreness, bleeding, and/or painful bowel movements. If an infection occurs in the throat, it may cause a soreness, but usually there aren't any symptoms.[6]

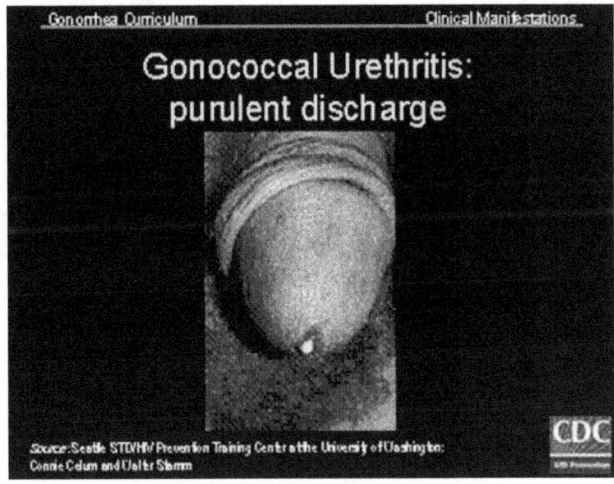

Figure 8.4: Discharge from contracting gonorrhea.

HUMAN PAPILLOMA VIRUS (HPV)

The human papilloma virus (HPV) causes warts in which there are many different strains of the virus. Some cause common warts, which can be found on places such as the hands, face, knees, feet, etc. The

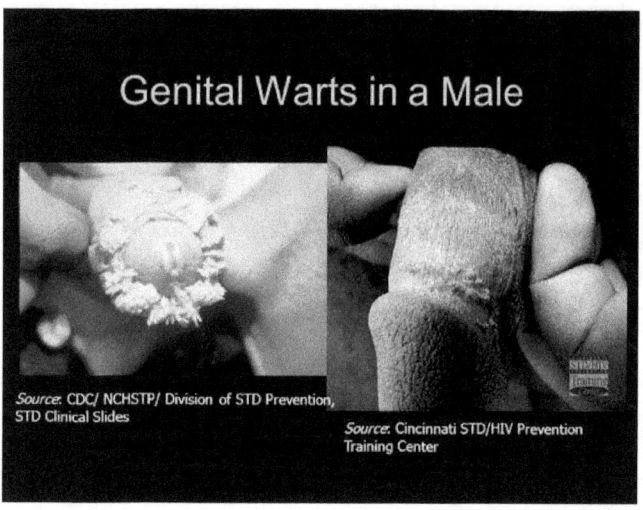

Figure 8.5: Male Genital Warts.

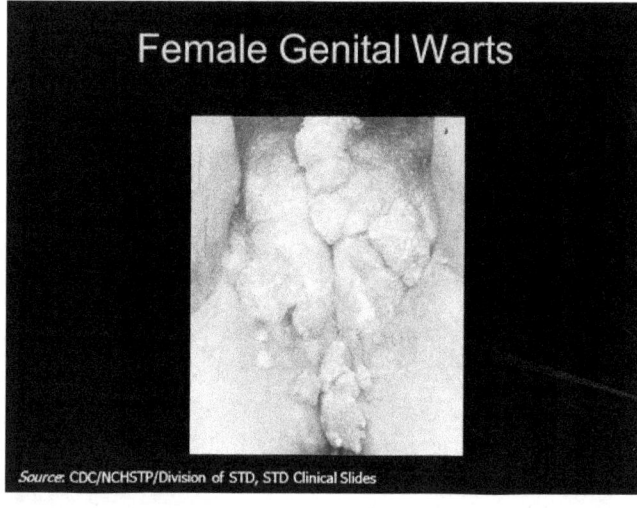

Figure 8.6: Female Genital Warts.

virus type we will discuss in this section is genital warts, which appear as a pinkish cauliflower design. This virus can be spread through vaginal, anal, or oral sex, and is one of the most common sexually transmitted infections (STI). It is believed that the incubation period for this virus is two to three months on average. The difficult part with HPV is that an individual can develop symptoms years after they had a sexual relation with someone who was infected, thus going undiagnosed for a long time. Many times the HPV virus will go away on its own, however, sometimes it does not go away and can cause significant health problems, such as genital warts or cancer (e.g., cervical, vulva, vaginal, penile, or anal cancer). If present in the back of the throat, it can also lead to oropharyngeal cancer. The warts generally disappear on their own once the body builds up enough resistance against them, but this can take months to years to accomplish. There are treatments out there such as surgery or cryotherapy to remove the warts. We currently have a vaccine to prevent individuals from contracting HPV and it is recommended that all boys and girls ages 11 or 12 should get vaccinated. If an individual did not get vaccinated at this age the CDC recommends a catch up vaccine for males through age 21, and females through age 26. Keep in mind there is no test to diagnose and find out if an individual has the virus; the only test available is one to screen for cervical cancer. This is what makes HPV dangerous—the warts may or may not be there, the incubation period can be long, an individual can be asymptomatic for years, and there is no test to diagnose the virus.[6]

HERPES

The herpes simplex virus has two different strains that we refer to as type 1 (HSV-1) or type 2 (HSV-2). Type 1 herpes affects the upper portion of the body, such as the lips and face (e.g., cold sores). Type 2 affects the lower portion, which is usually genital herpes, however both types can occur anywhere in the body depending on sexual activity and areas exposed. The virus has an incubation period of two to twelve days and it can be spread through the saliva of an infected person or through vaginal, anal, or oral sex of an infected person. This is why individuals with active cold sores on their lips/in their mouths are told to refrain from being close to young infants, or very careful not to get into close contact with their faces. The virus can spread through a break in the skin or via mucous membrane. This means coming into contact with a lesion, mucosal surfaces, genital secretions, or oral secretions. Both type 1 and 2 viruses can also be shed from skin that may look normal. In most cases, an individual can only contract HSV-2 during sexual contact with someone who has a genital HSV-2 infection, but both viruses can be transmitted by oral-genital or oral-anal contact. The majority of all adults worldwide have been exposed to HSV-1, about 70% to 90%. Once an individual contracts either virus (HSV-1 or 2), they are infected for life. The majority of those infected do not realize they have the infection, as many times the symptoms that occur are often mistaken for another skin condition. Symptoms may appear as one or more vesicle on or around the genital area, rectum, or mouth. Both HSV-1 and 2 have recurrent outbreaks; however, HSV-1 has more recurrences, which include symptoms that are shorter in duration that cause mild tingling or pain in the legs, hips, or buttocks. This tingling or pain usually occurs a few hours to days before the lesions occur. Symptoms of genital herpes include painful ulcers, and in some cases both HSV-1 and 2 can cause significant complications (e.g., blindness, inflammation of the brain, meningitis), however, this is very rare. There is no cure for the virus, only management techniques. Antiviral medications can help decrease the severity of the ulcers or shorten an outbreak. The only way to prevent contracting this virus is to abstain from sex or use condoms correctly, as there are no vaccines.[6]

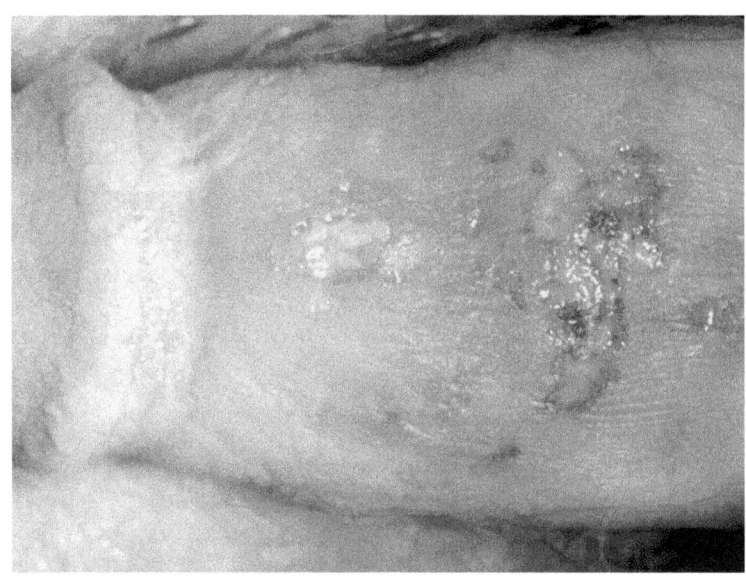

Figure 8.7: Genital Herpes.

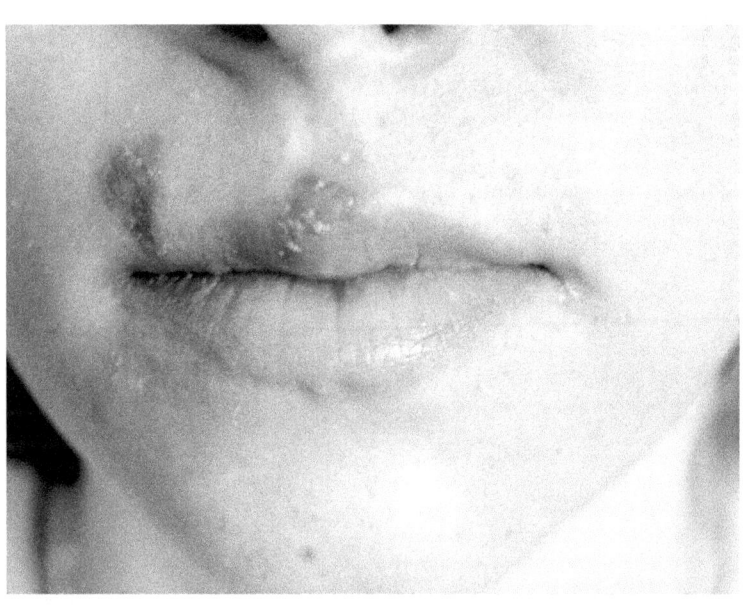

Figure 8.8: Oral Herpes.

PELVIC INFLAMMATORY DISEASE

We previously mentioned pelvic inflammatory disease (PID) when we discussed chlamydia. Let's go into more detail of what this disease is. This disease occurs when damaging microorganisms that oftentimes occur from bacterial STDs, such as chlamydia or gonorrhea, move their way from the vagina or cervix up the genital tract, towards the uterus and fallopian tubes. This disease can lead to permanent damage to the woman's reproductive organs and infertility. It can lead to chronic pelvic pain, or cause future ectopic pregnancies (i.e., egg attaches in the fallopian tube). Signs and symptoms of PID can range from mild to severe, and can include all or some of the following: lower abdominal pain, mild pelvic pain, increased vaginal discharge, irregular menstrual bleeding, fever, painful intercourse, dysuria and polyuria (i.e., painful and frequent urination), abdominal, pelvic, and uterine tenderness, cervical motion tenderness, and inflammation. Diagnosing PID includes getting a health history of signs and symptoms, biopsy, ultrasound, lab tests, and many other evaluative tools. To treat PID, the physician will prescribe antibiotics, but keep in mind that this does not undo the scarring damage the disease may have already caused to the reproductive organs. Any and all sexual partners should also be informed and treated, whether they have symptoms or not, as they could still be infected. The only way to prevent PID is to prevent contracting any STDs, so condom use and consistent STD screenings are important. A small amount of PID cases has been linked to vaginal douching and the intrauterine birth control device (IUD). Overall, multiple research studies have indicated that the prevalence of PID has been declining, however, education on safe sex practices needs to occur to continue preventing these diseases.[7]

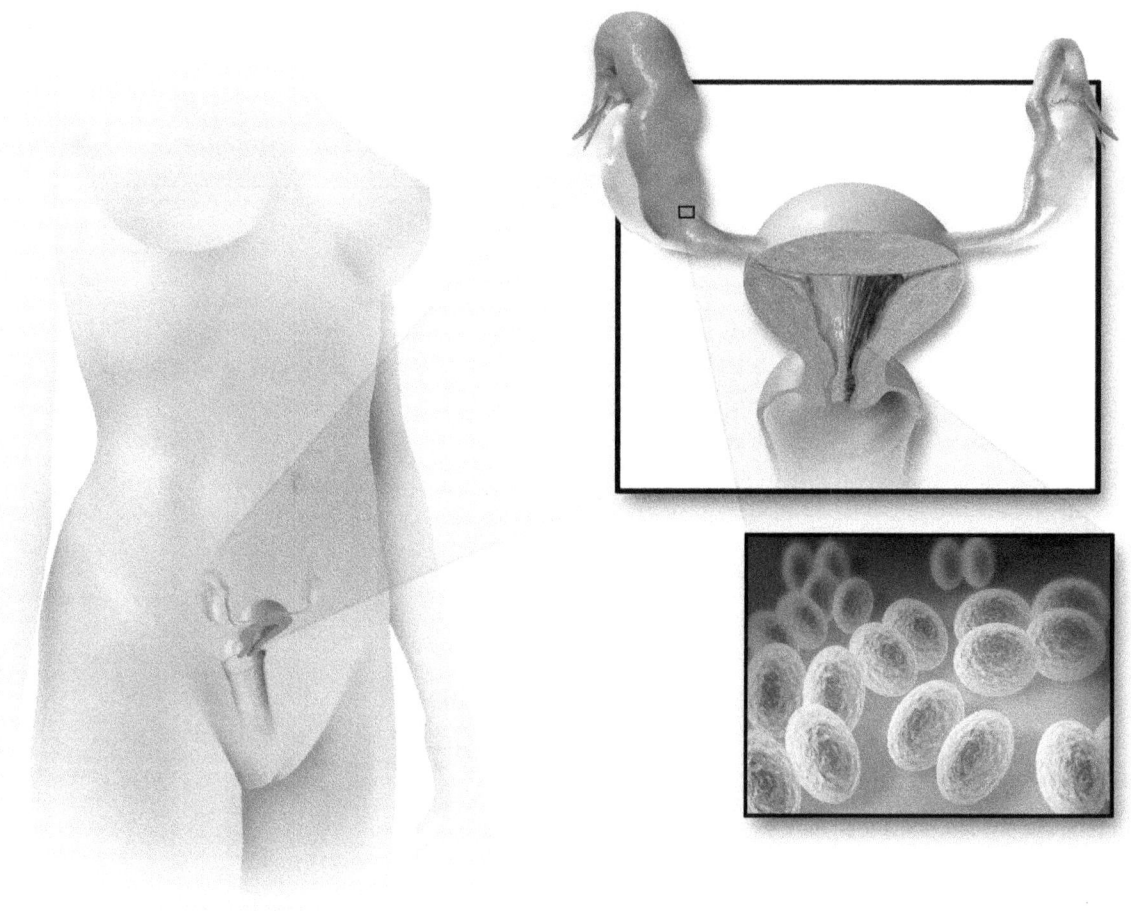

Figure 8.9: Pelvic Inflammatory Disease.

SYPHILIS

Syphilis is a bacterial infection that has been around forever; we have record of it being described by Hippocrates back in 460 B.C., and it is discussed in the Bible, as well as by a Roman physician in A.D. 25. This STD was a serious problem in the United States in the War of 1812, however, once we discovered penicillin, the cases dropped significantly. From then on we saw a rise, decline and rise in the STD, depending on different events that were occurring in the United States at the time. In 2014, the CDC reported only 63,450 new cases. **Chancres**, which are sores, can be found on the external areas of the vagina, penis, anus, or in the rectum, and transmission occurs with direct contact with a chancre or through mucous membranes contact via vaginal, anal, or oral sex. It can also be passed congenitally to a newborn through the birth canal. The average incubation period is 21 days after infection.

Syphilis occurs in three different stages. The first, or primary stage, is the chancre and there may be multiple sores. This chancre is usually round and painless and appears at the location where the infection entered the body. Many times individuals go undiagnosed because the chancre can be hidden and occur in the rectum or cervix. The secondary stage develops in a few days to weeks while the chancre(s) are healing and usually includes a rash that occurs on the palms of the hands and bottoms of the feet as well as other parts of the body. Other symptoms include enlarged lymph nodes, headache, general aches and pains, fever, hair loss, and fatigue. The symptoms of the secondary stage will diminish on their own with or without treatment, however, untreated it will progress to the last stage, known as the latent or tertiary stage. During this last stage, the individual will oftentimes not experience any symptoms and can take 10 to 20 years to develop after the infection was first contracted. The late stage is critically damaging as it is hidden, and can damage many internal organs including the brain, eyes, heart, blood vessels, liver, etc. The late stage may also cause lesions known as **gumma**, a soft, non-cancerous growth. Once an individual reaches this stage, they are no longer able to transmit the infection to others. This disease is an easy one to treat if it is diagnosed; penicillin is used in all three stages to cure the disease. If organ damage occurs, then that damage is irreversible.[8]

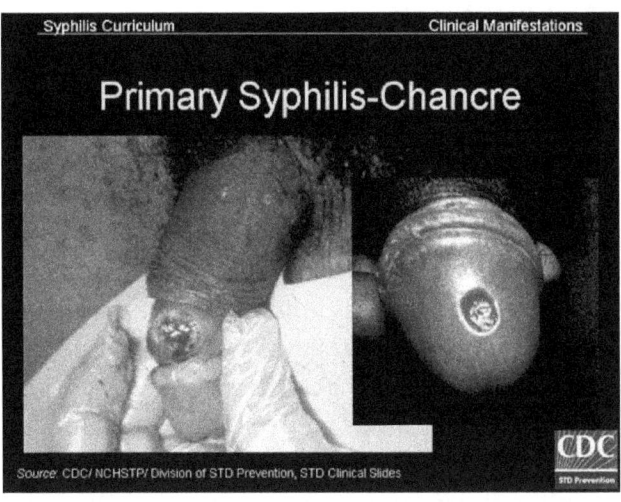

Figure 8.10: Aerobic Pilates Women Group With Stability Balls.

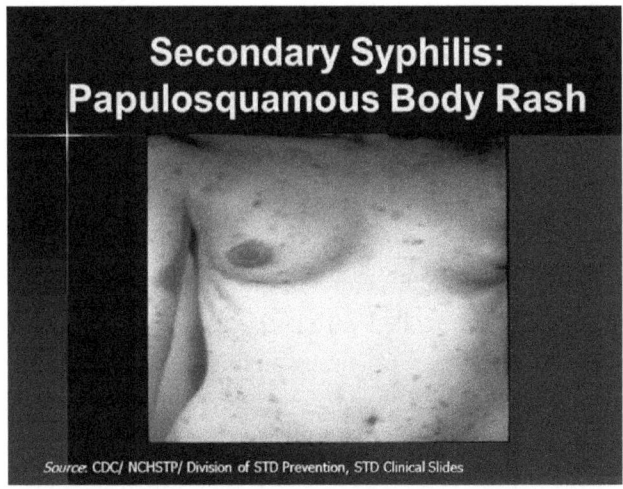

Figure 8.11: Moderate Syphilis Chancre.

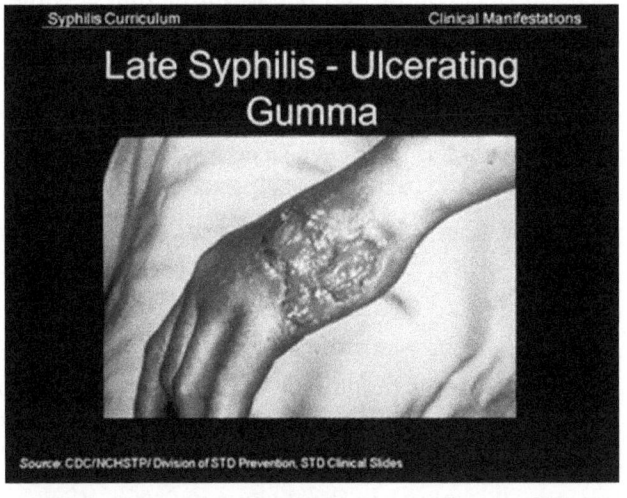

Figure 8.12: Late Syphilis Chancre.

TRICHOMONIASIS

The next STI we are going to discuss is one that you may or may not have heard of. It is an extremely common STI. Trichomoniasis, or "trich" is a bacterial infection and similar to previous STIs in that the majority of individuals are asymptomatic. The CDC estimates that 3.7 million people in the United States (yes, that reads MILLION), have the infection, however, only approximately 30% of those infected develop symptoms. Researchers cannot be sure on the incubation period as the majority (70%), of those infected do not have symptoms at all. This specific STI occurs more often in women, specifically older women. Similar to all other STIs, this infection is transmitted through vaginal, anal, or oral sex. It is generally uncommon for this parasite to cause infection in other body parts such as the hands, mouth, or anus. Mild to severe symptoms can occur if an individual does experience symptoms and includes men having an itching feeling inside the penis, a burning sensation after urination or ejaculation, and some discharge from the penis. Women with symptoms may also have an itching, burning, or soreness of the vaginal area, as well as discomfort with urinating, and discharge from the vagina. This STI can cause genital inflammation, which in turn can make it easier to get infected with HIV. Pregnant women with the infection have an increased chance of delivering their babies preterm, and the babies have a higher risk of having a low birth weight. Simple lab work is completed to diagnose the infection, and it is easily cured with a round of antibiotics. To prevent future infections, practice safe sex (condom use) and make sure your partner(s) also receive treatment.

HIV

Human immunodeficiency virus (HIV) is a virus that leads to acquired immunodeficiency syndrome (AIDS). Once an individual is infected with this virus, he will have it for life, as there is no cure. The infection can be controlled with antiretroviral therapy (ART). Presently, with the use of ART, those diagnosed with HIV can start treatment right away and many times have a normal life expectancy. This virus attacks a person's CD4, or T cells, which are a type of white blood cell in our bodies that help fight off infections. In a normal uninfected adult, the CD4 count ranges from 500 cells/mm^3 to 1,600 cells/mm^3. Once an HIV positive individual's CD4 count falls below 200 cells/mm^3 they become classified as progressed to the AIDS stage. There are three stages to the infection: acute HIV infection, clinical latency, and AIDS. Once an individual reaches the AIDs stage, it is expected that without treatment, he will only survive about 3 years. If they contract an opportunistic illness while in this stage, and are not receiving any treatment, then survivability decreases to about 1% year. An opportunistic infection is a secondary infection that the individual contracts while infected with HIV/AIDS, such as pneumonia, tuberculosis, and herpes simplex, among many others. According to the United States Department of Health and Human Services, if an individual is taking ART and avoids increasing his risk of obtaining an opportunistic infection, then most likely they will have a normal life span and never progress to the AIDS stage. HIV can be transmitted through vaginal, anal, or oral sex (e.g., semen, pre-seminal fluid, rectal fluids, vaginal fluids), sharing of needles for drugs (e.g., blood), and from mother-to-baby through birth or breastfeeding. These fluids must come into contact with a mucous membrane or damaged tissue, or be directly injected into the bloodstream for transmission to happen. Remember mucous membranes are found inside the vagina, penis, rectum, and mouth. It is NOT transmitted through air or water, saliva, sweat, tears or closed-mouth kissing, insects or pets, or sharing of toilets, food, or drinks. The only way to prevent an HIV infection is to abstain from sex, limit your sexual partners, use condoms, and avoid drug use or sharing of needles. If you are sexually active, you should be tested consistently, and if you think you have been exposed, you should see your physician immediately as there is a post exposure prophylaxis (PEP) medication that can prevent HIV, but must be started within 72 hours of exposure. If an individual has HIV, depending on what state he lives in, he must inform any and all partners of his infection. Many states have adopted HIV-specific criminal exposure laws, which penalize those living with the infection that are aware of their diagnoses, and potentially expose others to HIV, and this includes notifying needle-sharing partners. Depending on the state, those that potentially infect their partners without disclosing their HIV status can still be charged, even if the partner does not become infected. The only current federal legislation against HIV infection is in regards to banning blood donation.[10,11,12]

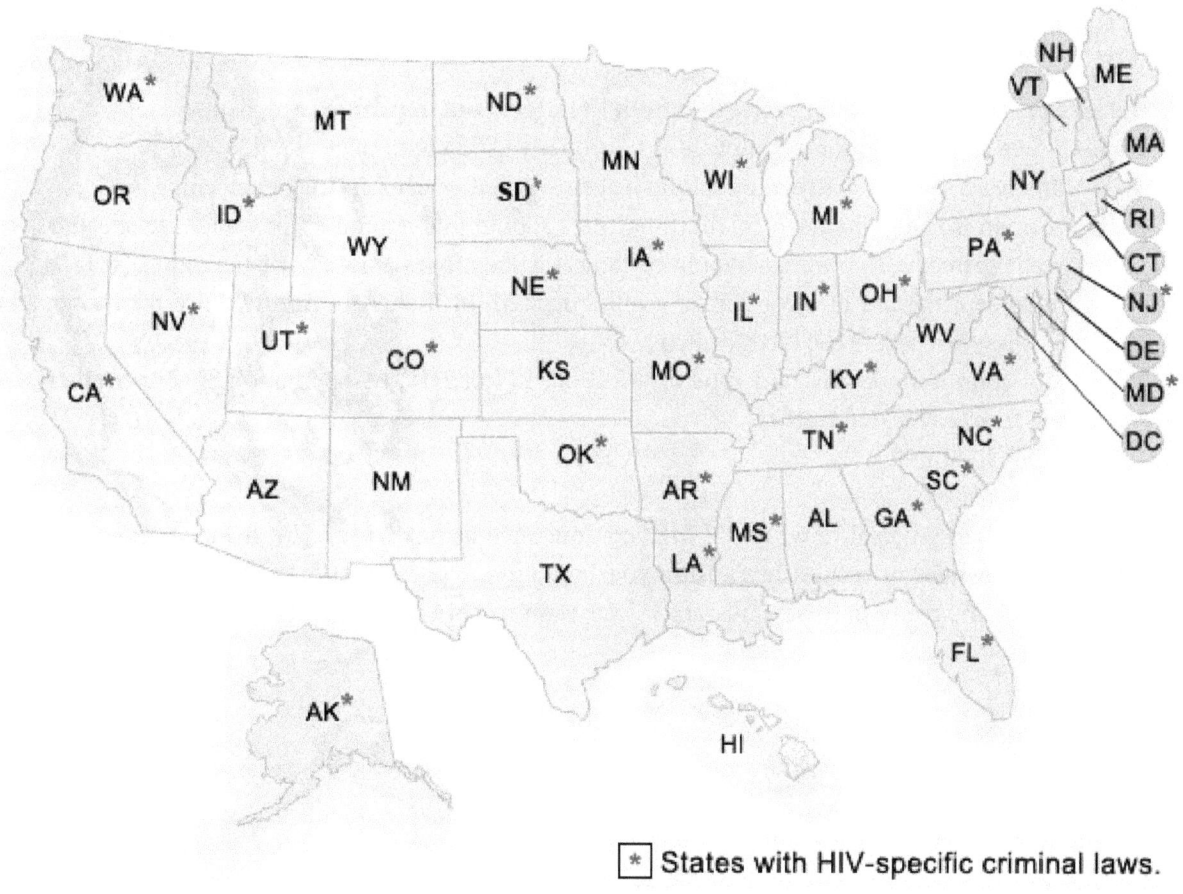

Figure 8.13: States with HIV Exposure Laws.

RESPONSIBILITY AND SEX

Now that we have discussed many of the dangerous side effects of unsafe sex, let's recap how to be responsible. It is up to each individual person to become educated and seek out resources available to him. Being responsible, sexually, is making informed decisions and choosing safer sex (or abstinence) options. It is taking precautions in regards to preventing STIs, HIV, and unplanned pregnancy. Each person must acknowledge that she controls her own sexuality and human rights, and has the ability to say no to sex at any point. Let's look at the following list of items that pertain to being sexually responsible and safe:

1. Understand it is your choice to be sexually active
2. Be informed on sexuality, sexual health, and all the components that make up a healthy relationship
3. Respect your partner and have open communication—this includes receiving consent every time you engage in sexual activity
4. Come to an agreement in a sexual relationship (male-female, male-male, or female-female) to pursue monogamy, or if multiple partners are involved, to agree upon routine screenings, proper protection, and to be open and honest of any infections contracted
5. Take precautions to protect each other from STIs, HIV, and unplanned pregnancy
6. Both men and women should know how to properly use a condom
7. If women are sexually active, they should be getting their yearly pap smear screening
8. If a woman is using birth control, both partners should understand all possible side effects as well as take it correctly. The woman should be honest if she misses a dose of birth control (missed pill), or implement the use of a condom if a pill is missed, or if she is currently on a medication that diminishes the effect of the birth control
9. And, of course, if you have any type of infection, STI or HIV, be open and tell your partner(s) or abstain from any sexual activity
10. BE RESPONSIBLE!

It isn't necessarily illegal to withhold information, such as having an STI, from a partner, but it is illegal if you knowingly or recklessly transmit your infection to your partner or another person. How do you know if you are ready to be sexually active? Or want to be? Here are some questions people should ask themselves:

- Why do you want to have sex?
- What kinds of sexual activity are you interested in?
- What types of protection or safe sex methods will you use?
- Will you use a contraceptive? If yes, what method of contraception will you use and why?
- How will you communicate all these answers to your partner?

Even if you go through the process of figuring out whether you are ready to be sexually active or not, remember it is always your choice and you should never let anyone try to force, persuade, or guilt you into engaging in sexual activity. Well, that's easier said than done, as many of you may be able to relate to this situation. If you've been with the same partner for a long time, how do you continue to say no, or how do you continue to make sure a condom is used? Let's look at Indiana University of Pennsylvania's safer sex comebacks. These practice answers are to help individuals who are with a partner who may be trying to convince someone into engaging in risky sexual behavior, such as not using a condom (Table 8.2).

Statement	Response
"I'm on the pill; you don't need a condom."	"The pill doesn't protect us from HIV or STIs."
"I know I'm clean, I haven't had sex in six months."	"I want to use protection anyways. We'll both be protected from any infections that we may not realize we have."
"Just this once..."	"Once is all it takes" *This can also relate to pregnancy...
"I love you. I would never hurt you. Just trust me."	"I love you too and I don't think you would hurt me on purpose. This is not about trust. Many people don't even know they have an infection."
"I tested negative for HIV."	"The test isn't perfect. *Besides*, there are other infections *besides* HIV."
"I don't have protection on me."	"Lucky for us, I do!"
"None of my other partners used protections."	"Please don't compare me to your other partners. If you want to have sex with ME we are going to practice safer sex."
"Sex doesn't feel good with a condom."	"Let's try another brand or style. Besides, I bet it feels better than an STI."
"Stopping to get protection spoils the mood."	"I can't enjoy sex if it's not safe. That spoils the mood for me. If that is what you're worried about, we can make it fun and enjoyable."
"I won't have sex then."	"Okay, let's not have sex."[15]

HOW TO PROTECT AGAINST STIS AND PREVENT UNPLANNED PREGNANCY

We've talked about sexual health, responsibility, infections and diseases, now we are going to look at the many different ways you can protect yourself from both STIs/HIV and unplanned pregnancy. First, let's look at the options available that protect against STIs and HIV. The following options also prevent pregnancy, but know that these are the ***ONLY*** options available that protect against sexually transmitted infections and HIV/AIDS.

STI, HIV, AND PREGNANCY PROTECTION

Condoms (male & female): the male condom covers the entire penis to prevent contact with any mucous membrane in the vagina, rectum, or mouth. The female condom is inserted and makes a tunnel barrier for intercourse, preventing contact with any mucous membranes. With the physical barrier covering the mucous membrane, it prevents contact with any possible infections. These physical barriers also block semen from entering the woman's uterus and thus preventing pregnancy.

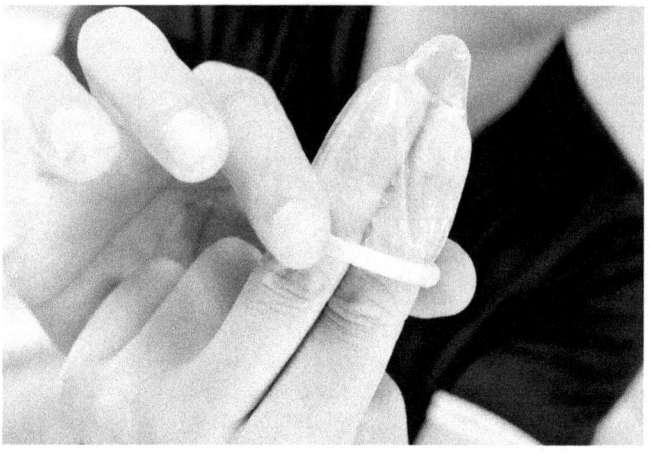

Figure 8.14: Male Condom.

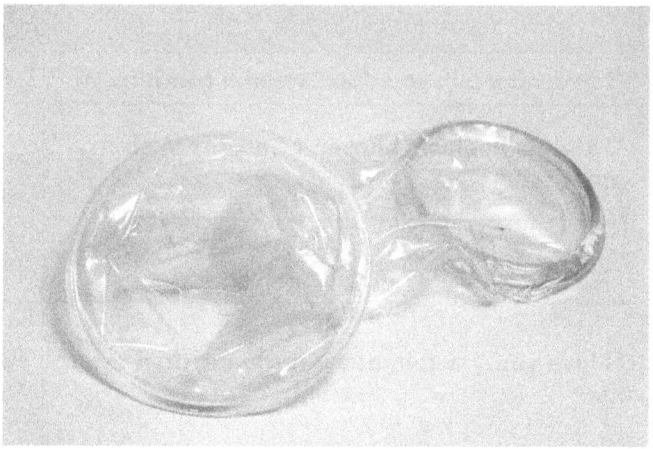

Figure 8.15: Female Condom.

FAQs CHECK!

What about abstinence-only education?

Repeated studies in multiple cities have shown that increased education in contraceptives, specifically condoms, helps decrease the amount of unprotected sex that occurs among students. However, the question that many who support abstinence-only education ask is if there is an increase in sexual activity by students if they are aware of how to use proper protection. A comparison of public high schools in New York City and Chicago found positive effects of condom availability programs. Sexual activity among senior high students in both cities was about the same (NYC, 59.7 percent; Chicago, 60.1 percent). Sexually active students in New York, where there was a condom availability program, were more likely to report using a condom during their last intercourse than were those in Chicago, where condoms were not available in school (60.8 to 55.5 percent).[12, 13] Similar studies found the same results in Philadelphia and other cities. Yet, do students increase their sexual activity as they have an increase in sexual education? A study of New York City's school condom availability program found a significant increase in condom use among sexually active students, but no increase in sexual activity. The World Health Organization review of studies on sexuality education found that access to counseling and contraceptive services did not encourage earlier or increased sexual activity. In Europe and Canada, where comprehensive sexuality education and convenient, confidential access to condoms are more common, the rates of adolescent sexual intercourse are no higher than in the United States.[14]

Dental dams: Are little square pieces of stretchy plastic or latex that are used to place over any mucous membrane areas (vulva, penis, or anus) to provide oral pleasure. Local health clinics and university wellness centers many times carry dental dams. These are used to prevent the spread of STIs and HIV, again preventing mucous membrane contact. If you do not have a dental dam available, you can create your own using plastic wrap or by cutting a condom into a flat rectangle.

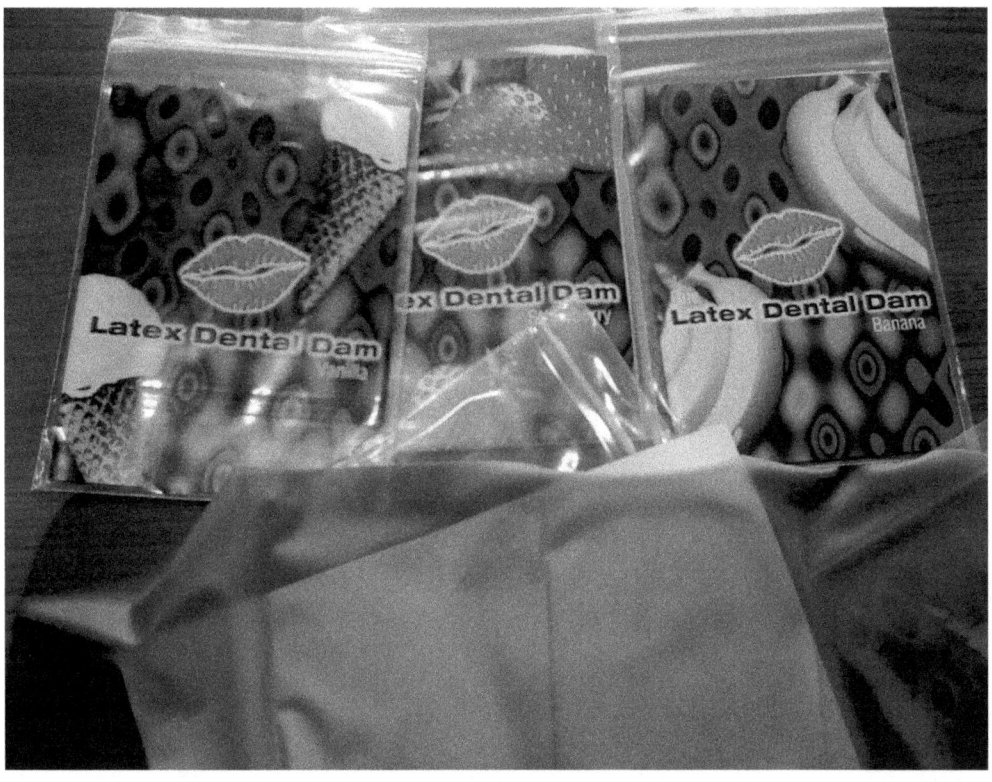

Figure 8.16: Dental Dam.

Gloves or finger cots: These items can be used to prevent the risk of getting an STI or HIV if you are providing pleasure to your partner by hand, but have a small cut on your finger(s).

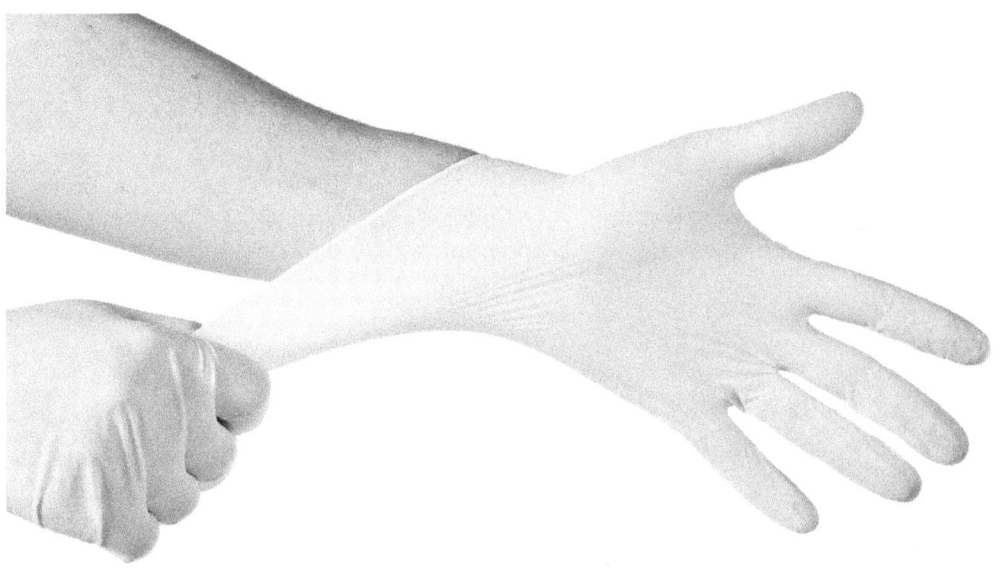

Figure 8.17: Gloves.

CONTRACEPTIVE METHODS

Physical Barriers: All physical barriers cover the cervix and block sperm from entering the uterus, or cover the penis and prevent sperm from entering the vagina. Many times spermicide is used in conjunction with a physical barrier to increase the effectiveness of pregnancy prevention. This can be done by adding spermicide to the inside of a condom, diaphragm, or cervical cap. Advantages include, ease of access and low cost. The main disadvantages for these options are a decrease in natural sensation, and the time it takes to prepare and put on or insert. Remember, only the male and female condoms prevent STIs and HIV; other barriers listed do not. The list below is the option available as physical barriers.

- Male & female condoms (as previously discussed)
- Diaphragm
- Cervical Cap (FemCap®)
- Sponge

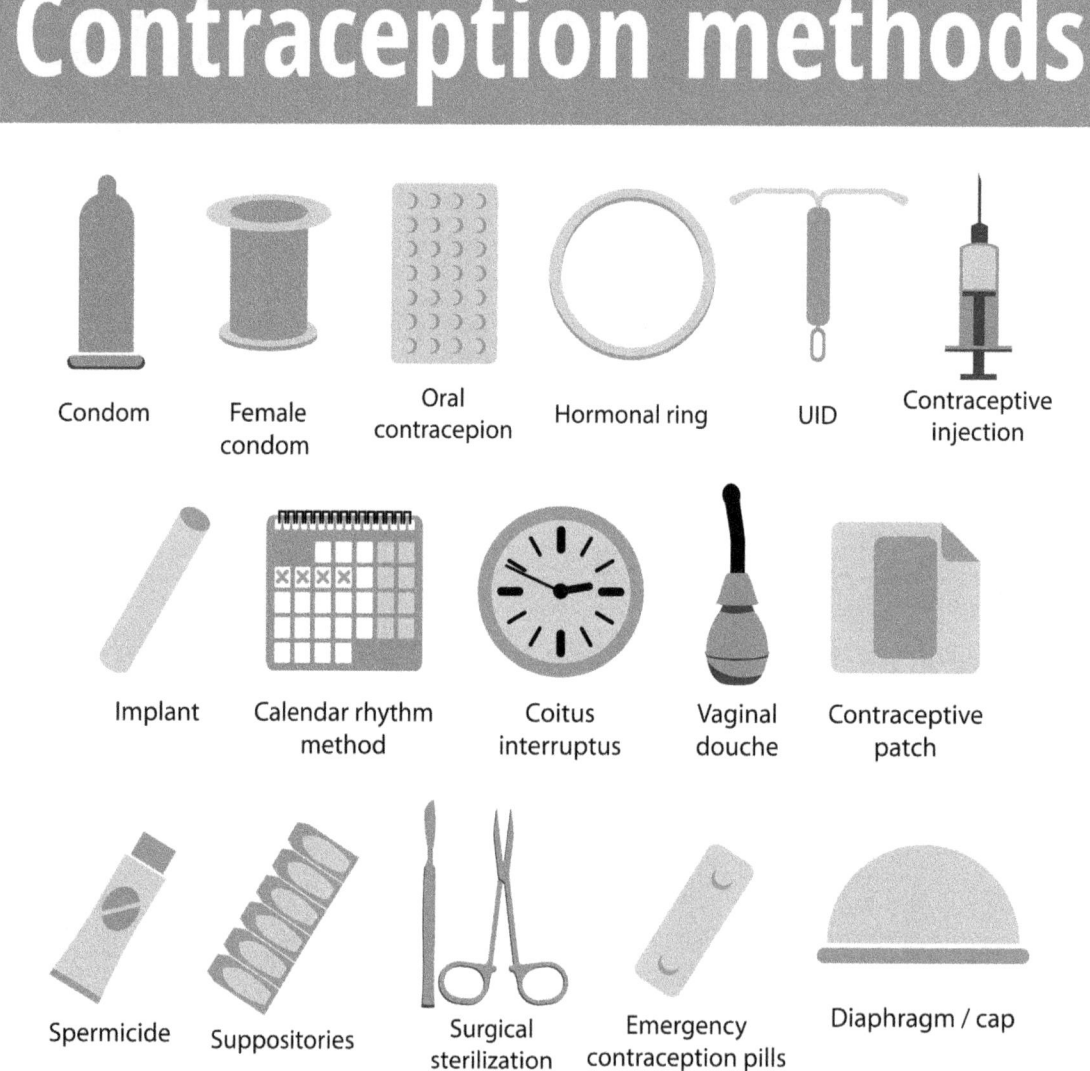

Figure 8.18: Illustrations of Contraceptives.

Chemical Barriers (Spermicides): Spermicide used on its own is only approximately 78% effective at preventing pregnancy. When used in conjunction with a physical barrier, and consistently, the effectiveness is 95% or greater. Spermicide is a chemical (i.e., nonoxynol-9) that kills and disables sperm so that it cannot cause pregnancy. A benefit of spermicide is that depending on the form chosen, it can also provide lubrication. One of the main disadvantages that may occur with spermicide is one of the partners having irritation or an allergic reaction to the chemical. Refer to the list below for chemical barrier options.

- Creams
- Jellies
- Foam
- Vaginal Contraceptive Film (VCF)
- Suppositories
- Sponge[16]

Hormonal Contraceptive Methods: Hormonal birth control is a prescribed medication that a woman takes. Each type releases different and varied amounts of multiple hormones and can do a variety of things, depending on the method to prevent pregnancy. Before we continue, we are going to make a disclaimer that women should always consult with their healthcare provider prior to deciding on a birth control method. Many factors play into whether or not you may use a specific birth control method, depending on your previous and current health history. First, let's look at the list of hormonal contraceptives, and then we will discuss each one in more detail:

- Oral contraceptive (pill)
- NuvaRing insert
- Patch
- Implant
- Injection
- IUD

Oral Contraceptives: There are multiple options available for oral birth control. For the purpose of this text, we will focus on the goal of the contraceptive, the advantages, and disadvantages. Before we get started, let's look at a quick picture of the female anatomy so you know what parts we are referring to.

There are two types of pill options: Combination pills which contain both estrogen and progestin hormones, and the minipill, which only contains the progestin hormone. With the combination pill, the

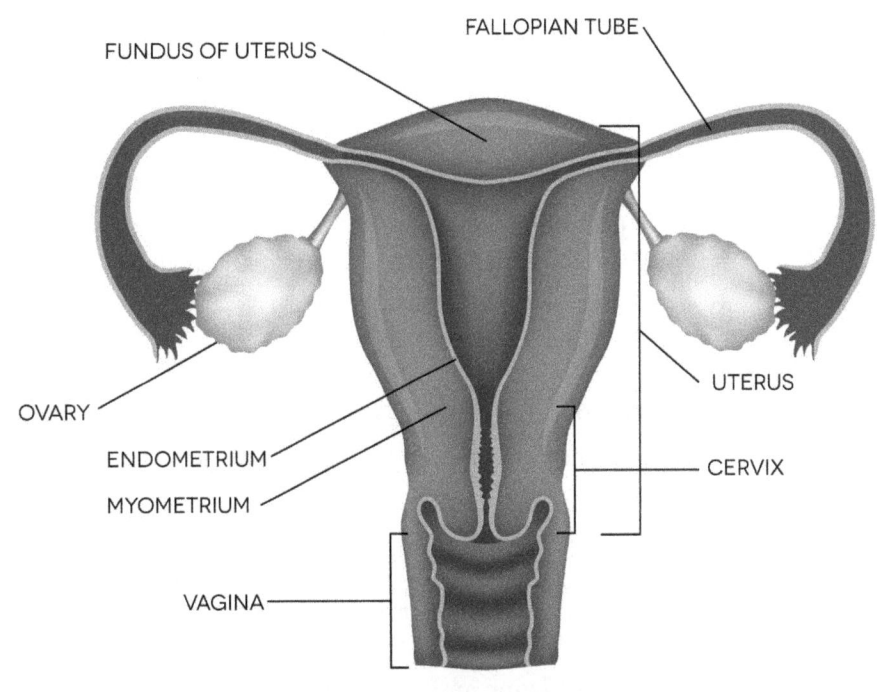

Figure 8.19: Female Anatomy.

hormones prevent ovulation; therefore the ovaries do not release an egg. The combination pill also thickens the cervical mucus, making it more difficult for the sperm to get past the cervix into the uterus. The last thing it does is thin the lining of the uterus, making it difficult for the sperm to join an egg and attach. The minipill's main goal is thickening the cervical mucous, and it only sometimes prevents ovulation.

Pros of the combination pill:

- Decreased risk of ovarian and endometrial cancers
- Improves acne
- Less severe menstrual cramping
- Reduction in heavy bleeding and related anemia
- Relief from premenstrual syndrome (PMS)
- Shorter, lighter, and more predictable periods

Cons of the combination pill:

- Does not protect against STIs or HIV
- Increased risk of heart attack and stroke
- Increased risk of blood clots
- Side effects: Irregular bleeding, bloating, breast tenderness, nausea, depression, weight gain, and headache

Pros of the minipill:

- Can be taken if you have current health problems such as a high risk of heart disease, blood clots, high blood pressure, or migraines
- Can be used during breastfeeding
- Offers a quick return to fertility

Cons of the minipill:

- No protection against STIs or HIV
- Potentially less effective than combination pills
- Must be taken at the same time every day (if taken more than three hours late then a backup birth control method is required)
- Side effects: Irregular bleeding, ovarian cysts, decreased libido (sex drive), headache, breast tenderness, acne, weight gain, depression and hirsutism (hair growth on face, chest and back)
- Slight increased risk if pregnancy occurs it will be an ectopic pregnancy (egg attaches outside of uterus)

NuvaRing: This hormonal method is a flexible, transparent plastic ring that is inserted into the vagina by the user. It is worn for three weeks, and then removed to allow the menstrual cycle to take place the fourth week. NuvaRing is similar to the combination pills, releasing both estrogen and progestin, suppressing ovulation and thickening cervical mucus.

Pros of the NuvaRing:

- Comfortable and easy to use
- Removable at any time with a quick return to fertility
- Do not need to interrupt sex for contraception
- Do not need to remember a daily pill
- Safe for women allergic to latex
- Does not require sizing
- Does not seem to cause weight gain
- Less likely to cause irregular bleeding

Cons of the NuvaRing:

- Breakthrough bleeding or spotting
- Vaginal infection or irritation
- Does not protect against STIs or HIV
- Increased vaginal secretion
- Headache
- Nausea
- Depression
- Decreased libido
- Breast tenderness
- Increased risk of blood-clotting, heart attack, stroke, liver cancer, gallbladder disease and toxic shock syndrome

Birth Control Patch: The patch, like the combination pill, contains both estrogen and progestin hormones. Similar to the NuvaRing, the patch is placed on the woman's skin once a week for three weeks and during the fourth week a patch is not used so menstruation can occur. Pregnancy is prevented through ovulation suppression and thickening of the cervical mucus. The only patch approved by the USFDA and available in the U.S. is Xulane.

Pros of the Patch:

- Eliminates the need to interrupt sex for contraception
- Doesn't require daily attention or remembering to take a pill every day
- Provides a steady dose of hormones
- Can be removed at any time and allows a quick return to fertility

Cons of the Patch:

- Increased risk of blood clotting problems, heart attack, stroke, liver cancer, gallbladder disease, and high blood pressure
- Breakthrough bleeding or spotting
- Skin irritation
- Does not protect against STIs or HIV

- Breast tenderness or pain
- Menstrual pain
- Headaches
- Nausea or vomiting
- Abdominal pain
- Mood swings
- Weight gain
- Dizziness
- Acne
- Diarrhea
- Muscle spasms
- Vaginal infections and discharge
- Fatigue
- Fluid retention

Contraceptive Implant: The implant is a small, flexible plastic rod that is about the size of a matchstick. It is surgically implanted under the skin of the upper arm. This method offers long-term birth control coverage. It releases a progestational hormone that thickens the cervical mucus and thins the lining of the uterus, and it suppresses ovulation as well. Nexplanon is the only implant approved by the USFDA available in the U.S., and is radio opaque, which allows for it to be seen on X-ray.

Pros of Implant:

- Offers long-term (up to 3 years) birth control coverage
- Can be removed at any time with a quick return to fertility
- Eliminates need to interrupt sex for contraception
- Provides relief from menstrual pain and pelvic pain due to endometriosis
- Does not contain any estrogen

Cons of Implant:

- Abdominal or back pain
- Does not protect against STIs or HIV
- Increased risk of noncancerous ovarian cysts
- Changes in vaginal bleeding patterns (possible absence of menstruation)
- Decreased sex drive
- Dizziness
- Headaches
- Mild insulin resistance
- Mood swings and depression
- Nausea or upset stomach
- Potential interaction with other medications
- breasts tenderness
- Vaginal inflammation or dryness
- Weight gain

Depo-Provera Injection: The Depo injection only uses the progestin hormone, and is given as an injection deep into the muscle every three months. The injection suppresses ovulation and thickens cervical mucus. It is also available in a lower dosage called Depo-SubQ Provera 104, and this lower dose is injected just beneath the skin and has similar benefits and risks.

Pros of Depo-Provera:

- Eliminates the need to take a daily pill
- Doesn't require daily attention
- Eliminates the need to interrupt sex for contraception
- Decreases menstrual cramps and pain
- Lessens menstrual blood flow, and in some cases stops menstruation
- Decreases the risk of endometrial cancer

Cons of Depo-Provera:

- There may be a delay in return to fertility, possibly 10 or more months
- Does not protect against STIs or HIV
- Potential for loss of bone mineral density
- Abdominal pain
- Acne
- Breast tenderness
- Decreased interest in sex
- Depression
- Dizziness
- Headaches
- Irregular period and breakthrough bleeding
- Brown discharge
- Nervousness
- Weakness and fatigue
- Weight gain

FAQs CHECK!

Free Condom Programs?

Some states allow non-profit organizations to ship condoms to anyone who requests them to reduce unplanned pregnancies and risk of disease. This is done entirely free of cost to the individual. Examples of states such as California, Arizona, and Nevada have allowed programs like Project Hard Hat to operate. Programs can be seen at www.projecthardhat.org and www.teensource.org/condoms/free

Intrauterine Device (IUD): Intrauterine devices are hormonal birth control methods shaped like a "T" that are inserted directly into the uterus (womb) through the vagina. The device is inserted during, or directly after a menstrual cycle. It is recommended the woman take a nonsteroidal anti-inflammatory drug (NSAID) such as Ibuprofen a couple hours before the procedure to help reduce cramping, which occurs shortly after the device is inserted. There are multiple brands available, including Mirena, Liletta, Skyla, and ParaGard. Both Liletta and Skyla provide three years of birth control coverage. Mirena provides up to five years, and ParaGard provides up to 10 years of coverage. The Mirena and Liletta both provide 52 mg of the female hormone levonorgestrel that slowly releases into the body, and Skyla provides 13.5 mg. These methods stop a woman's egg from fully developing each month, and therefore the egg can no longer accept a sperm and fertilization cannot occur. ParaGard is a copper wire and as the copper is released into the lining of the uterus, it causes an inflammatory response in the uterus that is toxic to sperm thus preventing fertilization. The IUD method of birth control is recommended to women who have had at least one child, due to the cervix having been stretched from pregnancy. A woman who has never been pregnant will have a closed cervix and it may be difficult or impossible to insert the IUD into the uterus. After insertion, the woman must check for the tail, or string, that hangs from the bottom of the IUD once a month to ensure its placement (preferably after your menstrual cycle). Some women will experience lighter or no periods while on the IUD.

Pros of Mirena, Liletta and Skyla:

- Eliminates need to interrupt sex for contraception
- Offers long term birth control coverage (3–5 years)
- Can be removed at any time with a quick return to fertility
- Decreases menstrual bleeding after several months of use
- Decreases menstrual pain and pain related to endometriosis
- Decreases risk of pelvic inflammatory disease (PID) caused by STIs by causing cervical mucus to thicken (barrier against bacteria and sperm)
- Decreases risk of endometrial cancer and cervical cancer
- Can be used while breastfeeding (recommended to wait at least six weeks after birth)
- Doesn't have side effects related to birth control with estrogen

Cons of Mirena, Liletta and Skyla:

- Does not protect against STIs or HIV
- Increased risk of PID if individual gets infections easily, has a certain cancer, has a pelvic infection, and persistent pelvic or abdominal pain
- Small risk of IUD slipping partly or all the way out (most likely to occur during first year); check the tail regularly for placement
- Rarely, IUD may make a hole in the wall or become embedded in the uterus after insertion
- May cause changes in blood sugar level as well as hide signs of low blood sugar
- Must notify physician of device prior to an MRI
- Headache
- Acne
- Breast tenderness
- Irregular periods or spotting

- Absence of periods (amenorrhea), especially after one year of use
- Mood changes
- Weight gain
- Ovarian cysts
- Cramping or pelvic pain[17,19,20,21,22]

Pros of ParaGard:

- Eliminates need to interrupt sex for contraception
- Long-term birth control, up to 10 years
- Can be removed at any time with a quick return to fertility
- Decreases risk of endometrial cancer and cervical cancer
- Can be used while breastfeeding
- No side effects that related hormonal birth control methods would have (copper only, no hormones)
- Can be used for emergency contraception if inserted within five days after unprotected sex

Cons of ParaGard:

- Does not protect against STIs or HIV
- Anemia
- Backache
- Bleeding between periods
- Cramps
- Inflammation of the vagina (vaginitis)
- Pain during sex
- Severe menstrual pain and heavy bleeding
- Vaginal discharge
- Small risk of IUD slipping partly or all the way out (most likely to occur during first year); check the tail regularly for placement
- Small risk of allergic reaction to the copper[18]

PERMANENT CONTRACEPTIVE METHODS

There are permanent sterilization methods available to both men and women (refer to list below). Women have one of two options; they may choose to have their tubes tied (i.e., tubal ligation) or to use the Essure system (i.e., tubal occlusion). Men may opt to have a vasectomy. With a tubal ligation, the fallopian tubes are cut and tied, or cauterized, to prevent the movement of the egg to the uterus for fertilization; it also prevents sperm from moving up to the fallopian tubes. A ligation does not affect a woman's menstrual cycle; she will still continue to have her monthly cycle. A tubal ligation can be reversed where the cur segments of the fallopian tubes are reconnected to allow eggs and sperm to travel back and forth to be able to join. Most physicians will not perform a tubal ligation unless the client is very sure she does not want to become pregnant as a reversal is very difficult; is not a guarantee, and not all physicians will attempt a ligation reversal.

Tubal occlusion, the Essure system, is a permanent birth control method for women that cannot be reversed. Essure is a procedure where a small flexible tube is inserted through the vagina, into the cervix, and up to the uterus with use of a small camera. Small metal and fiber coils are passed through the camera's scope into the fallopian tube that causes damage to the tissue, and creates scar tissue to form around the coils. With the coils in place, and the scar tissue built up around the coils, the fallopian tubes become blocked, therefore preventing eggs from dropping and sperm from going up. This method takes about three months to become effective to allow the scar tissue to completely form.

Vasectomy is the only available permanent birth control method for men. With this procedure, the vas deference (tubes that carry the sperm) are cut and sealed/tied, therefore preventing sperm from leaving the penis. This procedure is simple, low cost, and has a very minimal risk of problems. It is performed in the physician's office, many times by a urologist, under local anesthesia. This procedure can be reversed, but similar to tubal ligation, your physician will want to make sure you no longer want children, and see it as a form of permanent sterilization.

- Tubal ligation
  - Pros: Permanent birth control, decreased risk of ovarian cancer, possibility of reversal
  - Cons: Like most surgical procedures, damage to bowel, bladder or major blood vessels, adverse reaction to anesthesia, improper wound healing or infection, prolonged pelvic or abdominal pain, no protection against STIs or HIV[23,24]

- Tubal occlusion
  - Pros: Permanent birth control, highly effective, lack of significant long-term side effects, no incision or scarring of the skin, convenience (can be inserted at your health care provider's office)
  - Cons: Tubal blockage occurring on only one side, perforation of uterus or fallopian tubes from movement of the device, pelvic pain, infection, does not protect against STIs or HIV, increased risk of ectopic pregnancy[25]

- Vasectomy
  - Pros: It is nearly 100% effective in preventing pregnancy, completed as an outpatient surgery, low risk of complications or side effects, very low cost (sometimes just your copay)
  - Cons: Bleeding or a blood clot (hematoma) inside the scrotum, blood in the semen, bruising of your scrotum, infection of the incision site, mild pain or discomfort, swelling. Possible delayed complications include chronic pain which is rare, fluid buildup in the testicle causing a dull ache that worsens with ejaculation, inflammation caused by leaking sperm, abnormal cyst on epididymis, or fluid-filled sac around testicle[26]

MISCELLANEOUS CONTRACEPTIVE METHODS

The fertility awareness method (FAM) is a natural family planning birth control method that is used by many women. This method cannot be used unless the woman is disciplined and consistent on documenting a variety of items. This includes tracking when she has her cycle and her body temperature at varied points throughout each month, assessing her cervical mucus for consistency (it changes depending on whether a woman is ovulating or not), as well as watching for signs and symptoms she may experience pre, during, and post her menstrual cycle. The goal of this method is to know which days she is ovulating and to abstain from sex on those days to prevent pregnancy. There is a window of about 7 days during a woman's cycle that she can become pregnant, and this will vary per individual. There are also over the counter test kits women may use that will let them know if they are ovulating or not, however, this is not recommended as the only resource to use for determining ovulation. For FAM to be effective, both partners must be disciplined in doing all the proper checks and strictly using a back-up birth control, or abstaining from sex during the fertilization window. The effectiveness of FAM is low, and 25% of women will become pregnant using these methods. Some women use only cervical mucus, some use only basal body temperature, and some use both, which is called the symptom-thermal awareness method. A woman should check her body temperature every single day upon awakening and check her cervical mucus a couple times every day and to keep a log of the findings. These items help identify when a woman is ovulating.

The calendar or rhythm method is counting a woman's cycle on the calendar, and figuring out which days she will be ovulating based on when she had her last period and when she is expected to start her next. This is not an effective method, as every woman's cycle is different and each woman's cycle can change per month depending on stress, illness, etc. To use this in conjunction with FAM would increase effectiveness.

Another alternative method of birth control is the Withdrawal or pull-out method, also referred to as coitus interruptus. The withdrawal method occurs when a man removes his penis from the vagina prior to ejaculation. Approximately 35 million couples worldwide rely on withdrawal. With typical use, where partners do not always perform this method correctly, it is only 73% effective (27 out of 100 women will become pregnant). Assuming the man has complete control and knows exactly when to pull out, and does so consistently every time, this method is 96% effective (4 out of 100 women will become pregnant). Remember that this is complete trust in the male partner to be able to self-observe and assess and know when to remove prior to ejaculation.[27,28,28,30]

- Fertility Awareness Method
  - Basal body temperature
  - Cervical mucus
  - Symptom-thermal

  Pros: Inexpensive, no health risk and convenient, allows for development of respect, communication and responsibility between partners, helps a woman track and improve PMS symptoms

  Cons: High failure rate, difficulty in accurately predicting ovulation or fertile time, requires commitment from both partners, no protection against STIs or HIV

- Calendar/Rhythm method

  Pros: Free, no clinic visit necessary, no equipment or supplies, no side effects

  Cons: Not all women have regular cycles, stress and illness can affect a woman's cycle and throw off which days were supposed to be her ovulation days, does not protect against STIs or HIV

- Withdrawal "pull-out" method

  Pros: Free, no clinic visit necessary, no equipment or supplies, no side effects, increased sensation without a condom, can be used with other methods of contraception

  Cons: May be difficult for some men to know when they need to withdraw before the point of ejaculation, may cause increased anxiety for both partners around withdrawal time and therefore decrease enjoyment of sex, no protection against STIs or HIV, sperm may be present in the clear fluid that releases from the penis before ejaculation so pregnancy may still be possible

EMERGENCY CONTRACEPTIVE (EC) METHODS

Emergency contraception is available to couples as a backup method of birth control, for example if the condom breaks. The morning-after pill options (except Ella) can cost anywhere from $25 to $65 and can be obtained from health clinics or drug stores. The copper IUD must be prescribed and inserted by a physician and may cost anywhere from $0 to $900.

To prevent pregnancy after unprotected sex, a woman has two options; She may get the ParaGard IUD inserted within 120 hours, or 5 days after intercourse, which is the most effective emergency contraception, or she may choose to take a morning-after pill within 120 hours, or 5 days after intercourse. The copper in the IUD prevents pregnancy by making it difficult for sperm to swim to an egg (as previously discussed as a birth control method). This EC method is 99.9% effective, and an individual's weight and BMI does not effect the medication.

There are a couple of different options when it comes to the pill. Ella, a pill with ulipristal acetate, is the most effective morning-after pill, however, it requires a prescription from a physician. Other pill brands such as Plan B, Next Choice, My Way, etc., are available over-the-counter at pharmacies and provide a large dose of the hormone levonorgestrel. It is very important to keep in mind that these morning-after pills are not the same as an abortion pill; if you are already pregnant, the pill will not affect your pregnancy. These pills are preventative; they delay the release of an egg if taken up to 8 hours prior to ovulation. Ella is 85% effective and all other morning-after pill options are anywhere from 75–89% effective. Ella is the only morning-after pill that is not affected by a person's weight, as it is a prescribed medication—all other pills may have a decrease in effectiveness if an individual has a high BMI (e.g., more than 25).[31,32,33]

- ParaGard (Copper IUD)
  - Pros: Can be left in place up to 10 years as birth control coverage
  - Cons: Requires a visit to a health care provider and prescription to have an IUD inserted, possibly a high cost, possible side effects (see ParaGard previously in chapter), does not protect against STIs or HIV

- Ulipristal Acetate Pill
  - Ella
    - Pros: More effective than levonorgestrel pills, equally effective up to 120 hours following unprotected sex (just as effective on day 5 as day 1 after unprotected sex)
    - Cons: Only protection following a single unprotected event, does not work if ovulation already occurred, requires a prescription, possibly high cost, hormonal contraception cannot be started until 5 days after using this medication

- Progestin Pill (levonorgestrel)
  - Plan B, Contingency One, Next Choice, Option 2, My Way, etc.
    - Pros: Available without a prescription, can be purchased in advance to have "on hand," hormonal contraception can be started immediately afterwards
    - Cons: Only offers protection from a single unprotected event, effectiveness declines with delay in treatment (not as effective on day 5 as it would be on day 1 after unprotected sex), does not

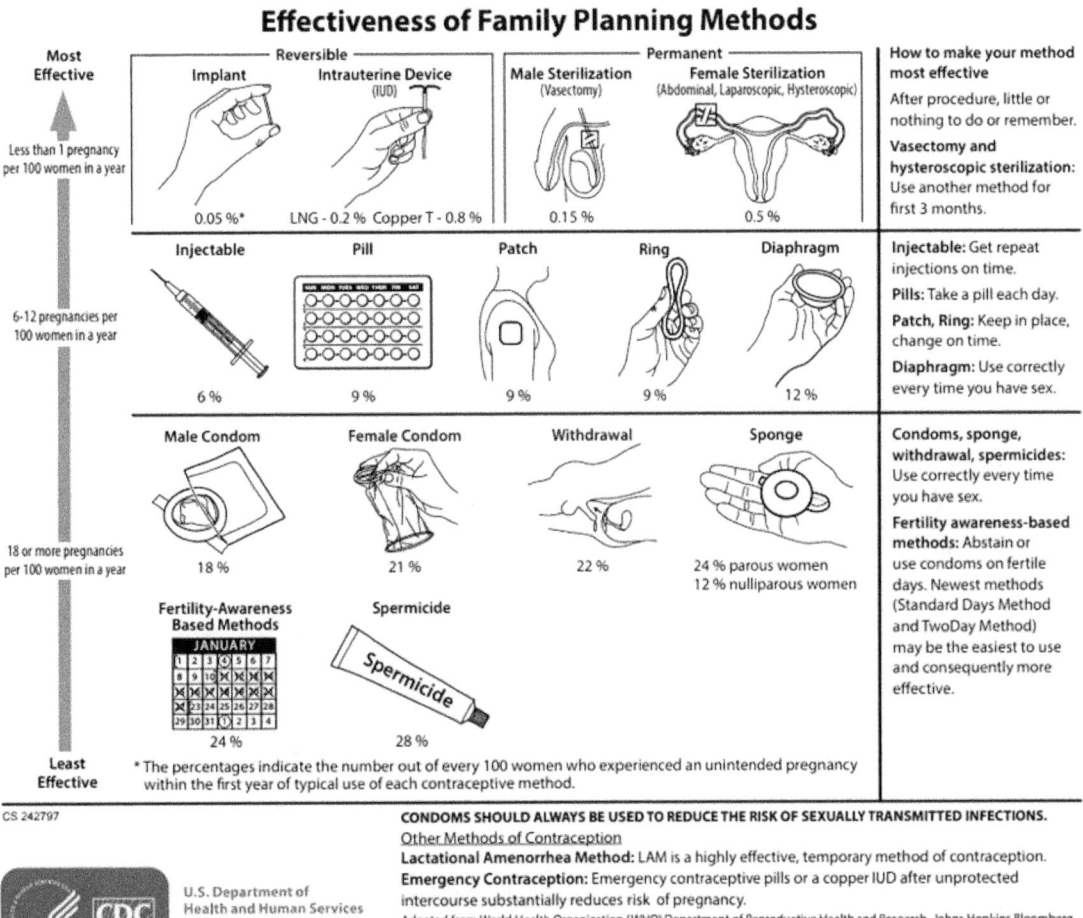

Figure 8.20: Methods of Family Planning[34].

Table 8.3: Contraceptive Method Effectiveness.

METHOD	USE EFFECTIVENESS (Actual Use)	THEORETICAL EFFECTIVENESS (Perfect Use)
EVRA PATCH	92%	99.7%
PILL–Combined –Progestin	92% 92%	99.7% 99.7%
NUVARING	92%	99.7%
IUD Copper T Levonorgenestrel (Mirena)	99.2% 99.9%	99.4% 99.9%
DIAPHRAGM & SPERMICIDE	84%	94%
SPERMICIDE & MALE CONDOMS**	no confirmed data	99%
FEMALE CONDOM ALONE	79%	95%
MALE CONDOM ALONE	85%	98%
SPERMICIDES***	71%	82%
TUBAL LIGATION	99.5%	99.5%
VASECTOMY	99.85%	99.9%
CERVICAL CAP Woman has had children Woman has not had children	68% 84%	74% 91%
DEPO-PROVERA	97%	99.95%
SPONGE Woman has had children Woman has not had children	68% 84%	80% 91%
FERTILITY AWARENESS METHOD	75%	95–97%
WITHDRAWAL	73%	96%
NO METHOD (CHANCE)	15%	15%

*Adapted from Contraceptive Technology, 19th Revised Edition, Hatcher, et al (New York: 2007).[35]
**Separate spermicide in addition to condoms.
***Foams, creams, gels, vaginal suppositories, and vaginal film.

work if ovulation already occurred, does not protect against STIs or HIV, may be less effective if person has an increased BMI

ABSTINENCE

Abstinence is a personal choice that prevents pregnancy and sexually transmitted infections. This method of birth control is safe, easy, convenient and 100% effective. But, how realistic is this method for the majority of teenagers and adults? Many may assume someone who practices abstinence is not sexually active at all, which isn't the case. Some identify as being abstinent, but may partake in other sexual activity such as oral sex; this is described as **outercourse**. There are many benefits to being abstinent, besides the ones already mentioned, it allows for individuals to wait to find the right partner, focus on school, careers or extracurricular activities, encourages couples to build relationships in other ways, etc. Some disadvantages can be if you end up in the heat of the moment and choose to have sex, then you and your partner may not have protection handy. We are all sexual in nature, and those who practice abstinence will still have a sex drive, and may have to find other ways to redirect their sexual energy. To be abstinent you do not have to be a virgin, but it should be an agreement in a relationship, be with someone you trust, and continue to have barrier or emergency contraception handy just in case.

Abstinence is a choice people must make on their own, whether it is religious-based, or just personal. It should be a thought process as to why they want to be abstinent, rather than deciding impulsively. Some questions to consider include being clear about why you want to be abstinent, being aware of situations that could make being abstinent difficult, being aware that alcohol and other drugs can alter your judgment in specific situations, finding people in your life who you can discuss your decision with, and who will support you, and most importantly, do you have information about methods of birth control and know where and how to access them if needed.

In many schools we teach abstinence only, however, there have been many studies disproving the benefit of these programs. For example, a study showed that abstinence-only programs have not produced sufficient evidence to even justify their widespread adoption; in most cases we do not implement programs until we have strong evidence that demonstrates efficacy. There is also not any strong evidence that abstinence-only programs actually delay the initiation of sex, hastens the return to abstinence, or reduces the number of sexual partners.[36] Bearman and Bruckner (2001) conducted a study on virginity pledges and found that pledges did in fact delay the onset of sexual intercourse, but only for an average of 18 months. They also discovered that these virginity pledges can do more harm than good, as those who pledged were one-third less likely to use contraception.[37] There are many more studies which can be found on the Sexuality Information and Education Council of the United States website in regards

Table 8.4: U.S. Teenage Pregnancy and Birth Rates are High Compared to Other Developed Countries.

Country	U.S.	France	Germany	Netherlands	Canada	U.K.
Pregnancy Rate (2002–2005)	72.2	25.7	18.8	11.8	29.2	41.3
Birth Rate (2006)	41.9	7.8	10.1	3.8	13.3	26.7

Rates are listed as numbers per 1000 girls 15–19 years old[39]

to abstinence-only education: *www.siecus.org*. Refer to the table below for pregnancy rates in multiple countries, including the United States, as of 2011, and you will note that we still have the highest occurring teen birth rate.[38,39, 40,41]

As of 2011, the U.S. ranked first out of developed nations in rates of teen pregnancy and STDs.[39]

REFERENCES

1. World Health Organization. "Sexual and Reproductive Health." http://www.who.int/reproductivehealth/topics/sexual_health/sh_definitions/en/.
2. American Sexual Health Association. "Understanding Sexual Health." http://www.ashasexualhealth.org/sexual-health/.
3. Merriam-Webster Dictionary. "Sexual Health." http://www.merriam-webster.com/.
4. American Sexual Health Association. "STDs/STIs." http://www.ashasexualhealth.org/stdsstis/.
5. O'Brien, S. "This App Makes Sure You Never Walk Home Alone." *CNN Money*. Retrieved from http://money.cnn.com/2015/09/18/technology/companion-safety-app/
6. Hamann, B. *Disease: Identification, Prevention & Control*. New York: McGraw Hill, 2001.
7. Rady's Children Hospital "Pelvic Inflammatory Disease (PID)." http://www.rchsd.org/health-articles/pelvic-inflammatory-disease-pid/.

8. CDC. "Sexually Transmitted Disease Surveillance." https://www.cdc.gov/std/stats14/surv-2014-print.pdf.

9. CDC. "Sexually Transmitted Diseases (STDs)." http://www.cdc.gov/std/default.htm.

10. Aids.gov. "Opportunistic Infections." https://www.aids.gov/hiv-aids-basics/staying-healthy-with-hiv-aids/potential-related-health-problems/opportunistic-infections/.

11. Aids.gov. "Stages of HIV Infection." https://www.aids.gov/hiv-aids-basics/just-diagnosed-with-hiv-aids/hiv-in-your-body/stages-of-hiv/.

12. Aids.gov. "CD4 Count." https://www.aids.gov/hiv-aids-basics/just-diagnosed-with-hiv-aids/understand-your-test-results/cd4-count/.

13. American College Health Association. "ACHA Pap Test and STI Survey." Retrieved from http://www.acha.org/ACHA/Resources/Pap_STI_Survey.aspx.

14. Advocates for Youth. "School Condom Availability." http://www.advocatesforyouth.org/publications/449-school-condom-availability.

15. Indiana University of Pennsylvania. "Safer Sex." http://www.iup.edu/healthawareness/campaigns/safer-sex/.

16. Options for Sexual Health. "Spermicides." https://www.optionsforsexualhealth.org/birth-control-pregnancy/birth-control-options/barrier-methods/spermicides.

17. Mayo Clinic. "Levonorgestrel (Intrauterine Route)." http://www.mayoclinic.org/drugs-supplements/levonorgestrel-intrauterine-route/precautions/drg-20073437.

18. Mayo Clinic. "ParaGard (copper IUD)." http://www.mayoclinic.org/tests-procedures/paragard/basics/how-you-prepare/prc-20013048.

19. Paragard. "What is Paragard?" http://paragard.com/What-is-Paragard.aspx?&utm_source=google&utm_medium=cpc&utm_term=iuds&utm_campaign=IUD&utm_content=sxQ66kQhn_pcrid_107545030745_pdv_c&gclid=CIHOo7zLj84CFUddMgodLL0PXQ&gclsrc=ds.

20. Skyla. "What is Skyla?" http://www.skyla-us.com/what-is-skyla.php.

21. Liletta. "About Liletta." https://www.liletta.com/?cid=sem_goo_43700009973935214.

22. Mayo Clinic. "Mirena (hormonal IUD)." http://www.mayoclinic.org/tests-procedures/mirena/basics/risks/prc-20012867.

23. Mayo Clinic. "Tubal Ligation." http://www.mayoclinic.org/tests-procedures/tubal-ligation/basics/definition/prc-20020231.

24. Mayo Clinic. "Tubal Ligation Reversal." http://www.mayoclinic.org/tests-procedures/tubal-ligation-reversal/basics/definition/prc-20020246.

25. Mayo Clinic. "Essure." http://www.mayoclinic.org/tests-procedures/essure/basics/risks/prc-20014310.

26. Mayo Clinic. "Vasectomy." http://www.mayoclinic.org/tests-procedures/vasectomy/home/ovc-20177726.

27. Options for Sexual Health. "Fertility Awareness Method (FAM)." https://www.optionsforsexualhealth.org/birth-control-pregnancy/birth-control-options/natural-methods/fam.

28. Planned Parenthood. "Fertility Awareness-Based Methods (FAMs)." https://www.plannedparenthood.org/learn/birth-control/fertility-awareness.

29. Fertility Aware "What is Fertility Awareness?" http://www.fertaware.com/faqs/what-is-fertility-awareness/.

30. Planned Parenthood. "Withdrawal (Pull Out Method)." https://www.plannedparenthood.org/learn/birth-control/withdrawal-pull-out-method.

31. Planned Parenthood. "Morning-After Pill (Emergency Contraception)" https://www.plannedparenthood.org/learn/morning-after-pill-emergency-contraception.

32. Options for Sexual Health. "What is Emergency Contraception?" https://www.optionsforsexualhealth.org/sites/optionsforsexualhealth.org/files/ec_fact_sheet_june_9_2016.pdf.

33. Options for Sexual Health. "Emergency Contraception (EC)." https://www.optionsforsexualhealth.org/birth-control-pregnancy/emergency-contraception-ecp.

34. CDC "How Effective are Birth Control Methods? http://www.cdc.gov/reproductivehealth/unintendedpregnancy/contraception.htm.

35. Options for Sexual Health. "RELATIVE EFFECTIVENESS OF BIRTH CONTROL METHODS*." https://www.optionsforsexualhealth.org/birth-control-pregnancy/birth-control-options/effectiveness.

36. Kirby, D. "Emerging Answers: Research Findings on Programs to Reduce Teen Pregnancy and Sexually Transmitted Diseases, Washington, DC: The National Campaign to Prevent Teen and Unplanned Pregnancy." http://www.thenationalcampaign.org/EA2007/EA2007_full.pdf.

37. Bearman, P & Brückner, H. "Promising the Future: Virginity Pledges and the Transition to First Intercourse." *American Journal of Sociology* 106, no. 4 (2001): 859–912.

38. Siecus.org. "Abstinence-Only-Until-Marriage Programs." http://www.siecus.org/index.cfm?fuseaction=Page.ViewPage&PageID=1195.

39. National Institute of Health. "Abstinence-Only Education and Teen Pregnancy Rates: Why We Need Comprehensive Sex Education in the U.S." http://www.ncbi.nlm.nih.gov/pmc/articles/PMC3194801/.

40. Options for Sexual Health. "What is Abstinence?" https://www.optionsforsexualhealth.org/birth-control-pregnancy/birth-control-options/natural-methods/abstinence.

41. Planned Parenthood. "Abstinence." https://www.plannedparenthood.org/learn/birth-control/abstinence

42. Lambda Legal "Answers to Some Common Questions about Equal Access to Public Restrooms." http://www.lambdalegal.org/know-your-rights/transgender/restroom-faq#Q8.

43. Glow-Ovulation Calculator. "An App for Fertility & Beyond." https://glowing.com/glow.

44. Merriam-Webster. http://www.merriam-webster.com/.

FIGURE CREDITS

Fig. 8.6: Ceners for Disease Control and Prevention, Chlamydia Curriculum, https://www2a.cdc.gov/stdtraining/Ready-To-Use/Manuals/Chlamydia/Chlamydia-Slides-2015.pdf. Copyright in the Public Domain.

Fig. 8.7: Bober275, https://commons.wikimedia.org/wiki/File:GenitalGerpes.gif. Copyright in the Public Domain.

Fig. 8.8: WarXboT, https://commons.wikimedia.org/wiki/File:Herpes_labialis_-_opryszczka_wargowa.jpg. Copyright in the Public Domain.

Fig. 8.9: Copyright © BruceBlaus (CC BY-SA 3.0) at https://commons.wikimedia.org/wiki/File:Blausen_0719_PelvicInflammatoryDisease.png.

Fig. 8.10: Ceners for Disease Control and Prevention, "[image]: Early Syphilis Chancre," Chlamydia Curriculum, https://www2a.cdc.gov/stdtraining/Ready-To-Use/Manuals/Chlamydia/Chlamydia-Slides-2015.pdf, ~1. Copyright in the Public Domain.

Fig. 8.11: Ceners for Disease Control and Prevention, "[image]: Moderate Syphilis Chancre," Chlamydia Curriculum, https://www2a.cdc.gov/stdtraining/Ready-To-Use/Manuals/Chlamydia/Chlamydia-Slides-2015.pdf, ~1. Copyright in the Public Domain.

Fig. 8.12: Ceners for Disease Control and Prevention, "[image]: Late Syphilis Chancre," Chlamydia Curriculum, https://www2a.cdc.gov/stdtraining/Ready-To-Use/Manuals/Chlamydia/Chlamydia-Slides-2015.pdf, ~1. Copyright in the Public Domain.

Fig. 8.13: Ceners for Disease Control and Prevention, "[image]: HIV Law," https://www.cdc.gov/hiv/policies/law/states/index.html, ~1. Copyright in the Public Domain.

Fig. 8.14: Copyright © Depositphotos/mariakarabella.

Fig. 8.15: Copyright © Depositphotos/nito103.

Fig. 8.16: Copyright © inga (CC BY-SA 2.0) at https://commons.wikimedia.org/wiki/File:Latex_Dental_Dam_near.jpg.

Fig. 8.17: Copyright © Depositphotos/wacpan.

Fig. 8.18: Copyright © Depositphotos/vadim-design.

Fig. 8.19: Copyright © Depositphotos/megija.

Fig. 8.20: Centers for Disease Control and Prevention, Adapted from World Health Organization (WHO) Department of Reproductive Health and Research. Copyright in the Public Domain.

9 CHRONIC WELLNESS

BY KACEY DIGIACINTO

WHAT IS A CHRONIC DISEASE?

A **chronic disease** is a health condition or disease that lasts for a long time. Usually, a condition or disease is considered chronic when symptoms and their treatments last for more than a year. According to the Centers for Disease Control and Prevention (CDC), chronic diseases are responsible for 7 out of 10 deaths every year and can account for 86% of the United States' health care costs. The most prevalent chronic diseases are: heart disease, stroke, type 2 diabetes, obesity, and arthritis. These diseases are preventable for a large part of the population. Nearly 48% of all deaths are attributed to either cancer or heart disease in the United States. Overweight and obesity are exhibited by 66.3% of adults in the United States. So, learning how to minimize your risk of developing a chronic disease is really important.[1,2,16]

TYPES AND CONSIDERATIONS

There are several categories of causes of chronic disease, however, they have similar risk factors: underlying socioeconomic, cultural, political, and environmental determinants included globalization, urbanization, and population ageing. Lifestyle choice risk factors include unhealthy diet (e.g., low in fruits and vegetables and/or high in sodium and saturated fats), physical inactivity, and tobacco use. Non-modifiable risk factors include age and heredity. Finally, intermediate risk factors include: raised blood pressure, raised blood glucose, abnormal blood lipids, and overweight/obesity.[3]

CARDIOVASCULAR DISEASE

According to the World Health Organization, cardiovascular disease is the number one cause of death in the world. There are many forms of heart disease such as: coronary heart disease, hypertension, atherosclerosis, stroke, and rheumatic heart disease. In Western countries, cardiovascular disease accounts for 30% of deaths for men and 25% of deaths for women, and is the primary killer of African-American and white men and women[4].

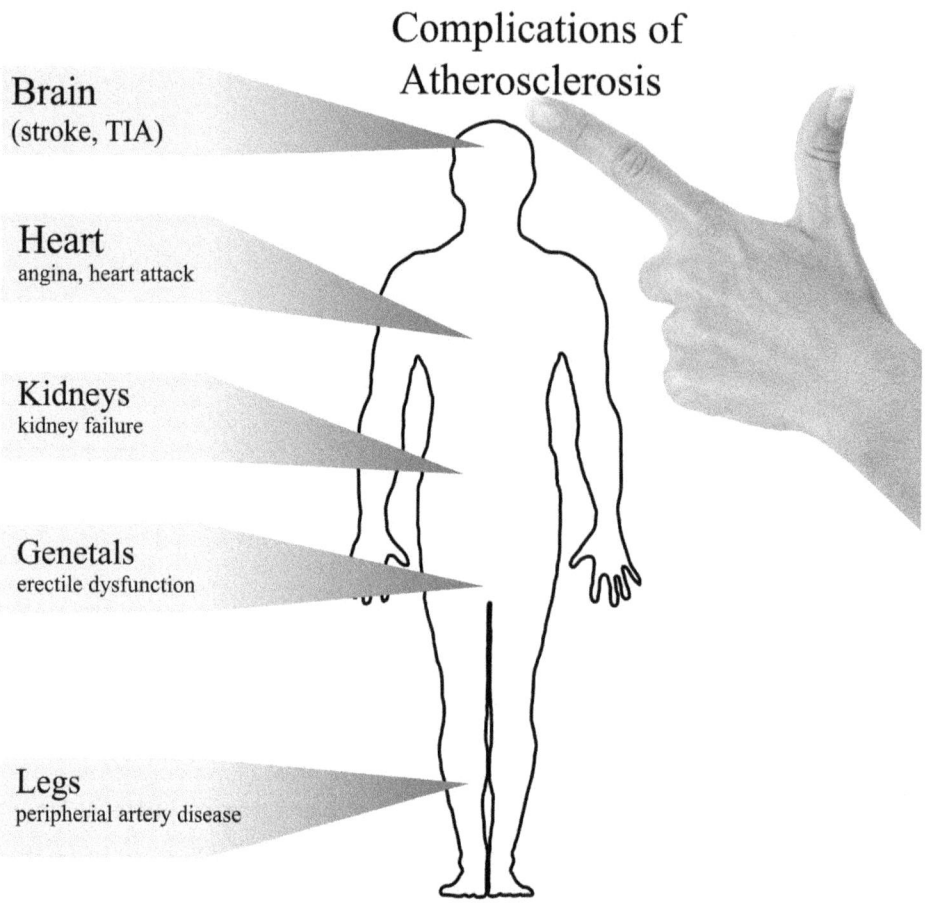

Complications of Atherosclerosis

Brain
(stroke, TIA)

Heart
angina, heart attack

Kidneys
kidney failure

Genetals
erectile dysfunction

Legs
peripherial artery disease

Figure 9.1: CVD.

Atherosclerosis, a buildup of fatty plaques in the lining of arteries, is one of the main causes of cardiovascular disease in the United States. This build up prevents blood from flowing properly through the arteries, to the rest of the body. A heart attack can occur when the coronary arteries (in the heart) can't supply oxygen and nutrients to the heart due to a build-up of plaques in the arteries. Quitting smoking, reducing fat intake, managing one's weight and blood cholesterol levels, reducing stress, and participating in regular physical activity are known ways to improve the overall health of the cardiovascular system, and help protect it from chronic disease. To prevent atherosclerosis, it is important to follow the nutritional guidelines set by the USDA, pay extra attention to limiting the intake of saturated fat, minimize intake of drinks and foods that contain excess sugar, lower sodium intake, and consume alcohol in moderation.

Hypertension is asymptomatic in most individuals; this means most people show no symptoms of the disease, until it is often too late to seek treatment. Hypertension can cause a lot of damage to the heart, kidneys, and nervous system without the individual knowing that something is wrong. To protect against hypertension, it is important to maintain a diet that is low in sodium.

Cerebrovascular Disease, which can result in stroke, is at the top of the list for leading causes of death in all developed countries, not just the United States. Stroke is a sudden impairment of the body that results in the disruption of blood flow to the brain. While stroke usually occurs in middle age to old age, individuals can take steps while they are young, to lead a healthy lifestyle, which can reduce

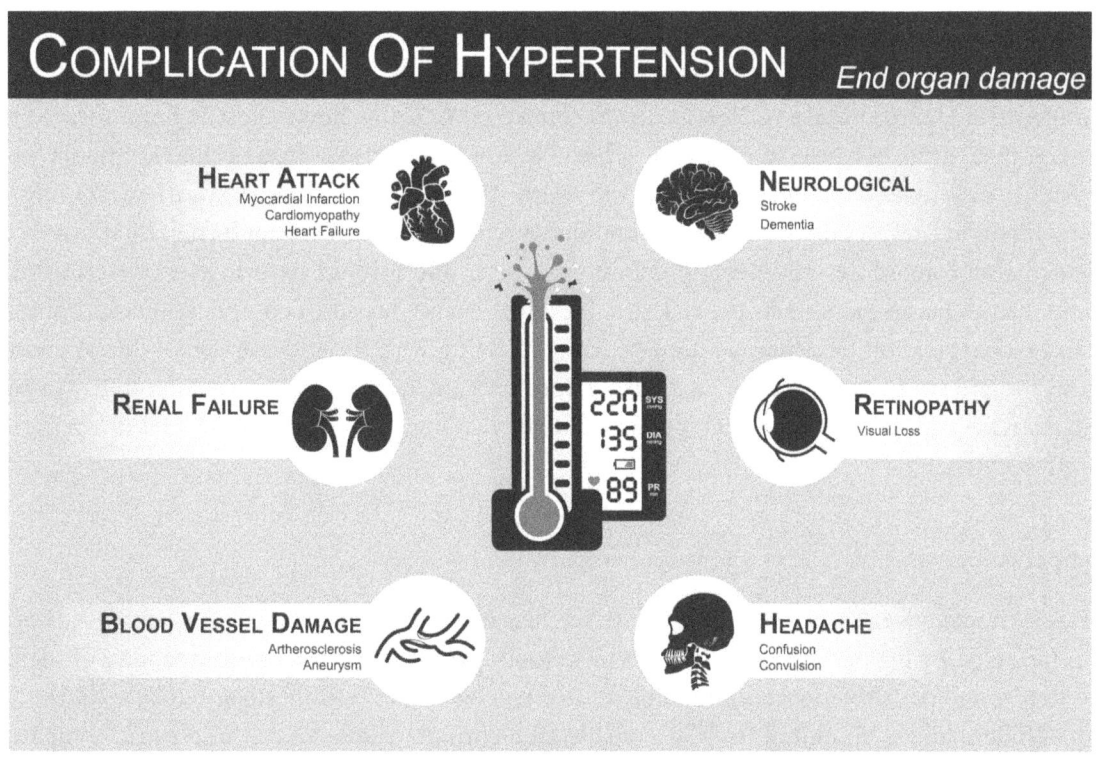

COMPLICATION OF HYPERTENSION
End organ damage

HEART ATTACK
Myocardial Infarction
Cardiomyopathy
Heart Failure

NEUROLOGICAL
Stroke
Dementia

RENAL FAILURE

220 SYS
135 DIA
89 PR

RETINOPATHY
Visual Loss

BLOOD VESSEL DAMAGE
Artherosclerosis
Aneurysm

HEADACHE
Confusion
Convulsion

Figure 9.2: Damage from High Blood Pressure, Hypertension.

the risk for developing a stroke later on in life. Even if an individual survives a stroke his or her quality of life is often diminished substantially. That individual often needs a lot of physical and/or occupational therapy, and usually does not return to full his pre-stroke condition. Men are at a higher risk for having a stroke than women, and African-Americans are at a higher risk of developing a stroke than any other racial group.

Congestive Heart Failure (CHF) is when the muscle of the heart does not pump as efficiently as it should. This typically occurs when issues like high blood pressure, or hardening of the arteries due to plaque buildup, begin to weaken the heart, keeping it from being able to pump well. This can become severe and require a physician if there is chest pain, fainting or severe weakness, rapid or irregular heartbeat associated with shortness of breath, and/or sudden, severe shortness of breath. However, basic lifestyle changes, including increased

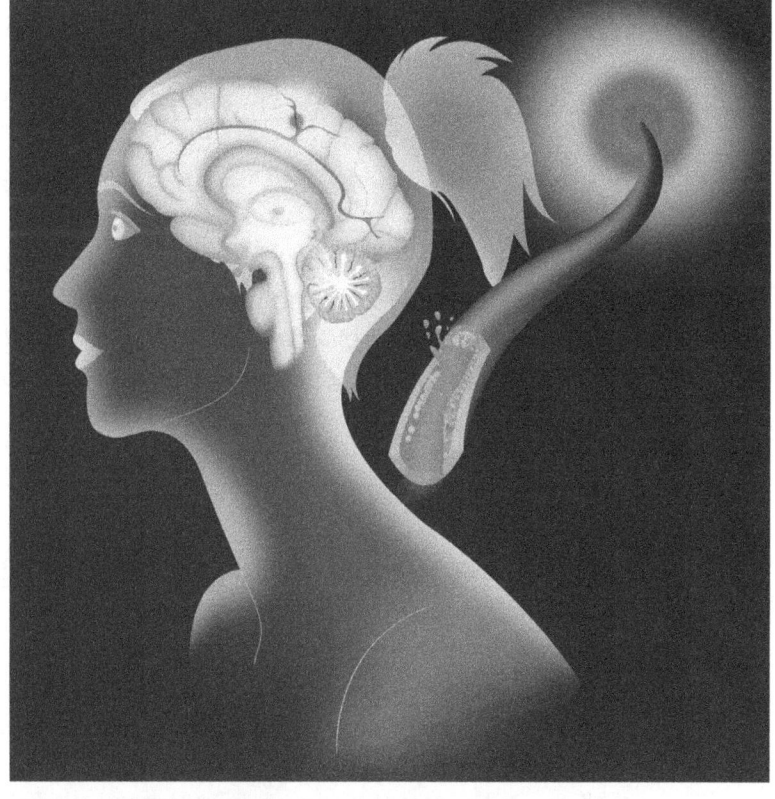

Figure 9.3: When a stroke occurs.

exercising, reducing salt in your diet, managing stress, and losing weight can greatly reduce the risk of developing CHF.[5]

Congenitial Heart Disease (CHD) is also a concen chronically, however, it is not a disease that is developed over time, but instead a person is born with it. This affects around 40,000 infants who are born with it. Examples of CHD are holes in the heart, defects in the valves, or even overlapping blood vessels which can cause a mix of oxygenated and deoxygenated blood. This can be hereditary, and caused by abnormal chromosomes and genetic issues. Also drug and alcohol use, or even infections during pregancy can cause an increase in the risk of CHD. This is very broad in complications and physicians need to be consulted on what can be done to assist in living with these conditions, which can involve medications and surgeries. There are large discussions on how this may alter a person's ability to participate in exercise and sports, since it can pose a risk, but also may allow a person's heart to strengthen to better protect itself.[6,7]

DIABETES

Diabetes is characterized by raised blood glucose (i.e., sugar) levels. This results from a lack of the hormone insulin (secreted by the pancreas), which controls blood glucose levels, and/or an inability of the body's tissues to respond properly to insulin. When cells stop responding to insulin, sugar builds up in the bloodstream. While diabetes, in and of itself, is considered a chronic disease, it can also cause complications including heart disease, blindness, kidney failure, and lower-extremity amputations.

FAQs CHECK!

Why are some diabetics missing limbs?

Individuals with diabetes can also develop **neuropathy**. This is damage to the peripheral nerves, located in the arms, legs, hands and feet. It can often cause weakness, numbness, and pain. It can also affect other areas of the body, including the digestive system, urinary tract, blood vessels, and heart. The problem is that the symptoms, like numbness, occur due to restricted blood flow. As this continues to occur, the lack of blood flow causes tissue to die. This is **tissue necrosis**, where the area turns black, and since this cannot be healed, surgical amputation is usually required.[24]

Type 1 diabetes (i.e., juvenile diabetes) most often presents at a young age, but can develop in adults. If a person develops type 1 diabetes her body does not produce insulin, or if it does produce insulin, the body's immune systems attacks and destroys the cells that make insulin. The treatment options for type 1 diabetes include: taking shots or injections of insulin, sometimes taking medicines by mouth, eating a healthy diet, participating in regular physical activity, controlling blood pressure levels, and controlling cholesterol levels.

Type 2 diabetes (i.e., non-insulin-dependent diabetes mellitus) develops when a body's cells stop responding to insulin. Type 2 diabetes accounts for 90 to 95% of all diagnosed cases of diabetes. Type 2 diabetes used to be known as adult-onset diabetes, however, more and more children are developing this chronic disease. Older age, obesity, family history of diabetes, prior history of gestational diabetes, impaired glucose tolerance, physical inactivity, and race and ethnicity are all risk factors for type 2 diabetes. African Americans, Hispanic and Latino Americans, American Indians, and some Asian Americans and Pacific Islanders are at a higher risk for type 2 diabetes than other ethnicities. Individuals with Diabetes can often benefit from a low-glycemic diet that contains foods with a low glycemic index, so foods are digested slower and cause a smaller glucose increase. This ensures a steady level of glucose in the bloodstream, instead of levels that spike and dip. Treatment for type 2 diabetes includes: using diabetes medicines, eating a healthy diet, participating in daily physical activity, controlling your blood pressure, and controlling your cholesterol levels.[17]

What are the signs and symptoms of diabetes?

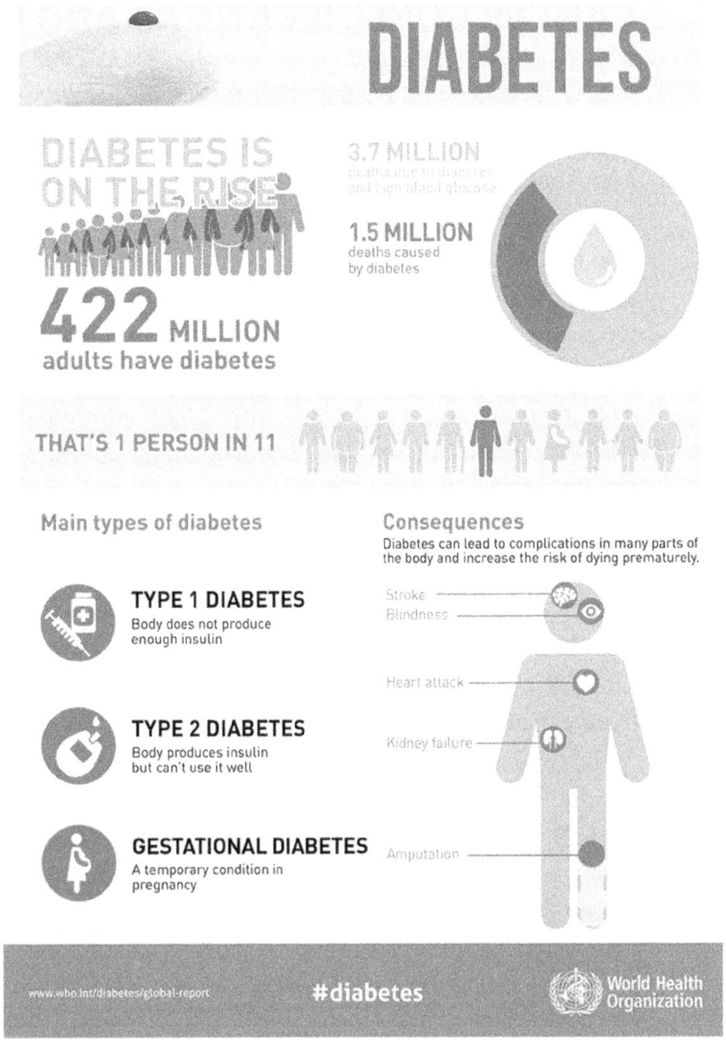

- Extreme thirst
- Frequent urination
- Feeling very hungry
- Feeling extremely tired
- Losing weight without trying
- Sores that won't heal or heal slowly
- Dry, itchy skin
- Having the feeling of pins and needles in your feet
- Loosing feeling in your feet
- Blurry eyesight.

Figure 9.4: Diabetes Inforgraph.

Gestational diabetes can develop in a woman who is pregnant, due to the hormones produced during pregnancy, which can lead to insulin resistance. According to the National Institute of Health, all women have insulin resistance late in their pregnancies. Diabetes develops when the pancreas can't produce enough insulin during pregnancy. Women who are overweight or obese are at a higher risk for developing gestational diabetes. Also, gaining a significant amount of weight during pregnancy increases the likelihood of developing gestational diabetes. Fortunately, gestational diabetes often goes away after the baby is delivered. As stated earlier, a woman who develops gestational diabetes is more likely to develop type 2 diabetes. Unfortunately, babies who are born to mothers who had gestational diabetes are more likely to develop obesity and type 2 diabetes.

CANCER CONSIDERATIONS AND PREVENTIONS

Cancer is second on the list of leading causes of death in the United States. Cancer is a collection of over 100-related diseases that share the main characteristic of rapid and uncontrolled cell growth. While there is hope that if a tumor or other cancers are found, it is **benign**, meaning not continuously growing. However, cancer can be found to be **malignant,** meaning infectious and spreading. This can lead to the cancer going into **metastasis**, where there are secondary sites of cancer that are due to, but located away from the primary site where the original cancer was found. The American Cancer Society reports that in 2016, 8 more cancer types have been linked to being overweight or obese. They are: stomach, liver, gallbladder, pancreatic, ovarian, thyroid, multiple myeloma (i.e. malignant plasma cells), and meningioma (i.e., a tumor of the lining over the brain and spinal cord). These eight additional types join the already existing cancers: esophagus, colon and rectum, breast (i.e., in postmenopausal women), kidney, and endometrium. Being overweight or obese may also raise the risk of breast cancer, diffuse large B-cell lymphoma, and prostate cancer in men.

Anyone is at risk for developing cancer, however, there are certain groups who are at a higher risk. According to the CDC, in 2011, those most at risk for developing cancer were (in order): African-Americans, whites, Hispanics, American Indians/Alaska Natives, and lastly, Asian/Pacific Islanders. Men have a 1 in 2 (42.05%) risk of developing cancer, but only a 1 in 4 (22.62) risk of dying from cancer (Table 9.1). Females have a 1 in 3 (37.58%) risk of developing cancer, and a 1 in 5 (19.13%) risk of dying from cancer (Table 9.2).

Table 9.1: Risk of Developing and Dying from Cancer among Males.

	Risk of developing		Risk of dying from	
	%	1 in	%	1 in
All invasive sites	**42.05**	**2**	**22.62**	**4**
Bladder (includes in situ)	3.84	26	0.92	109
Brain and nervous system	0.69	145	0.51	196
Breast	0.13	769	0.03	3,333
Colon and rectum	4.69	21	1.99	50
Esophagus	0.80	125	0.79	127
Hodgkin disease	0.24	417	0.04	2,500
Kidney and renal pelvis	2.03	49	0.62	161
Larynx (voice box)	0.59	169	0.20	500
Leukemia	1.75	57	1.03	97
Liver and bile duct	1.31	76	0.94	106
Lung and bronchus	7.19	14	6.33	16
Melanoma of the skin	2.62	38	0.43	233
Multiple myeloma	0.85	118	0.47	213

(Continued)

	Risk of developing		Risk of dying from	
	%	1 in	%	1 in
Non-Hodgkin lymphoma	2.37	42	0.86	116
Oral cavity and pharynx	1.55	65	0.40	250
Pancreas	1.54	65	1.37	73
Prostate	13.97	7	2.58	39
Stomach	1.07	93	0.48	208
Testicles	0.38	263	0.02	5,000
Thyroid	0.59	169	0.06	1,667

Table 9.2: Risk of Developing and Dying from Cancer among Females.

	Risk of developing		Risk of dying from	
	%	1 in	%	1 in
All invasive sites	37.58	3	19.13	5
Bladder	1.14	88	0.34	294
Brain and nervous system	0.54	185	0.40	250
Breast	12.32	8	2.69	37
Cervix	0.64	156	0.23	435
Colon and rectum	4.35	23	1.81	55
Esophagus	0.22	455	0.21	476
Hodgkin disease	0.20	500	0.03	3,333
Kidney and renal pelvis	1.20	83	0.34	294
Larynx (the voice box)	0.13	769	0.05	2,000
Leukemia	1.22	82	0.72	139
Liver and bile duct	0.54	185	0.49	204
Lung and bronchus	6.04	17	4.89	20
Melanoma of the skin	1.63	61	0.21	476
Multiple myeloma	0.64	156	0.39	256
Non-Hodgkin lymphoma	1.89	53	0.68	147
Oral cavity and pharynx	0.67	149	0.18	556
Ovary	1.31	76	0.97	103
Pancreas	1.50	67	1.34	75
Stomach	0.66	152	0.32	313
Thyroid	1.72	58	0.07	1,429
Uterine corpus	2.78	36	0.58	172[8]

There are lots of ways to lower one's risk of developing cancer.

- Avoid tobacco
- Limit alcohol intake
- Limit exposure to ultraviolet rays (including tanning beds)
- Eat healthy (consume lots of fruits and vegetables and limit red meat consumption)
- Maintain a healthy weight
- Participate in regular physical activity
- See a physician regularly

Seeing a physician regularly for screenings will help identify any problems early. For example, the earlier a lesion can be detected, the sooner it can be treated before cervical or colorectal cancer fully develops. There are routine screenings that can be performed by your doctor to detect cancers such as cervical, colorectal, and breast cancers. Because of healthy living, early cancer detection, and advances in treatment, more and more individuals diagnosed with cancer are surviving.

FAQs CHECK!

Vaccines and Cancer?

There are vaccines that can help reduce the risk of developing certain types of cancer. The occurrence of cervical, vaginal, vulvar, and other cancers can be severely reduced by taking the vaccine for the Human Papillomavirus (HPV). And the Hepatitis B vaccine can help reduce the risk of developing liver cancer.

MELANOMA

Melanoma is also known as skin cancer, and there are three types of skin cells that can be affected, and the first type is **melanocytes**. Most melanoma cells continue to make melanin, the pigment responsible for tanning the skin in the sunlight. This tends to make melanoma tumors brown or black. Occasionally though, some melanomas do not make melanin and can appear pink, tan, or even white. While melanomas may develop anywhere on the body's skin, they are more likely to start on the trunk area (chest, stomach, and back) in men, and on the breast and legs in women. The neck and face are also not uncommon. While skin with darker pigment may lower the chance of melanoma development in the most common areas of the body, this form of cancer occurs enough that it is still a major concern regardless of skin color.

The second type, **squamous cells**, are flat cells located in the outer part of the epidermis, which we shed often, as our body continuous to form new ones. The third type of skin cells, **basal cells,** are located in the lower part of the epidermis, known as the basal cell layer. In this layer, the cells consistently divide to form new cells to replace the squamous cells that wear off the skin's surface. As these cells move up in the epidermis, eventually they get flatter and flatter, becoming squamous cells. While melanoma cancer is much less common than cancer in the basal and squamous cells, melanoma is considered more dangerous due to it being likely to spread to other parts of the body if not caught early. The best recommendation is routine screenings performed by your doctor, and to note any changes in the skin coloration, or alteration of a mole's color or size.[9,]

When tracking the potential changes in a mole on the skin, use the following technique to look for these specific alterations that could occur:

A—*Asymmetrical Shape*, melanoma lesions are often irregular, or not symmetrical, in shape. Benign moles are usually symmetrical.

B—*Border*, typically, non-cancerous moles have smooth, even borders. Melanoma lesions usually have irregular borders that are difficult to define.

C—*Color*, the presence of more than one color (blue, black, brown, tan, etc.) or the uneven distribution of color can sometimes be a warning sign of melanoma. Benign moles are usually a single shade of brown or tan.

D—*Diameter*, melanoma lesions are often greater than 6 millimeters in diameter (approximately the size of a pencil eraser).

E—*Evolution*, the evolution of your mole(s) is the most important factor when worrying about melanoma. This means knowing what is normal for you.[25]

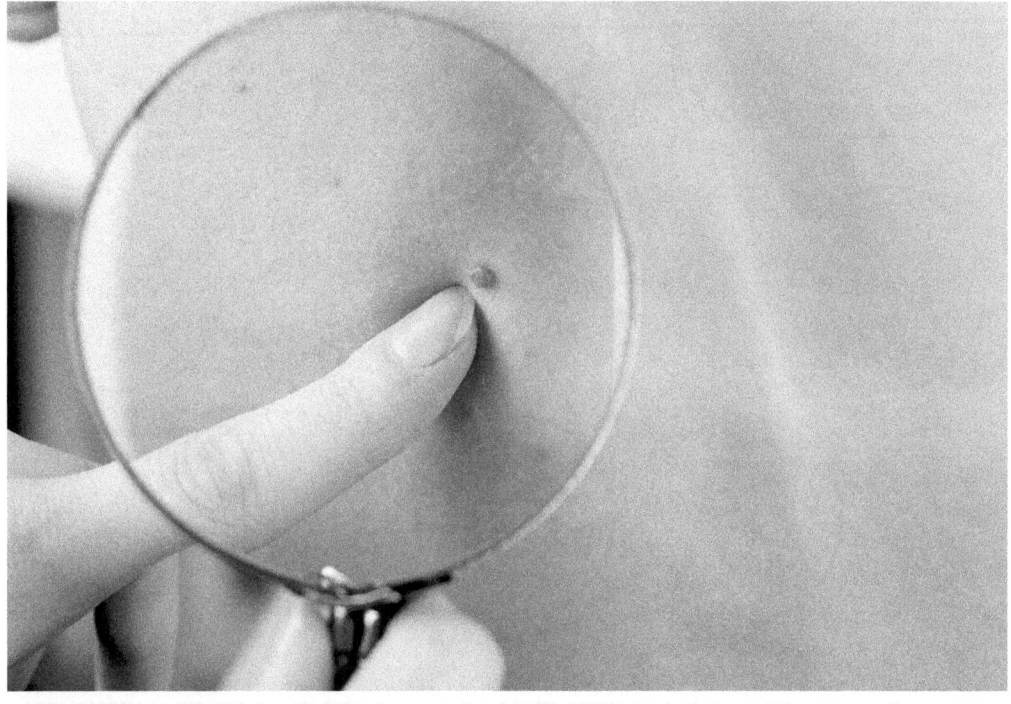

Figure 9.5: Watch for changes in moles.

BREAST CANCER

Over the past several years, there has been a massive increase in breast cancer awareness, and understandably so. It may affect one out of every eight women inside their lifetimes. Each year there are about 230,000 new cases in women, at least that we know about. It isn't just a woman's problem though, with 2,300 new cases a year reported for breast cancer in men. For women, it is the second most fatal cancer after melanoma. However, the five year survival rate is around 90% if immediately acted upon.

Some common issues that lead to an increased risk are:
- Age
- Genetics
- Personal choices (alcohol consumption, exercise, etc.)
- Using hormonal therapy

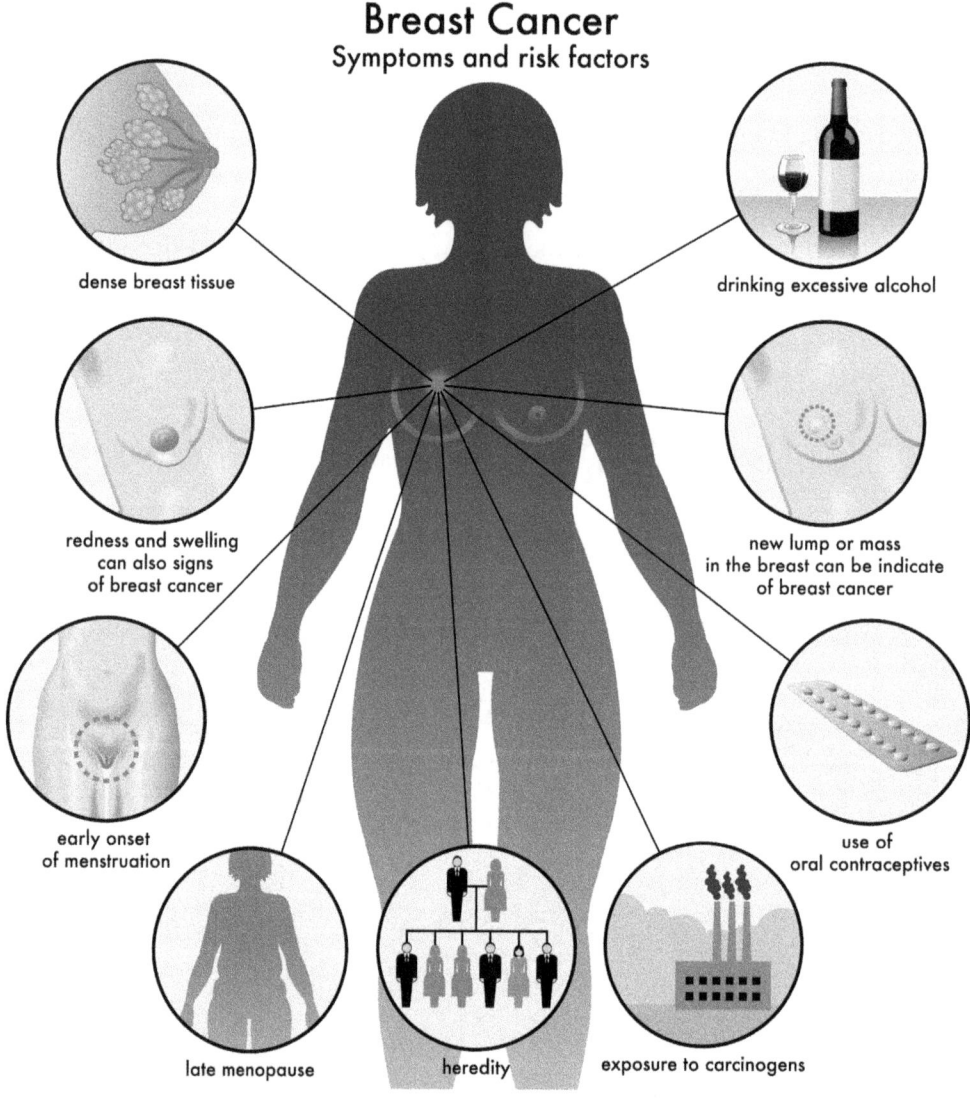

Figure 9.6: Breast Exam.

Symptoms of breast cancer may include a lump in the breast, also a change in size or shape of the breast can be an indication. There may also be a discharge from one or both nipples. The recommendation is to perform breast self-exams and mammography screening to help find breast cancer early. Early treatment, removal of the cancerous proteins, is usually the only successful method. A possible treatment is having a surgery, such as a lumpectomy or a mastectomy (i.e., removal of the entire breast). Additional treatments may include radiation therapy, chemotherapy, hormone therapy, and targeted therapy. There are targeted therapies that use various substances that attack cancer cells without harming normal cells.[10,11]

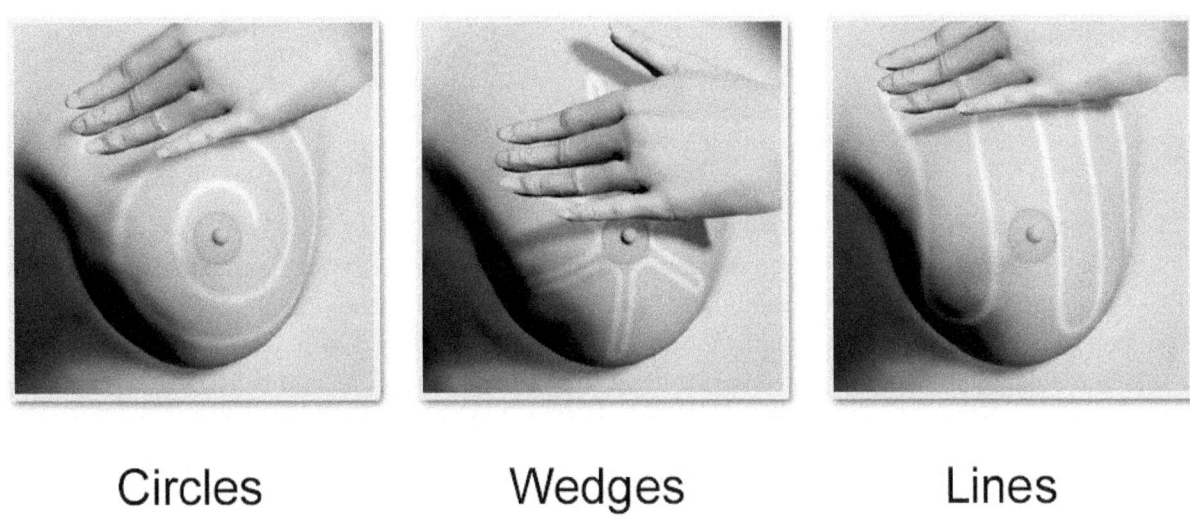

Circles   Wedges   Lines

Figure 9.7: Breast Self Exam.

LUNG CANCER

Lung cancer is believed to affect more than 200,000 Americans every year, and is a leading cause of death in the U.S. Cigarettes make up the most *preventable* cause of lung cancer. Second-hand smoke is also a major concern in leading to potential lung cancer, so much so that many states have enacted laws to keep smoking away from the general populace, and they have outlawed smoking in closed spaces, inside cars for example, with children.

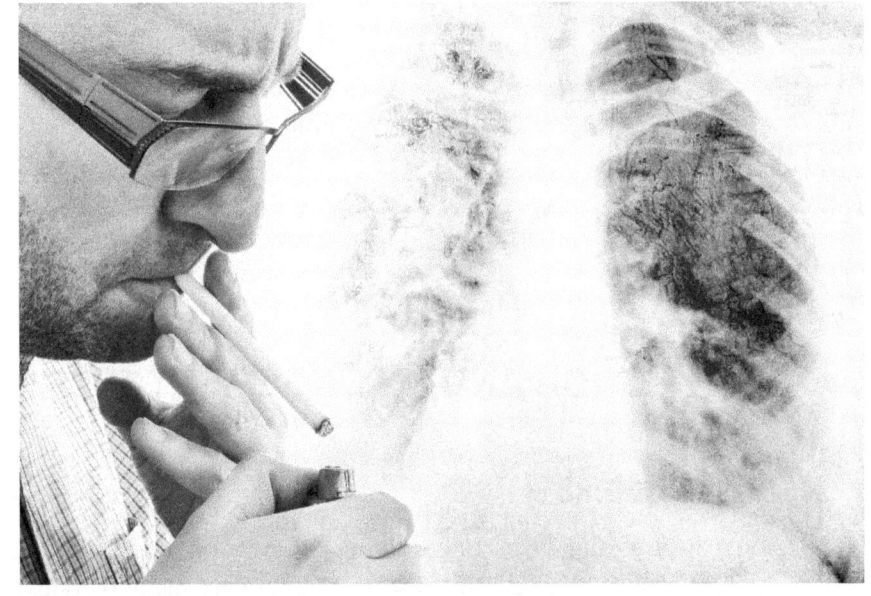

Figure 9.8: Lung Cancer.

There are three different types of lung cancer:

- **Non-Small Cell Lung Cancer**: Most common type of lung cancer. Makes up about 85% of lung cancers diagnoses. Squamous cell **carcinoma** (i.e., those lining the inner/outer surface of the body), adenocarcinoma, and large cell carcinoma are all examples of non-small cell lung cancer.
- **Small Cell Lung Cancer**: Small cell lung cancer sometimes is known as "oat-cell cancer." It typically makes up 10% to 15% of lung cancers. The major concern with small cell lung cancer is that it tends to spread rapidly.
- **Lung Carcinoid Tumor**: Less than 5% of lung cancers are diagnosed as lung carcinoid tumors. It may also go by the name "lung neuroendocrine tumors." The majority of these tumors grow slowly and rarely spread far.

Signs and systems that might indicate a concern for lung cancer:

- A new cough developed in a smoker or a former smoker
- A cough that does not go away or gets worse over time
- Coughing up blood (i.e., hemoptysis) occurs in a significant number of people who have lung cancer. Any amount of coughed-up blood should be evaluated by a health care provider.
- Pain in the chest area is a symptom that can occur in one-fourth of people who have lung cancer. It described as dull, aching, and persistent pain.
- Shortness of breath, which usually results from a blockage in a part of the lung, a potential collection of fluid around the lung, or the spread of tumor through the lungs
- Wheezing or hoarseness, which may signal blockage or inflammation, that commonly go along with cancer
- Repeated respiratory infections, such as bronchitis or pneumonia, can be a sign of lung cancer.

Unfortunately, the five year survival rate is only 54% when found and acted upon. Potential treatment of lung cancer usually involves some combination of surgery, chemotherapy, and radiation. It may also include new experimental methods since there is a low survival rate. The biggest priority is to engage smokers in smoking cessation programs to reduce their risk for lung cancer.[12,13,14]

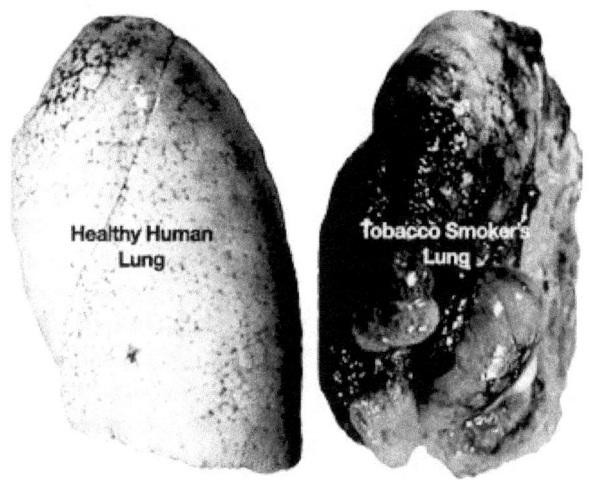

Figure 9.9: Healthy Lung compared to a Smoker's Lung.

PREVENTION AND MANAGEMENT TECHNIQUES

THE BIG PICTURE

You may be asking, "Where does all this information come from?" and "What is being done to prevent the development of more chronic diseases?" There are many private, public, and government organizations that have contributed to the CDC's recommendations for coordinating chronic disease prevention. There are 4 domains the CDC recognizes as contributing to disease prevention:

- Epidemiology and surveillance: to monitor trends and track progress
  - Provides data
- Environmental approaches: to promote health and support healthy behaviors
  - Fosters change to policies, education, and physical surroundings
- Health care system interventions: to improve the effective delivery and use of clinical and other high-value preventive services
  - Improvements to health care that lead to better treatment and diagnosis for all individuals
- Community programs linked to clinical services: to improve and sustain management of chronic conditions
  - Provides access to programs that individuals can participate in to improve their health and reduce their risk of developing chronic disease or help them manage an existing disease

So, there are organizational efforts, policies, and individual approaches to helping prevent the development of chronic diseases. Some examples of where you can see these four domains in everyday life are as follows:[18]

- Epidemiology and surveillance
  - Data found on the CDC website is an example of spreading information related to the trends in chronic disease prevention, development, and treatment
- Environmental approaches
  - Laws created to make workplaces, restaurants, and bars smoke-free to protect non-smokers
  - Bans on artificial trans fats
  - Water fluoridation
  - Soda taxes
- Health care system interventions
  - Expanded population coverage
  - Involvement of a large number and broader range of health care professionals, who can deliver care
  - Rural health care initiatives
- Community programs linked to clinical services to improve and sustain management of chronic conditions
  - Education and outreach programs such as smoking cessation and weight management
  - Linking tobacco cessation call lines to the overall health care system.

INDIVIDUAL EFFORTS: LOOKING BACK AT THE TRANSTHEORETICAL MODEL IN ACTION

What can you do to help yourself? There are *four* major health risk behaviors that you can change that will decrease your risk of developing chronic diseases: lack of exercise or physical activity, poor nutrition, tobacco use, and consuming alcohol. While this is good information to know, many individuals struggle with making significant changes to lead a more active and healthy lifestyle. An important factor to remember is an individual's readiness to make change. As discussed in chapter one, the transtheoretical model (TTM) of behavior change, better known as the stages-of-change model, can be applied to many different types of health behavior change including: increasing physical activity, eating healthier, quitting tobacco use, or decreasing alcohol consumption. One reason there are so many different types of health behavioral change programs is because not everyone is ready to change at the same time or in the same way. So, there is not a simple one-size-fits-all model for health behavior based programs.

For many, it may help if the stages-of-change model are thought of as a stairway. Each time a person takes a step up the stairway and transitions to the next stage, he or she is closer to leading a healthier lifestyle. It is important to remember that an individual must decide for himself if he is ready to change. No one can force another individual to progress to the next step. While it is important to have supportive friends, family, and colleagues, an individual will not progress or remain in a stage if she is not ready for it, or willing to commit to the work involved in the change. For example, an individual might agree to go to the gym with her friend, but if she spends all her time texting, taking pictures, and chatting, and puts a minimal amount of effort into actually exercising (e.g., maybe she is lifting weight way too light for herself, or walking way slower on a treadmill than her fitness level dictates), she is not really in the action stage. She is still stuck in the preparation stage.

FAQs CHECK!

Transtheoretical Model in Action?

Let's pretend you and one of your classmates are both tobacco users. You both read the information in this chapter. You both know that smoking is bad for you and can lead to a long list of chronic diseases. However, due to your individual readiness to change, one of you is ready to take action immediately and go out and buy a smoking cessation patch program from your local pharmacy, and start tomorrow (this student would fall in the Preparation stage). On the other hand, one of you is not as ready to change. Even though this student finds the information valuable, he has some reservations and wants to take some time to evaluate several smoking cessation programs (this student would fall in the Contemplation stage).

PHYSICAL ACTIVITY

The CDC recommends 150 minutes of moderate intensity activity or 75 minutes of vigorous intensity activity weekly to maintain health benefits associated with leading a physically active lifestyle.[19,20,21]

HEALTHY EATING

As you have read in your other chapters, eating healthy has a major impact on so many elements of your overall health and well-being. It helps control your weight, BMI, body fat percentage, and minimizes your risk of developing many diseases. "Choose My Plate" recommends the following servings per day to maintain a healthy diet.

Specifically, to prevent or reduce your risk of developing chronic diseases, you need to eat a diet that is:

- Rich in fruits and vegetables
- Minimizes sodium intake
- Controls portion sizes
- Low in fat
- Rich in whole grains instead of processed grains
- Promoting drinking plenty of water
- Following the United States Department of Agriculture guidelines[15]

ALCOHOL CONSUMPTION

Alcohol consumption is a common link between all the chronic diseases discussed in this chapter, and it will be discussed further in the Acute Health Detriments chapter. However, it is important to note in this chapter that alcohol can raise blood pressure levels, which will increase your risk for developing heart disease and it increases your triglycerides, which can harden an individual's arteries. The CDC recommends that women limit their alcohol consumption to no more than 1 drink per day, and men should consume no more than 2 drinks per day.

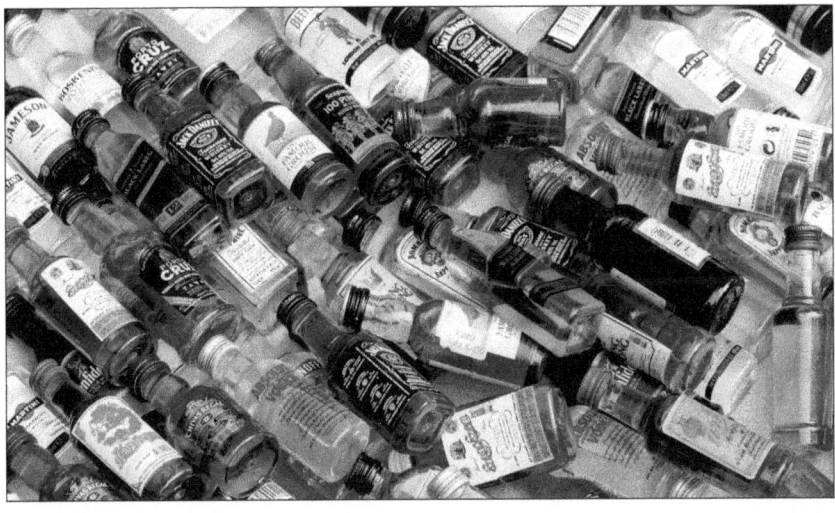

Figure 9.10: Alcohol Bottles.

TOBACCO USE

We will talk about tobacco more in the Acute Health Detriments chapter, however, it is a prime risk factor for heart and blood vessel disease, chronic bronchitis, and emphysema. It is known that cigarette smoking is responsible for more cancers and more cancer deaths than any other known agent. Even passive smoke, also known as side stream smoke or secondhand smoke, can adversely affect a person's health and raise his risk factor for developing a chronic disease. Along with being linked to cancer, cigarette smoking can damage the heart and blood vessels, which increases your risk of developing atherosclerosis and heart attack. The nicotine in tobacco raises blood pressure, and the presence of carbon monoxide in the blood lowers the amount of oxygen the blood can carry. Avoiding contact with tobacco products is the only way to reduce this risk factor.

HEALTH SCREENINGS

We mentioned earlier that routine screenings by a physician are important. Since 1991, the National Breast and Cervical Cancer Early Detection Program (NBCCEDP) exists to help low-income, uninsured, and underinsured women access diagnostic services like: mammograms, Pap tests, clinical breast exams, and pelvic exams. In the event that a screening results in an abnormal result, there is follow-up care and treatment referrals in the event that cancer is found. The NBCCEDP also provides important public health activities like: outreach, education, case management, quality assurance, and program evaluation.

ACCESS

Many other programs exist to help marginalized individuals gain access to health information and health care. There are programs available for individuals and families who are considered: low-income, individuals who live in rural areas (and must travel a great distance to gain access to health care), migrant workers, illegal immigrants, African-Americans, Hispanic-Americans, Native Americans, the uninsured, and gender-specific health care programs. A number of these programs vary by state. Many of these programs can be found by visiting the Chronic Disease Prevention and Health Promotion section of the CDC website at http://www.cdc.gov/chronicdisease/index.htm.

REFERENCES

1. Centers for Disease Control and Prevention.http://www.cdc.gov/chronicdisease/resources/publications/aag/dcpc.htm.
2. Centers for Disease Control and Prevention. http://www.cdc.gov/chronicdisease/.
3. Centers for Disease Control and Prevention. http://www.cdc.gov/chronicdisease/overview/.
4. Centers for Disease Control and Prevention. http://www.cdc.gov/heartdisease/behavior.htm.
5. Mayo Clinic. "Heart Failure Symptoms." http://www.mayoclinic.org/diseases-conditions/heart-failure/basics/symptoms/con-20029801.
6. WebMD. "Congenital Heart Disease Explained." http://www.webmd.com/heart-disease/congenital-heart-disease#1.
7. Children's Heart Foundation. "Facts Sheet." http://www.childrensheartfoundation.org/about-chf/fact-sheets.
8. American Cancer Society. "Risk of Developing and Dying from Cancer among Males and Females." http://www.cancer.org/cancer/cancerbasics/lifetime-probability-of-developing-or-dying-from-cancer.
9. American Cancer Society. "Skin Cancer." http://www.cancer.org/cancer/skincancer-melanoma/detailedguide/melanoma-skin-cancer-what-is-melanoma.
10. MedlinePlus. "Breast Cancer." https://medlineplus.gov/breastcancer.html.
11. National Cancer Institute. "Breast Cancer-Patient Version." https://www.cancer.gov/types/breast.

12. WebMD. "Lung Cancer Health Center." http://www.webmd.com/lung-cancer/.
13. American Cancer Society. "Lung Cancer." http://www.cancer.org/cancer/lungcancer/.
14. Stoppler, M. "Lung Cancer." http://www.medicinenet.com/lung_cancer/article.htm.
15. USDA. www.ChooseMyPlate.gov.
16. World Health Organization. http://www.who.int/chp/chronic_disease_report/media/Factsheet1.pdf.
17. United States Department of Health and Human Services, National Institute of Health, National Institute of Diabetes and Digestive and Kidney Diseases. https://www.niddk.nih.gov/health-information/diabetes/types.
18. Centers for Disease Control and Prevention. http://www.cdc.gov/chronicdisease/resources/publications/four-domains.htm.
19. American Council on Exercise. *ACE's Essentials of Exercise Science for Fitness Professionals.* San Diego, CA: American Council on Exercise, 2012.
20. American Council on Exercise. *ACE Lifestyle & Weight Management Coach Manual.* San Diego, CA: American Council on Exercise, 2011.
21. American Council on Exercise. *ACE Personal Trainer Manual.* San Diego, CA: American Council on Exercise, 2010.
22. Reagan, P. and Brookins-Fisher, J. *Community Health in the 21st Century..* San Francisco, CA: Benjamin Cummings, 2002.
23. American Cancer Society. http://www.cancer.org/cancer/news/news/world-health-organization-links-8-more-cancer-types-to-excess-weight.
24. Mayo Clinic. "Diabetic Neuropathy." http://www.mayoclinic.org/diseases-conditions/diabetic-neuropathy/basics/symptoms/con-20033336.
25. Melanoma Research Foundation. "The ABCDEs of Melanoma." https://www.melanoma.org/understand-melanoma/diagnosing-melanoma/detection-screening/abcdes-melanoma?gclid=CNfZ27yXo88CFYkjgQodsEQF7w.

FIGURE CREDITS

10 ACUTE WELLNESS

BY KACEY DIGIACINTO

COMMON RISK FACTORS

While there are some things that may be legal in other countries, it doesn't make them necessarily safe or healthy. In the United States, smoking, alcohol, and some drugs are legal, but that doesn't mean that they don't have adverse effects on one's health. As you will see in this chapter, even participating in legal activities could put your health at risk, and decrease not only the amount of years in your life, but also the quality of your life.

THE NATURE OF ADDICTION

Many behaviors that we engage in daily that can affect our health may be poor habits, but they may also be addictions. This can be familiar addictions like smoking, or addictions severe as drugs, and for many it can be common behaviors, like daily caffeine consumption. Often people do not realize that addiction is a complex disease, and quitting typically takes significantly more than good intentions or a strong will. Various chemicals repeatedly consumed in drugs, smoking, caffeine, etc., make alterations to the brain, and therefore, make quitting extremely hard. Individual items that are common addictions are discussed throughout this chapter.

While many of these addictive items have acute concerns, some of the general long-term effects of addiction are:

- Learning
- Judgment
- Decision-making
- Stress
- Memory
- Behavior[1]

SMOKING

One in six adults in America currently smokes cigarettes, however, smoking is on the decline. In 2005, 20.9% of adults smoked cigarettes; by 2014 that number had dropped to 16.8%.[2] Even though cigarette smoking is on the decline, currently one of every five deaths is related to cigarette smoking, which is the leading cause of preventable disease death in the United States,[3] which has increased over the last 50 years. Research has shown that the more education you have, the less likely you are to smoke cigarettes. Meanwhile, those who live below the poverty level (at a rate of 26.3%) smoke more than those who live at or above the poverty level (around 15.2%). States located in the South and the Midwest are more likely to have higher amounts of their population smoke. This coincides with states who have the highest poverty rates and least educated population. Individuals living in rural areas are also more likely to use tobacco than those living in urban areas. Meaning education and socio-economic status are big risk factors for cigarette smoking, which can be linked to cultural factors, policies, and lack of appropriate health care (especially in rural areas).

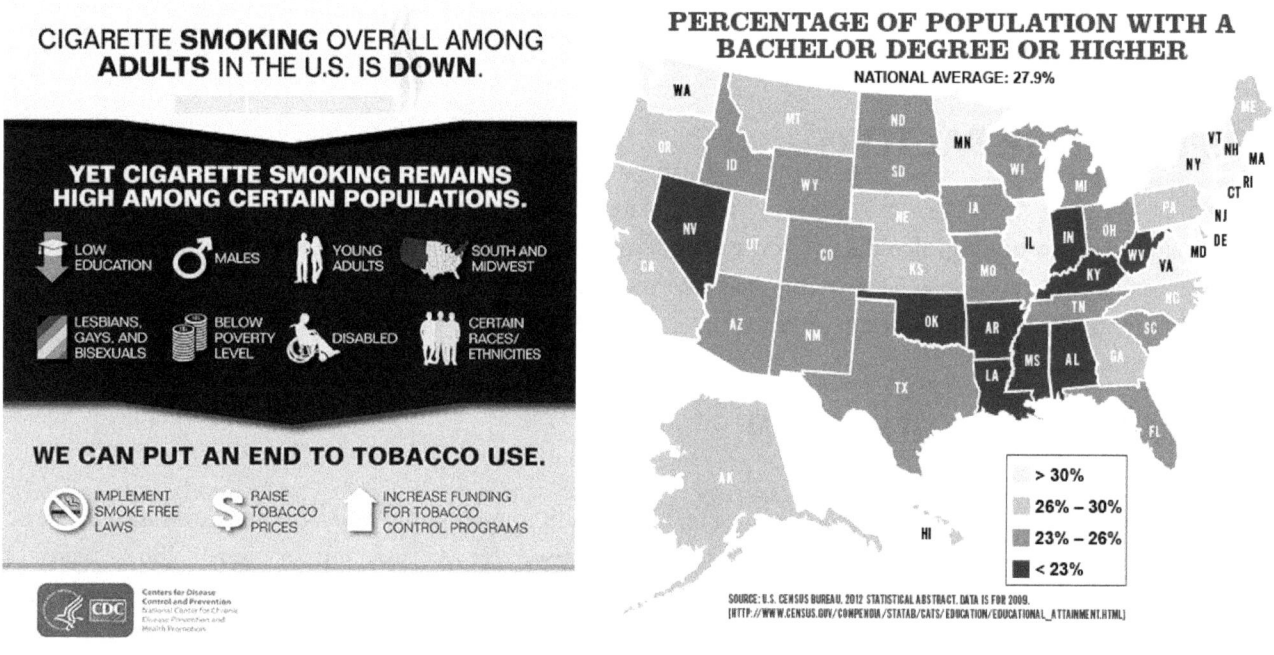

Figure 10.1: Smoking Infograph.

Smoking can shorten your life by at least 10 years. Smoking causes more deaths each year than the following causes combined: HIV, illegal drug use, alcohol use, motor vehicle injuries, and firearm-related incidents. The CDC noted that, "More than 10 times as many U.S. citizens have died prematurely from cigarette smoking than have died in all the wars fought by the United States during its history."[4] Smoking is the cause of about 90% of all lung cancer deaths and 80% of all deaths from chronic obstructive pulmonary disease (COPD). Even if you smoke as few as five cigarettes a day, you can experience early signs of cardiovascular disease. Smoking is linked to an increased risk of: coronary heart disease, stroke, cataracts, type 2 diabetes mellitus, increased inflammation in the body, bone health issues, teeth and gum health issues, tooth loss, cancer, rheumatoid arthritis, and decreased immune function. Smoking affects your health to such a degree that your overall quality of life is greatly impacted due to increased absenteeism from work and school, and increased health care utilization and cost. The more you miss work, the less money you make to cover medical and other expenses. Even if you are a salaried employee, the excess medical costs can quickly add up, especially when you add in the cost of the cigarettes themselves[7].

Risks from Smoking

Smoking can damage every part of the body

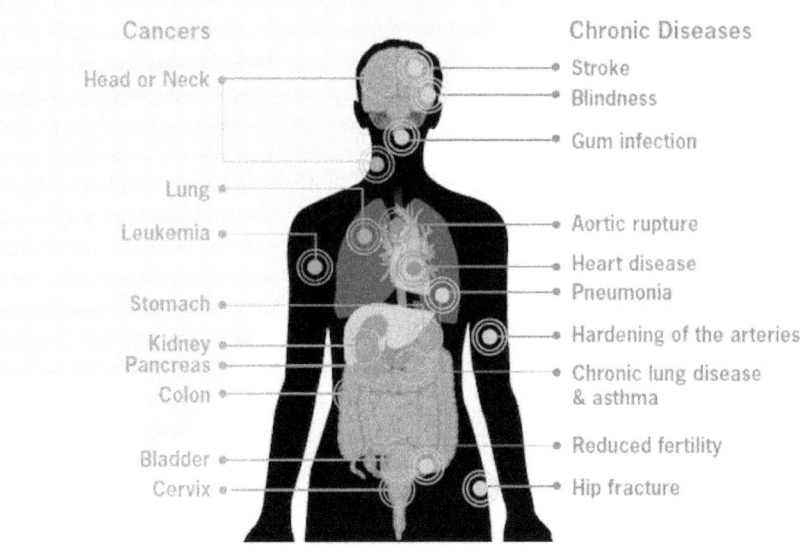

Cancers

- Head or Neck
- Lung
- Leukemia
- Stomach
- Kidney
- Pancreas
- Colon
- Bladder
- Cervix

Chronic Diseases

- Stroke
- Blindness
- Gum infection
- Aortic rupture
- Heart disease
- Pneumonia
- Hardening of the arteries
- Chronic lung disease & asthma
- Reduced fertility
- Hip fracture

Figure 10.2: Cancer and related Chronic Diseases.

FAQs CHECK!

Cost of a Pack?

The national average for a pack of cigarettes is $5.51. In some states like New York, they can cost as much as $12.85. For the sake of this exercise, we will use the national average of $5.51 and 20 cigarettes per pack. If you have a pack a day smoking habit, you will be spending $2,011.15 a year on cigarettes. Do you really want to spend that much money on something that could cost you even more in medical bills throughout your now shortened lifetime?

SMOKING AND PREGNANCY

If you are a woman who is trying to get pregnant, smoking can make it difficult to become pregnant. Once pregnant, smoking during pregnancy can increase the risk of: preterm delivery, stillbirth (i.e., death of the baby before birth), low birth weight, sudden infant death syndrome (i.e., SIDS or crib death), ectopic pregnancy, and orofacial clefts in infants. Smoking can also affect men's sperm, which can reduce fertility and increase risks for birth defects and miscarriage.

SECONDHAND SMOKE EXPOSURE

While many states have some kind of law against smoking in public places, such as bars, restaurants, and government buildings, many do not. These laws are put in place to try to deter individuals from smoking, and to protect non-smokers from the adverse health effects of second hand and side-stream smoke. Socio-economic status and education play a role in these smoke-free laws. According to the CDC, in some states, communities with less-educated and lower-income residents are less likely to be covered by comprehensive smoke-free laws that prohibit smoking in all areas of workplaces, restaurants, and bars. In some states, urban areas and areas with high per-capita income are more likely to have strong smoke-free laws. Residents of rural areas are more likely to allow smoking in the presence of children, such as in their homes and cars.[7] Unfortunately, the percentage of children in small rural areas who live in a household with a smoker is 35%; this is greater than the percentage of children in urban areas who live with a smoker (24.4%). Many Southern states have no statewide laws that prohibit smoking in worksites, restaurants, and bars.

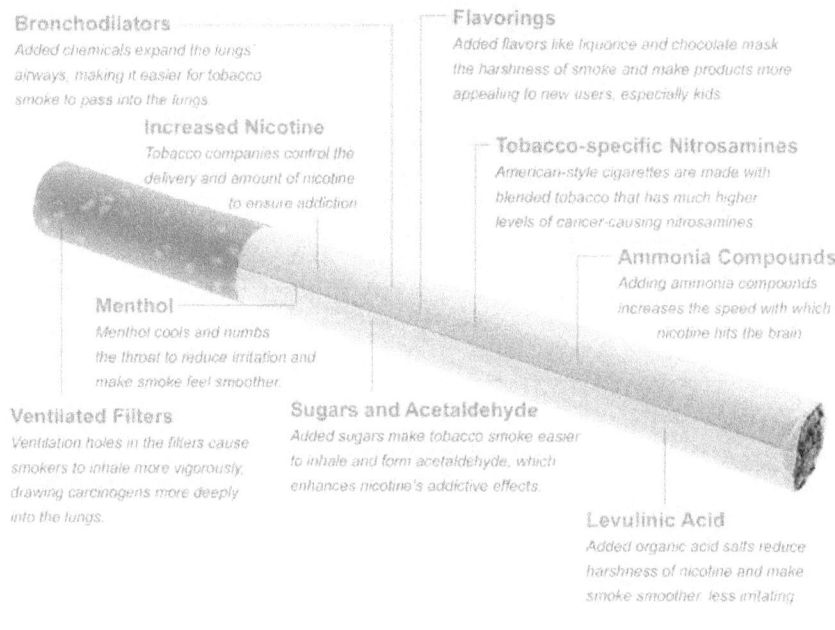

Figure 10.3: What is in a cigarette?

WHAT'S IN A CIGARETTE?

Tar

Tar is found in all tobacco products that are burned. Tar in the smoke of tobacco products enters the lungs, and affects the ability of the cilia in the lungs to operate. This can lead to emphysema, asthma, chronic bronchitis, and lung cancer. Aesthetically, tar is the substance in tobacco products that turns your fingers and teeth brown. When it comes to tobacco smoke, the last puffs of a cigarette contain twice as much tar as the first puffs. This is because as you draw the smoke through the cigarette, the tar collects through the whole cigarette and filter, and some of it is blocked. However, as you burn more of the cigarette, you are pulling in smoke from where the tar was being collected, bringing more in to your lungs.

Tobacco Industry and Marketing

The tobacco industry has historically glorified smoking. Using imagery of successful businessmen in some advertisements, and rugged, manly men in others, they are hoping to appeal to young men. These images imply that if you smoked, you would become a successful businessman, or a rugged man—two images that appeal to a large majority of young men. Meanwhile, young women look at ideal, slim, models smoking. This made young women think if they smoked, they could be slim and desirable like the women in the advertisements. This information, combined with the fact that rural children have less access to anti-smoking messages in the media, can help us better understand how the Midwest and South have higher incidences of smoking than other regions of the United States. Targeting buying habits for demographics is also common. An example is African-American communities marketed for the high number of exterior and interior point-of-sale successful advertising (purchases made at a register) for tobacco products.[7]

WHAT ABOUT OTHER FORMS OF TOBACCO?

Hookah

Hookahs are water pipes that allow you to smoke flavored tobacco. They have been around for centuries, starting in ancient Persia and India. People assume that because it is typically flavored and tastes good, like apple, mint, cherry, coconut, etc., it is somehow less harmful than cigarette smoking. Smoking hookah for one hour produces the same amount of smoke as several packs of cigarettes. Smoking hookah also produces high levels of carbon monoxide, metals, and cancer-causing chemicals and is known to cause lung, bladder, stomach, esophageal, and oral cancers. Smoking hookah tobacco can also lead to decreased fertility, reduced lung function, and clogged arteries and heart disease. Even studies of nontobacco products, like shisha and herbal shisha, show that the smoke produced contains carbon monoxide and other toxic agents, which are known to increase the risks for developing cancer, heart disease, and lung disease.[8]

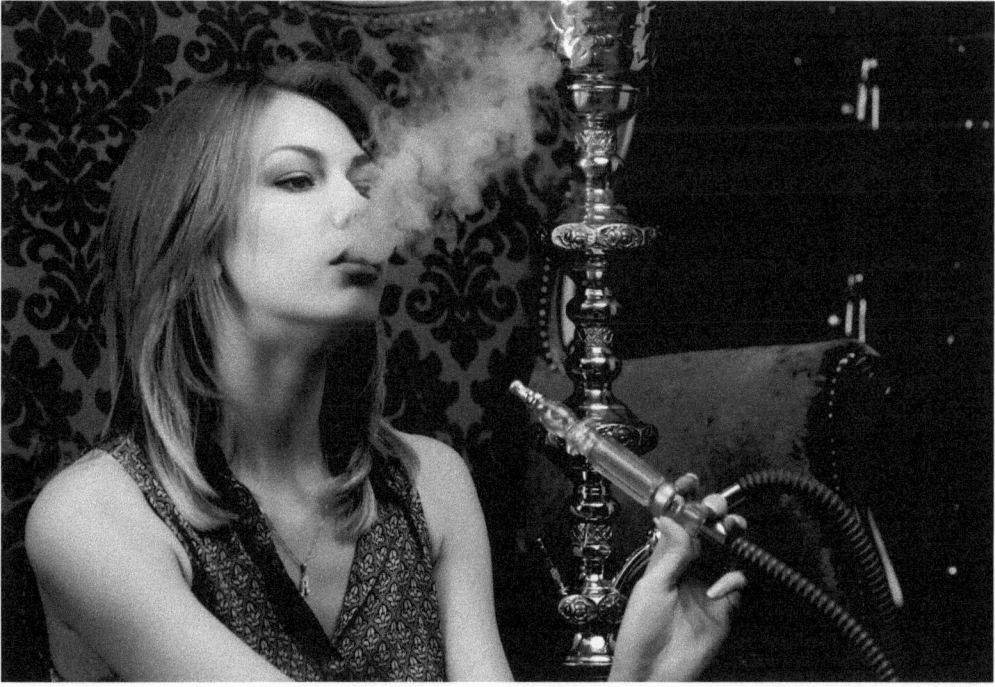

Figure 10.4: Hookahs have increased in popularity over the years.

ALCOHOL

Alcohol is considered a psychoactive substance with serious dependence-producing properties.[20] Ethyl alcohol, or ethanol, is the intoxicating ingredient in beer, wine, and liquor, which is produced by the fermentation of yeast, sugars, and starches. Categorized as a central nervous system depressant, alcohol is absorbed through the stomach and small intestine into the bloodstream. While the liver commonly metabolizes alcohol, the liver can only metabolize a small amount of alcohol at a time, leaving the remaining alcohol to circulate throughout the body via the bloodstream.[9] Why do some people react differently to alcohol than others?

Individual reactions to alcohol vary, and are influenced by many factors; such as:

- Age
- Gender
- Race or ethnicity
- Physical condition (e.g., weight, fitness level)
- Amount of food consumed before drinking
- How quickly the alcohol was consumed
- Use of drugs or prescription medicines
- Family history of alcohol problems

Consuming alcohol too often can lead to many short-term and long-term health problems. Over 200 diseases and injury-related health conditions can be attributed to alcohol.[20] Short-term health risks include: unintentional injuries (e.g., motor vehicle crashes, falls, drownings, burns), violence (e.g., homicide, suicide, sexual assault, and intimate partner violence), alcohol poisoning, and reproductive health (e.g., risky sexual behaviors, unintended pregnancy, sexually transmitted diseases, including HIV, miscarriage, still birth, and fetal alcohol spectrum disorders).[4] Long-term health risks include: chronic diseases (e.g., cirrhosis and pancreatitis), cancers (e.g., liver, mouth, throat, larynx, and esophagus), learning and memory problems, mental health, social problems, and alcohol dependence. Until 1984, each state had the ability to decide the legal drinking age to purchase or publically consume alcohol. However, in 1984 the National Minimum Drinking Age Act dictated that the legal drinking age in the United States was 21 years of age. According to the CDC, states that increased the legal drinking age to 21 saw a 16% decline in car crashes.[4] If you plan on enjoying alcohol, you should know that according to the Dietary Guidelines for Americans, moderate drinking is defined for women as having one drink per day for women, or two drinks per day for men.

FAQs CHECK!

Alcohol limit.

Every state has adopted 0.08% as the legal limit for drinking alcohol and operating any motor vehicle. In some states this extends to tractors, riding lawn mowers, and bicycles. In some cases, just driving anything on a designated road with wheels may count.

The term "injury" has replaced "accident" when it comes to reporting public health data. This is because unintentional injuries can be prevented with proper public health initiatives.[12]

Perhaps the most well known problem associated with long-term alcohol use is cirrhosis of the liver. Alcoholism is the second most common cause of cirrhosis. **Cirrhosis** affects the liver, slowly, over time, by replacing healthy liver tissue with scar tissue. This scar tissue blocks the flow of blood through the liver. When the flow of blood is blocked, the liver processes nutrients, hormones, drugs, and other naturally produced toxins. The National Institutes of Health reports that cirrhosis is the 12th leading cause of death by disease.[10]

BINGE DRINKING

Binge drinking occurs when a man consumes five or more drinks, or a woman consumes four or more drinks on one occasion. Heavy drinking is defined as consuming 15 or more drinks per week for men, and 8 or more drinks per week for women. Excessive alcohol use can shorten your life by an average of 30 years.[4] It should be noted that most people who drink excessively are not necessarily considered alcoholics or alcohol dependent. You might be thinking, "How do you define one drink?" The picture below shows the equivalent of one drink of beer, wine, liquor, and malt liquor. There is no single drink that is better for you to consume than another, when it comes to alcohol: 12 ounces of beer = 8 ounces of malt liquor = 5 ounces of wine = 1.5 ounces or a "shot" of distilled spirits or liquor.

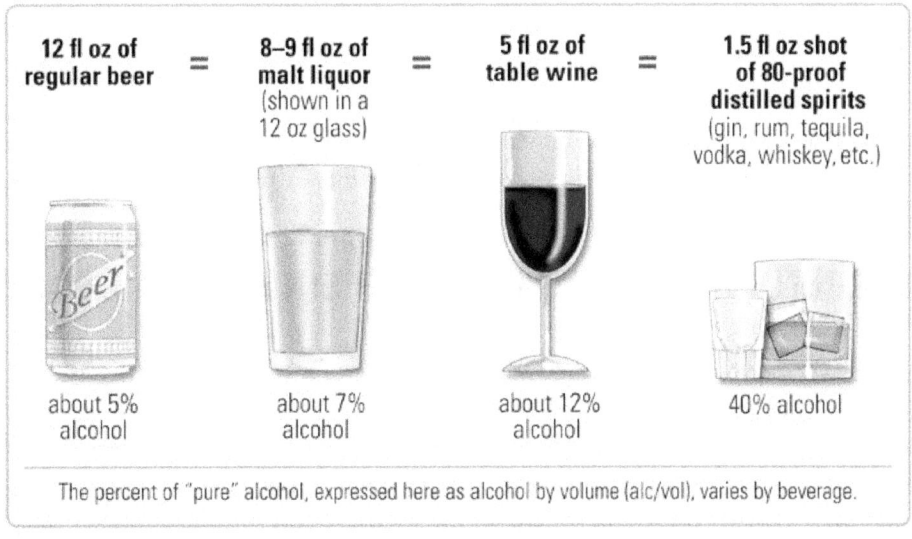

Figure 10.5: Watch for changes in moles.

Binge drinking is a large problem for many segments of the population. The age group with the most binge drinkers is 18 to 34 years old. However, what may be surprising to find out is that the age group that binge drinks the most often is the 65 and older group. The income group that binge drinks the most often, and drinks most per binge makes less than $25,000 a year. There are many evidence-based interventions to prevent binge drinking related issues: increasing alcoholic beverage costs and excise taxes, limiting the number of retail outlets that sell alcoholic beverages in a given area, holding alcohol retailers responsible for the harms cause by their underage or intoxicated patrons, restricting access to alcohol by maintaining limits on the days and hours of alcohol retail sales, consistent enforcement of laws against underage drinking and alcohol-impaired driving, maintaining government controls on alcohol sales, and screening and counseling for alcohol misuse[4].

UNDERAGE DRINKING

Alcohol is the most commonly used and abused drug among youth in the United States.[4] Excessive drinking is responsible for more than 4,300 deaths every year among underage youth. According to the CDC, "People aged 12 to 20 years drink 11% of all alcohol consumed in the United States. More than 90% of this alcohol is consumed in the form of binge drinks." It is not surprising that underage drinkers consume more drinks per occasion than adult drinkers, since we know 90% of underage drinks are consumed by binge drinking. There are many consequences of underage drinking: it changes brain development that may have life-long effects, abuse of other drugs is common, memory problems, social problems like increased absences from classes or work, disagreements or fights, legal issues resulting from arrest for driving or physically hurting someone while drunk, unwanted, unplanned, and unprotected sexual activity, disruption of normal growth and sexual development, physical and sexual assault, higher risk for suicide and homicide, and higher risk of death from alcohol poisoning.[4]

Drinking by those under the age 21 is a public health problem.

- Excessive drinking contributes to more than 4,300 deaths among people below the age of 21 in the U.S. each year.
- Underage drinking cost the U.S. economy $24 billion in 2010.
- There were about 189,000 emergency department visits by people under age 21 for injuries and other conditions linked to alcohol in 2010.
- More than 90% of the alcohol consumed by those under age 21 is consumed by binge drinkers (defined as 5 or more drinks per occasion for men; 4 or more drinks per occasion for women).

WHAT HAPPENS WHEN YOU MIX CAFFEINE AND ALCOHOL?

Energy drinks are very popular. They usually contain large amounts of caffeine, added sugars, other additives, and legal stimulants such as guarana, taurine, and L-carnitine. These energy drinks have the same effect on the body as other stimulants including increases in alertness, attention, energy, blood pressure, heart rate, and breathing. You or your friend probably use them regularly to help you stay up to study at night, or wake up for class in the morning. Energy drinks can have a very harmful effect on the nervous system, of which many people are unaware. Those dangers include: dehydration, seizure, heart complications (e.g., irregular heartbeat and heart failure), anxiety, and insomnia. Many may not realize that anyone can overdose on caffeine. It is recommended that adults do not consume more than 400 milligrams of caffeine, with some overdoses occurring with just 450 milligrams consumed in a 24-hour period. Symptoms of a caffeine overdose are: dizziness, diarrhea, increased thirst, insomnia, headache, fever, and irritability. When more severe symptoms are observed, medical treatment should be sought immediately if a person has trouble breathing, is vomiting, hallucinating, confused, has chest pain, is experiencing irregular or fast heartbeat, has uncontrollable muscle movements, or is in convulsions.[5]

You might be asking, "Why did I just have to learn about caffeine when I am learning about the effects of alcohol?" Many individuals mix energy drinks and alcohol, or drink caffeinated alcoholic beverages. When alcoholic beverages are mixed with energy drinks, the caffeine in these drinks can mask the depressant effects of the alcohol. At the same time, caffeine has no effect on the metabolism of alcohol by the liver, and thus does not reduce breath alcohol concentrations, or reduce the risk of alcohol-attributable issues. Individuals who consume alcohol mixed with energy drinks are three times more likely to binge drink than individuals who do not report mixing alcohol with energy drinks. Sadly, drinkers who consume alcohol with energy drinks are about twice as likely to report taking advantage of someone else sexually and to report riding with a driver who was under the influence of alcohol, compared to drinkers who do not report mixing alcohol with energy drinks to report being taken advantage of sexually. Caffeinated alcoholic beverages are premixed beverages that combine alcohol, caffeine, and other stimulants. These drinks can be malt or distilled-spirits, and usually have a higher alcohol content than beer. Meanwhile, the caffeine content in these drinks is often not reported. If the caffeine content is not reported, it could be quite easy to overdose. These drinks are marketed heavily to young audiences. In 2010, with the caffeine content being unknown, among other reasons, the Food and Drug Administration (FDA) told the manufacturers of seven caffeinated alcoholic beverage companies that their drinks need to be removed from the market, in their current forms. The reason cited was, "FDA does not find support for the claim that the addition of caffeine to these alcoholic beverages is 'generally recognized as safe,' which is legal standard."[6]

Individuals who should avoid alcohol?

- Pregnant women
- Individuals with medical conditions that can be aggravated by alcohol
- Individuals who take medications that interact with alcohol
- Individuals who plan to drive a vehicle or operate machinery

DRUG USE

GENERAL DRUG KNOWLEDGE

Something that all drugs have in common is they all affect the central nervous system (i.e., the brain and the spinal cord). Drugs can block, alter production, release, reuptake, or affect storage of **neurotransmitters** (i.e., chemicals found in the body), and there are at least two dozen neurotransmitters in the human body. Drugs appeal to people because of the effect they have on neurotransmitters. For example, **dopamine** is the neurotransmitter that stimulates the reward center of the brain. If a drug releases dopamine, you get a feeling of happiness and satisfaction. When you use drugs, your body becomes accustomed to the drugs and you build up a tolerance to them. That is why someone who uses drugs eventually needs more and more of a given drug to enjoy the same side effects, as the first time they took the drug. Eventually, this increased tolerance can lead to an overdose. A person can overdose on over-the-counter drugs, prescribed medication, and illicit drugs (i.e., illegal drugs). Drug addiction develops when a person's body cannot feel "normal" (i.e., physically and/or psychologically) without the drug. Drug dependency can develop when a person needs a specific drug to function normally, as a result of a physiological or a psychological effect it has on a person (Table 10.1). We say someone is abusing drugs when they take them outside of cultural norms.

Specific Drugs and Their Potential for Dependence		
Drug	Potential for Physical Dependence	Potential for Psychological Dependence
Morphine	High	High
Codeine	Moderate	Moderate
Heroin	High	High
Methadone	High	High
Barbiturates	High	Moderate
Cocaine	Possible	High
Amphetamines	Possible	High
Methamphetamine	Possible	High
LSD	None	Unknown
Mescaline, peyote	None	Unknown
Ecstasy	Unknown	Unknown
Marijuana	Unknown	Moderate
Alcohol	Possible	Possible
Steroids	Possible	Possible
Nicotine	High	High[11]

HALLUCINOGENS OR PSYCHOACTIVE DRUGS

Hallucinogens or psychoactive drugs cause users to experience sensations that are intensified, or cause the user to feel, hear, or see things that are not there. Marijuana, cocaine, ecstasy, alcohol, and tobacco are the most commonly abused drugs in the United States among individuals in the 19 to 24 age group.[10]

Marijuana. Marijuana is most often smoked in pipes, hand-rolled cigarettes (i.e., joints) or cigars (i.e., blunts), however, if prepared properly, it can be edible. The effects can be felt in as few as 15 minutes and last up to three hours. Marijuana is also classified as a stimulant, so increased heart rate and blood pressure, bloodshot eyes, and dry mouth and throat are all side effects of use. Smoking marijuana in joint form is the equivalent of smoking four cigarettes. The major chemical in marijuana that causes the hallucinogenic experience is delta-9-tetrahydrocannabinol or THC. THC works on nerve cells in the brain, specifically the hippocampus, affecting memory and concentration, motor coordination, and the way we sense the passage of time. Studies have shown that in the first hour of smoking marijuana, a person's risk of heart attack may increase by as many as four times that of a non-smoker.

Ecstasy. Ecstasy comes in the form of a crystalline powder or in pill or tablet form. It is usually taken sublingually, and because of this, it reaches the brain almost immediately. Signs of an ecstasy overdose include: rapid heartbeat, muscle cramping, panic attacks, seizures, and stroke.

OVER-THE-COUNTER DRUGS (OTC)

OTC drugs can be purchased without a prescription and can be taken orally or topically. The way your body breaks down a drug and converts the medication into an active chemical substance in the body is known as metabolism. In OTC drugs you have active and inactive ingredients. The active ingredients are the ones that produce the physical effects on the body. Unfortunately, some individuals misuse OTC drugs in order to achieve a temporary "high" or euphoric feeling. Continued misuse of OTC drugs can lead to drug dependence and have long-term adverse health effects.

Crystal Methamphetamine. Also known as crystal meth, it is a form of methamphetamine. It is produced with items that can be collected by individuals. Since it is not found in nature, crystal meth is often made in makeshift labs and sold relatively inexpensively. It is made using toxic chemicals including: pseudo ephedrine, red phosphorous, iodine, ammonia, paint thinner, ether, drain cleaner, and the lithium from batteries. When mixed, these toxic chemicals can cause damage to the brain, lungs, and eyes of the person mixing the chemicals. These chemicals are extremely unstable, when combined, and often produce dangerous reactions when improperly mixed or stored. Children who live in households where crystal meth is made usually exhibit increased aggression, paranoia, and violence, due to the chemical toxins they are exposed to during manufacturing. Because people were using pseudo ephedrine to make crystal meth, it is no longer sold as over-the-counter in an attempt to cut down on crystal meth production.

STIMULANTS AND DEPRESSANTS

Stimulants. Stimulants speed up bodily processes such as heart rate and respiration. Caffeine, cocaine, and amphetamines are all types of stimulants. As you read earlier in this chapter, you can become addicted to caffeine and overdose on it if you consume more than 400 milligrams in one day.

Cocaine. Cocaine is an anesthetic and a stimulant which causes: increased heart rate and blood pressure, feelings of euphoria, heightened self-confidence, and increased alertness. Cocaine comes in three main types, depending on the extraction process: rock cocaine, "crack" cocaine, and freebase cocaine, and can be smoked, injected, snorted, or ingested. Cocaine is rapidly absorbed, however, it produces a short-lived high lasting only 5 to 20 minutes. The side effects of cocaine use are: depression, irritability, and fatigue. Cocaine addicts often suffer psychological damage, which can affect work and school, and contributes to job loss. The high price of cocaine, combined with the short-lived high, leads to high spending, which can result in financial ruin if a person loses his or her job due to side-effects of becoming addicted to the drug. Long-term use of cocaine can cause: irregular heart-beat, heart attack, respiratory issues, neurological problems including strokes, seizures, and headaches, as well as gastrointestinal problems, including abdominal pain and nausea.[10]

Methamphetamine. Methamphetamine (i.e., meth) is a very addictive stimulant that is related to amphetamines, but it lasts longer, is more potent, and damages the central nervous system quicker than amphetamines. The short-term effects of meth are increased wakefulness, increased physical activity, decreased appetite, increased respiration, increased heart rate, increased blood pressure, and hypothermia. Even if you take meth only once, you can experience a cardiovascular collapse and death. Meth is extremely volatile. Long-term meth use is associated with: paranoia, aggressiveness, anorexia, memory loss, visual and auditory hallucinations, delusions, and dental problems.[10]

Amphetamines. Amphetamines can be snorted, injected, smoked, or ingested, and their effects can last between 8 to 24 hours.

Depressants. Depressants slow down bodily processes such as heart rate and respiration. Barbiturates are a type of depressant and long-term use of them can cause: bone pain, unexplained excitement, and jaundice.

Opioids. Opioids are a type of depressant. They cross the blood-brain barrier quickly and are particularly potent. Opioids are often used as short-term pain suppressants by hospitals. The two most prevalent alkaloids in opium are morphine and codeine, which cause the pain relieving effect.

Benzodiazepines. Benzodiazepines are commonly used in date rapes. Rohypnol and GHB are used to cause drowsiness, confusion, dizziness, blurred vision, weakness, and a lack of coordination in victims to make it easier for the rapist to take advantage of the victim. Some individuals take benzodiazepines for other reasons, and they can experience additional symptoms in less than two weeks of consistently taking the drug.

SPORT DRUGS

Sport drugs are becoming more and more popular as individuals try to gain an athletic advantage in their performance in a given discipline. The phrase, "Bigger, Faster, Stronger" seems to be engrained in every athlete's head. In trying to gain a competitive edge, many are turning to over-the-counter supplements and illicit drugs to try to gain an advantage. Some might be looking for a way to boost their energy, so they seek a supplement that has an ergogenic effect, or an energy producing effect.

ANABOLIC STEROIDS

Anabolic steroids can be legally obtained by individuals suffering from low testosterone. However, some individuals take them to try to gain an athletic or aesthetic advantage. Steroids can come in tablet or capsule form, injection, or topical cream or ointment. A common practice in steroid usage is "stacking." Stacking involves using more than two to three types of steroids, at one time. One potential side effect of steroids is probably well known to you as "Roid Rage;" this side effect is includes uncontrolled outbursts of anger, frustration, or combativeness, however, research in this area is inconsistent. Major side effects from abusing anabolic steroids include: liver tumors and cancer, jaundice, and kidney tumors. The anabolic effect of steroid use involves a drug-induced growth or thickening of the body's non-reproductive tract tissues, including skeletal muscles, bones, the larynx, and vocal cords, and a decrease in body fat. Androgenic effects involve the growth of the male reproductive tract and the development of male secondary sexual characteristics. Men, who abuse anabolic steroids, can expect to experience: shrinking of the testicles, development of breasts, and prostate cancer. Meanwhile, women who abuse anabolic steroids can expect to experience: growth of facial hair, enlargement of the clitoris, and cessation of the menstrual cycle. If adolescents take anabolic steroids before they experience a typical adolescent growth spurt, they can stunt their growth by confusing the body to not go through a normal growth spurt.

ASSESSING BEHAVIOR AND PREVENTION PLANNING

WHY SHOULD YOU QUIT USING TOBACCO?

Quitting smoking is difficult, and usually requires several attempts, but it is worth it. People often relapse when trying to quit smoking because of the withdrawal symptoms: feeling irritable, angry, or anxious, having trouble thinking, craving tobacco products, and feeling hungrier than usual, which can lead to

---

FAQs CHECK!

Various addictions?

Addiction is a compulsive psychological need for a drug or other behavior. In addition to drugs, alcohol and tobacco, people can also become addicted to video games, gambling, shopping, the internet, and a vast array of other behaviors. Addictions develop as a compulsive psychological need for a drug and/or behavior, and results from poor coping skills, genetics, as well as psychological and social issues.

---

weight gain. If you are thinking of quitting smoking, you can recover many health benefits. Just one year after quitting smoking, your risk for heart attack drops dramatically. Within two to five years after quitting smoking, your risk for stroke could fall to about the same risk as that of a nonsmoker's risk. If you quit smoking, you can look forward to your risks for cancers of the mouth, throat, esophagus, and bladder dropping by half within five years of quitting; at the 10-year mark, your risk for lung cancer can drop by half.[7] Quit lines can be very helpful in supporting an individual as they try to quit smoking. The most popular quite line, supported by the Department of Health and Human Services, is 1-800-QUIT-NOW. The help line provides you with options to support you while you are quitting and even offers Quit Coaching to support your efforts.

DO YOU OR SOMEONE YOU KNOW NEED HELP WITH A DRINKING PROBLEM?

You might be thinking, "How do I know if I have a drinking problem?" If your drinking has caused you to have issues at school, in social activities, in your relationships with friends, family, or a significant other, or in how you think and feel, then you may have a drinking problem. If you think you or someone you know has a drinking problem, you can consult your health care provider, or call the National Drug and Alcohol Treatment Referral Routing Service at 1-800-662-HELP. The National Drug and Alcohol Treatment Referral Routing Service will put you in contact with treatment programs in your local community as well as allow you to speak with someone about alcohol problems.

HOW CAN I KICK A DRUG HABIT?

Like smoking and alcohol cessation programs, quitting using drugs is difficult due to the withdrawal symptoms, and many individuals who try to quit using drugs often relapse. Recovering from drug addiction is difficult and can sometimes be specific to the drug to which you are addicted. The National Institute on Drug Abuse website, www.nida.nih.gov has excellent resources to aid you in finding the help you or a love one might need.

REFERENCES

1. National Institute on Drug Abuse. "DrugFacts: Understanding Drug Use and Addiction." https://www.drugabuse.gov/publications/drugfacts/understanding-drug-use-addiction
2. Centers for Disease Control and Prevention. http://www.cdc.gov/alcohol/fact-sheets/alcohol-use.htm.
3. Centers for Disease Control and Prevention. http://www.cdc.gov/alcohol/pdfs/alcoholyourhealth.pdf.
4. Centers for Disease Control and Prevention. http://www.cdc.gov/alcohol/fact-sheets/minimum-legal-drinking-age.htm.
5. Centers for Disease Control and Prevention. http://www.cdc.gov/alcohol/fact-sheets/caffeine-and-alcohol.htm.
6. Thombs, D.L., O'Mara, R.J., Tsukamoto, M., Rossheim, Me, Wheiler, R.M., Merves, M.L., & Goldberger, B.A. "Event-Level Analyses of Energy Drink Consumption and Alcohol Intoxication in Bar Patrons. *Addictive Behaviors* 35 (2010): 325–330.
7. Centers for Disease Control and Prevention. http://www.cdc.gov/tobacco/data_statistics/fact_sheets/adult_data/cig_smoking/index.htm.
8. Centers for Disease Control and Prevention. http://www.cdc.gov/tobacco/data_statistics/fact_sheets/tobacco_industry/hookahs/index.htm#compare.
9. Centers for Disease Control and Prevention. http://www.cdc.gov/alcohol/fact-sheets/underage-drinking.htm.

10. Department of Health and Human Services. *Results from the 2005 National Survey on Drug Use and Health: National Findings.* Rockville, MD: Substance Abuse and Mental Health Services Administration, Office of Applied Studies.

11. Powers, S.K. & Dodd, S. *Total Fitness & Wellness.* San Francisco, CA: Pearson, 2009.

12. Reagan, P. & Brookins-Fisher, J. *Community Health in the 21st Century.* San Francisco, CA: Benjamin Cummings, 2002.

13. Centers for Disease Control and Prevention. http://www.cdc.gov/tobacco/disparities/geographic/index.htm.

14. United States Department of Health and Human Services and U.S. Department of Agriculture. (2015). 2015–2020 Dietary Guidelines for Americans (8th ed.). Washington, DC.

15. United States Department of Health and Human Services, National Institute of Health, National Institute on Alcohol Abuse and Alcoholism. https://www.niaaa.nih.gov/alcohol-health/overview-alcohol-consumption/moderate-binge-drinking.

16. United States Department of Health and Human Services, National Institute of Health, National Institute on Alcohol Abuse and Alcoholism. https://www.niaaa.nih.gov/alcohol-health/overview-alcohol-consumption/what-standard-drink.

17. United States Department of Health and Human Services, National Institute of Health, National Institute of Diabetes and Digestive and Kidney Diseases. https://www.niddk.nih.gov/health-information/health-topics/liver-disease/cirrhosis/Pages/facts.aspx.

18. United States Department of Health and Human Services, National Institute of Health, National Institute on Drug Abuse. https://www.drugabuse.gov/drugs-abuse/commonly-abused-drugs-charts.

19. United States Food and Drug Administration. http://www.fda.gov/NewsEvents/PublicHealthFocus/ucm234900.htm.

20. World Health Organization (WHO). "Global Status Report on Alcohol and Health." p. XIV. http://www.who.int/substance_abuse/publications/global_alcohol_report/msb_gsr_2014_1.pdf?ua=1.

IMAGE CREDITS

Lab 1: Lifestyle Survey and Resting Heart Rate

Name: _____   Date: _____

Gender: _____   Age: _____   Section: _____

I. Lifestyle Survey

Please circle or highlight the appropriate response to the questions below.

	Always	Nearly always	Often	Seldom	Never
1. I perform aerobic exercise for 20 minutes three times a week and moderate activity for 30 minutes two additional days a week.	5	4	3	2	1
2. I perform strength training exercises, with a minimum of eight exercises, two or more days a week.	5	4	3	2	1
3. I perform flexibility exercises two days a week.	5	4	3	2	1
4. I am my recommended body weight.	5	4	3	2	1
5. I eat three regular meals with a variety of food daily.	5	4	3	2	1
6. I limit my intake of saturated and trans fats.	5	4	3	2	1
7. I eat five servings of fruits and vegetables daily.	5	4	3	2	1
8. I avoid snacking.	5	4	3	2	1
9. I avoid tobacco use of any kind.	5	4	3	2	1
10. I avoid alcohol or use in moderation (one or two drinks)	5	4	3	2	1
11. I avoid drugs that are addicting.	5	4	3	2	1
12. I rarely use prescription drugs, follow the directions, and only when prescribed to me.	5	4	3	2	1
13. I can recognize when I am under stress.	5	4	3	2	1
14. I perform stress management techniques.	5	4	3	2	1
15. I have individuals who are close enough to discuss life's problems with.	5	4	3	2	1
16. My free time is usually spent in fun, relaxing, leisure activity.	5	4	3	2	1
17. I sleep seven to eight hours a night.	5	4	3	2	1
18. I floss my teeth every day and brush them twice daily.	5	4	3	2	1
19. I use safe sun exposure practices.	5	4	3	2	1
20. I avoid unscientifically proven products.	5	4	3	2	1

(Continued)

	Always	Nearly always	Often	Seldom	Never
21. I am aware of the warnings for a heart attack, stroke, and cancer.	5	4	3	2	1
22. I can practice self-exams and get health screenings.	5	4	3	2	1
23. I have a dental checkup once a year.	5	4	3	2	1
24. I am not sexually active or practice safe sex.	5	4	3	2	1
25. I am able to handle feelings of sadness and disappointment.	5	4	3	2	1
26. I handle emotional problems without drugs, alcohol, or aggression.	5	4	3	2	1
27. I enjoy being with people who have a positive attitude.	5	4	3	2	1
28. I don't let setbacks get me down.	5	4	3	2	1
29. I wear a seat belt when driving.	5	4	3	2	1
30. I do not drive under the influence of alcohol and/or drugs.	5	4	3	2	1
31. I avoid being alone after dark in public places.	5	4	3	2	1
32. I attempt to keep places I live and work clean and accident-free.	5	4	3	2	1
33. I try to minimize environmental pollution.	5	4	3	2	1
34. I practice energy conservation (minimize water/ electric use).	5	4	3	2	1
35. I work in a clean environment.	5	4	3	2	1
36. I participate in recycling.	5	4	3	2	1

How to Score

Enter a score beside each question number below and total up each section (i.e., the number 19 below means question 19. You then write down your answer for question 19 next to it under the personal hygiene column).

	Health related	Nutrition	Avoiding chem. dep.	Stress manage- ment	Personal hygiene	Disease prevention	Emotional	Personal safety	Environmental
	1.	5.	9.	13.	17.	21.	25.	29.	33.
	2.	6.	10.	14.	18.	22.	26.	30.	34.
	3.	7.	11.	15.	19.	23.	27.	31.	35.
	4.	8.	12.	16.	20.	24.	28.	32.	36.
Total									
Rating									

Rating Categories

Category Rating	Score
Excellent	≥17
Good	13–16
Need to improve	≤12

II. Computing the Effects of Aerobic Activity on Resting Heart Rate

Make sure to **ROUND** your **FINAL ANSWER** to the nearest whole number. It is highly recommended you check all of your calculations more than once, as one wrong answer can result in multiple wrong answers.

Resting Heart Rate

Resting heart rate:	
Rating (see Table 1 below):	

Table 1: Rating Based on Beats per Minute

Rating	Beats per minute
Excellent	59
Good	60–69
Average	70–79
Fair	80–89
Poor	≥90

A. Beats per day = ☐ (RHR bpm) × 60 (min per hour) × 24 (hours per day) = ☐ beats per day

B. Beats per year = ☐ (use item A) × 365 = ☐ beats per year

*If your RHR dropped by 20 beats per minute (bpm) through an aerobic exercise program, determine the number of beats that your heart would save each year at that lower RHR:

C. Beats per day = ☐ (Current RHR) – 20 × 60 × 24 = ☐ beats per day

D. Beats per year = ☐ (use item C) × 365 = ☐ beats per year

E. Number of beats saved per year (B – D) = ☐ – ☐ = ☐ beats saved per year

*Assuming that you will reach the average U.S. life expectancy of 80 years for women or 75 for men, determine the additional number of "heart rate life years" available to you if your RHR was 20 bpm lower:

F. Years of life ahead = ☐ (use 81 for women & 76 for men) – ☐ (current age) = ☐ years

G. Number of beats saved = ☐ (use item E) × ☐ (use item F) = ☐ beats saved

H. Number of heart rate life years based on the lower RHR = ☐ (use item G) ÷ ☐ (use item D) = years ☐

Lab 2: Behavior Modification

Name: _____   Date: _____

Gender: _____   Age: _____   Section: _____

Stages of Change/Transtheoretical Model
First, identify two current behaviors you have (positive or negative); for example, smoking and exercise.

Behavior #1: _____   **Behavior #2:** _____

Next, figure out which stage each behavior is currently in on the Stages of Change Model (see Table 1) using the sentences below. Remember, the goal of a Behavior Model is to make a change and to work from the first stage to the last; therefore, you can only be in ONE stage at a time.

If your behavior is a negative or a problem behavior, you will use one of the first three sentences/stages 1–3. For example, "I currently <u>smoke</u>; I currently <u>do not exercise</u>."

If your behavior is positive, or you have already started to make changes, you will use one of the last three sentences/stages 4–6. For example, "I currently <u>do not smoke</u>; I currently <u>exercise three times a week</u>."

Behavior #1 (Check only one)

__ 1. I currently _____, and I do not intend to change in the foreseeable future.

__ 2. I currently _____, but I am contemplating changing in the next six months.

__ 3. I currently _____ regularly, but I intend to change in the next month.

__ 4. I currently _____, but I have only done so within the last six months.

__ 5. I currently _____, and I have done so for over six months.

__ 6. I currently _____, and I have done so for over five years.

Current Stage: _____ (see Table 1)

Behavior #2 (Check only one)

___ 1. I currently _____ , and I do not intend to change in the foreseeable future.

___ 2. I currently _____ , but I am contemplating changing in the next six months.

___ 3. I currently _____ regularly, but I intend to change in the next month.

___ 4. I currently _____ , but I have only done so within the last six months.

___ 5. I currently _____ , and I have done so for over six months.

___ 6. I currently _____ , and I have done so for over five years.

Current Stage: _____ (see Table 1)

Processes of Change
Processes of Change are used to help individuals advance from one stage to the next. There are 14 processes; however, not all can be used in all stages. Refer to Table 2 and list all the processes that apply to the stages your behaviors are in.

Behavior #1:

_____

_____

_____

Behavior #2:

_____

_____

_____

Behavior #1

Process #1: _____

Technique:

_____

_____

Process #2: _____

Technique:

_____

_____

Behavior #2

Process #1: _____

Technique:

_____

_____

Process #2: _____

Technique:

_____

_____

Table 1: Stages of Change

Stage	Classification
1	Pre-contemplation
2	Contemplation
3	Preparation
4	Action
5	Maintenance
6	Termination/Adoption

Table 2: Processes with Their Corresponding Stages

Pre-contemplation	Contemplation	Preparation	Action	Maintenance	Termination/ Adoption
Consciousness-raising	Consciousness-raising				
Social liberation	Social liberation				
Dramatic Relief	Dramatic Relief				
Environmental Reevaluation	Environmental Reevaluation				
	Self-Reevaluation	Self-Reevaluation			
		Self-liberation	Self-Liberation		
		Helping Relationships	Helping Relationships	Helping Relationships	Helping Relationships
		Counter Conditioning	Counter Conditioning	Counter Conditioning	Counter Conditioning
			Reinforcement	Reinforcement	Reinforcement
			Stimulus Control	Stimulus Control	Stimulus Control

Table 3: Processes of Change

Process	Technique Examples
Consciousness-Raising (Increasing awareness)	Become aware that there is a problem, read educational materials (for example a brochure, nutrition label, etc.) about the problem behavior or about people who have overcome this same problem, find out about the benefits of changing the behavior, visit a therapist, talk and listen to others, ask questions, take a class. Other intervention examples: feedback, confrontations, media campaigns
Social Liberation (Environmental opportunities)	Seek out advocacy groups (Overeaters Anonymous, Alcoholics Anonymous), join a health club, buy a bike, join a neighborhood walking group, and work in nonsmoking areas. Goal is to increase social opportunities. Advocacy and legislation can also empower people to change (e.g. smoke-free zones, salad bars in school lunches, etc.).
Dramatic Relief (Emotional arousal)	This process produces an initial increased emotional response which in turn reduces distress. Examples include role-playing, grieving, personal testimonies, media campaigns, all of which can move people emotionally.
Environmental Reevaluation (Social Reappraisal)	The individual stops and assesses how the presence or absence of their behavior or habit affects their social environment (internally or externally). This includes how the individual can serve as a positive or negative role model. Some ways an individual might become aware and stop to assess their influence on their environment could be through empathy training, documentaries, or family interventions.
Self-Reevaluation (Self reappraisal)	The individual assesses their self-image, picturing their self with or without a particular healthy or unhealthy habit (image as a physically active person or as a couch potato). Some example techniques include the individual clarifying their values, looking up to healthy role models, and mental imagery.

(Continued)

Process	Technique Examples
Self-Liberation (Committing)	This includes the belief that one can change and makes the commitment and/or recommitment to act on that belief. Some examples include New Year's resolutions (setting goals), signing a behavioral contract, public testimonies, setting start and completion dates, and telling others about goals for accountability. Research has shown that those with more than once choice have a stronger commitment, the greater the amount of choices the more likely the commitment due to increased willpower. For example, to quit smoking the individual sets a start date as well as tells their best friend who will help hold them accountable.
Helping Relationships (Supporting)	Having caring and supportive relationships has a great impact on whether or not the individual makes the change. Trust, openness and acceptance, as well as support for the healthy behavior change is very important. This can include buddy systems, counselor calls, etc.
Counter Conditioning (Substituting)	This process includes learning positive/healthy behaviors which can substitute for problem behaviors. Some examples are carrying gum to chew to replace smoking, using relaxation to counter stress, using assertion/confidence to counter peer pressure, chewing gum rather than smoking, etc.
Reinforcement Management (Rewarding)	This process is used to help manage and reinforce your behavior change. It provides consequences for taking steps in a particular direction; however it is much more effective when rewards are utilized more frequently than punishments. By having contingency contracts, positive self-statements and using group recognition procedures increase the likelihood that positive behavior will be repeated.
Stimulus Control (Re-engineering)	Avoid environments that may stimulate your unhealthy behavior. Surround yourself with people and or environments that will provide stimuli to support your behavior change and reduce your risk of relapsing. Some examples include choosing to park far away in a parking lot to get an extra walk in, choosing stairs over the elevator, you are removing cues for those unhealthy behaviors.

Adapted from Auburn University and Virginia Tech

http://www.auburn.edu/academic/education/sences/classinfo/transtheortical.html

http://www.cpe.vt.edu/gttc/presentations/8eStagesofChange.pdf

Lab 3: Food Diary and Estimated Energy and Protein Requirement

Name: _____ Date: _____

Gender: _____ Age: _____ Section: _____

Day 1 Date: _____

Time	Food	Amount	Calories	Protein (g)	Fat (g)	Sat. Fat (g)	Cholesterol (mg)	Carbs (g)	Fiber (g)	Calcium (mg)	Iron (mg)	Sodium (mg)
6:30AM	Starbucks Coffee	1 cup										
	Creamer	1 tsp.										
8:20AM	Toast	1 slice										
	Peanut Butter	1 Tbsp.										
	Milk	1 cup										
	Banana	1 whole										
10:00AM	Trail mix	¼ cup										
12Noon	Hamburger	1 patty										
	Bun	1 whole										
	Lettuce	2 leaves										
	Pickle	2 slices										
	Mustard	1 Tbsp.										
TOTALS												

THIS PORTION IS AN EXAMPLE ONLY
CONTINUE ONTO AVAILABLE SPACES BELOW FOR DAY 1

Day 2 Date: _____

Time	Food	Amount	Calories	Protein (g)	Fat (g)	Sat. Fat (g)	Cholesterol (mg)	Carbs (g)	Fiber (g)	Calcium (mg)	Iron (mg)	Sodium (mg)
TOTALS												

Day 3 Date: _____

Time	Food	Amount	Calories	Protein (g)	Fat (g)	Sat. Fat (g)	Cholesterol (mg)	Carbs (g)	Fiber (g)	Calcium (mg)	Iron (mg)	Sodium (mg)
TOTALS												

Totals for each day:

Day	Calories	Protein (g)	Fat (g)	Sat. Fat (g)	Cholesterol (mg)	Carbs (g)	Fiber (g)	Calcium (mg)	Iron (mg)	Sodium (mg)
One										
Two										
Three										
Total (All 3 days)										
Average (Divide totals by 3)										

Estimated Energy Requirement

This formula uses your height, weight, and age to give you an estimated caloric intake amount that is individualized for you. This is the amount of calories you should be consuming on a daily basis to meet your body's needs, have energy to function, and to maintain your current weight. **Round all to the second decimal place throughout and round your final answer to the nearest whole number.**

1. Calculate your weight in kilograms, **show all work** (pounds of body weight divided by 2.2046):

2. Calculate your height in meters, **show all work** (height in inches multiplied by .0254):

A. Now Estimate Energy Requirements (EER). Use the formula below to fill in the boxes, **all boxes must be filled in.**

For Men: EER = 663 − (9.53 × Age) + (15.91 × body weight) + (539.6 × height)

For Women: EER = 354 − (6.91 × Age) + (9.36 × body weight) + (726 × height)

EER = [663 or 354] − ([ ] × [ ]) + ([ ] × [ ]) + ([ ] × [ ])

EER = [663 or 354] − [ ] + [ ] + [ ] = [ ]

Estimated Protein Requirement

This is the basic formula for the general population to use to calculate how much protein they should be consuming on a daily basis according to their weight. *Weight must be in kilograms.*

Weight (kg) × 0.8

[ ] (kg) × 0.8 = [ ]

Once you've completed both calculations, go back up to compare your answers to your average daily totals for calories and protein to see whether you are short what your body needs or are above. Discuss your findings in detail here:

_____

_____

_____

_____

_____

Lab 4: Disease Risk with BMI and Recommended Body Weight

Name: _____   Date: _____

Gender: _____   Age: _____   Section: _____

Body Mass Index

Weight: [_____] lbs

Height: [_____] inches

BMI = Weight (lbs) × 705 ÷ Height (in) ÷ Height (in)

BMI = [_____] (lbs) × 705 ÷ [_____] (in) ÷ [_____] (in)

BMI = [_____] Disease Risk: (use Table 1): [_____]

Target Body Weight in pounds if BMI is ...

BMI of 25 = 25 × [_____] (in) × [_____] (in) ÷ 705 = [_____] lbs
(recommended weight for a BMI of 25)

BMI of 22 = 22 × [_____] (in) × [_____] (in) ÷ 705 = [_____] lbs
(recommended weight for a BMI of 22)

Recommended Body Weight Using Current Percent Fat and Desired Percent Fat

1. Body weight in pounds: [_____] lbs (BW)

2. Current percent fat: [_____]

3. Percent fat (%F) in decimal form: [_____] %F → **Convert your percent fat to a decimal (for example 25% = .25)**

A. Calculate how many pounds of fat (FW) make up your body weight using the formula below. Use the decimal form for your %F:

$$FW = BW \times \%F$$

FW = [＿＿＿] × [＿＿＿] = [＿＿＿] lbs

B. Calculate how many pounds of lean body mass (LBM) on your body (muscle, skeletal tissue, etc.) make up your body weight using your FW answer to fill in the formula below:

LBM = BW – FW

LBM = [＿＿＿] – [＿＿＿] = [＿＿＿] lbs of LBM

C. Recommended body weight (RBW) in pounds to reach the percent of fat you would like to achieve:

Desired fat percent (DFP). See **Table 2** below, find your gender and age and look for your **CURRENT** percent fat. Write your **CURRENT** classification below:

Current percent fat classification:

Now, using the same table, write down what percent fat you would like to achieve. Write the percentage amount in the first box, then change the percent to a decimal to use in the recommended body weight formula below.

[＿＿＿] → Convert to decimal [＿＿＿] (DFP)

RBW = LBW ÷ (1.0 – DFP)

RBW = [＿＿＿] ÷ (1.0 – [＿＿＿]) = [＿＿＿] lbs of total recommended body weight

---

Discussing Body Composition Results and Goals

State your feelings about your body composition results and your recommended body weight **using both BMI and percent body fat**. Do you plan to reduce your percent body fat and to increase your lean body mass? If so, why? In detail, write the goal(s) you would like to achieve by the end of the school year and indicate how you plan to achieve them.

_____

_____

_____

_____

_____

Table 1 Disease Risk According to Body Mass Index (BMI)

BMI	Disease Risk	Classification
<18.5	Increased	Underweight
18.5–24.9	Acceptable/Low	Normal
25.0–29.9	Increased	Overweight
30.0–34.9	High	Obesity I
35.0–39.9	Very High	Obesity II
40.0+	Extremely High	Extreme Obesity III

*Adapted from National Heart, Lung, and Blood Institute (2015)

Table 2 Body Composition Classification Based on Percent Body Fat

	Age	Underweight	Excellent	Good	Moderate	Overweight	Obese
MEN	≤19	<3	12.0	12.1–17.0	17.1–22.0	22.1–27.0	≥27.1
	20–29	<3	13.0	13.1–18.0	18.1–23.0	23.1–28.0	≥28.1
	30–39	<3	14.0	14.1–19.0	19.1–24.0	24.1–29.0	≥29.1
	40–49	<3	15.0	15.1–20.0	20.1–25.0	25.1–30.0	≥30.1
	≥50	<3	16.0	16.2–21.0	21.1–26.0	26.1–31.0	≥31.1

	Age	Underweight	Excellent	Good	Moderate	Overweight	Obese
WOMEN	≤19	<12	17.0	17.1–22.0	22.1–27.0	27.1–32.0	≥32.1
	20–29	<12	18.0	18.1–23.0	23.1–28.0	28.1–33.0	≥33.1
	30–39	<12	19.0	19.1–24.0	24.1–29.0	29.1–34.0	≥34.1
	40–49	<12	20.0	20.1–25.0	25.1–30.0	30.1–35.0	≥35.1
	≥50	<12	21.0	21.1–26.0	26.1–31.0	31.1–36.0	≥36.1

▓ High physical fitness standard   ░ General health fitness standard

Lab 5: How Many Calories do I Need per Day?

Name: _____   Date: _____

Gender: _____   Age: _____   Section: _____

1. Calculate your weight in kilograms (pounds of body weight divided by 2.2046):

2. Calculate your height in meters (height in inches multiplied by .0254):

A. Now Estimate Energy Requirements (EER). Use the formula below to fill in the boxes.

> *For Men:*   EER = 663 − (9.53 × Age) + (15.91 × body weight) + (539.6 × height)

> *For Women:*   EER = 354 − (6.91 × Age) + (9.36 × body weight) + (726 × height)

EER = [663 or 354] − ([ ] × [ ]) + ([ ] × [ ]) + ([ ] × [ ])

EER = [663 or 354] − [ ] + [ ] + [ ] = [ ]

B. Select a physical activity[1] .... [ ]

C. How many exercise sessions per week .... [ ]

D. How long will each session last (duration in minutes) .... [ ]

E. Total weekly exercise time (C × D) .... [ ]

F. Average exercise time per day (E ÷ 7) .... [ ]

G. Calorie expenditure (cal/lb/min) of physical activity (**use Table 1**) ..... [ ]

H. Body weight (in pounds) .... [ ]

I. Calories burned per minute of physical activity (G × H) .... [ ]

J. Average calories burned from exercise program (F × I) .... [ ]

---

1   If there is more than one physical activity, you will need to estimate the average daily calories burned as a result of each additional activity (steps B through I) and add all these figures to J above.

K. Daily energy requirement with exercise to **maintain current body weight** (A + J) .... ☐

Stop here if no weight loss is required; otherwise, proceed to items L and M.

L. Calories to subtract from daily requirement to achieve a negative caloric balance (H × 5) .... ☐

M. Target daily calorie intake with current exercise program to lose weight (K – L)² .... ☐

Table 1: Physical Activities and Caloric Expenditures

Activities	Cal/lb./min burn	Activities	Cal/lb./min burn
Aerobics		–13 mph	.071
–Moderate	.065	Dance	
–Vigorous	.095	–Moderate	.030
Archery	.030	–Vigorous	.055
Badminton		Elliptical Training	
–Recreation	.038	–Moderate	.070
–Competition	.065	–Vigorous	.090
Baseball	.031	Golf	.030
Basketball		Gymnastics	
–Moderate	.046	–Light	.030
–Competition	.063	–Heavy	.056
Bowling	.030	Handball	.064
Calisthenics	.033	HIIT (High Intensity Interval Training)	.120
Cross-Country Skiing		Hiking	.040
–Moderate	.090	Martial Arts	.086
–Vigorous	.120	Jogging	
Circuit Training		–11.0 min per mile	.070
–Moderate	.070	–8.5 min per mile	.090
–Vigorous	.100	–7.0 min per mile	.102
Cycling		–6.0 min per mile	.114
–5.5 mph	.033	Jumping Rope	.060
–10 mph	.050	Racquetball	.065

---

2 This result should never be below 1,200 calories for small women or 1,500 for everyone else.

Activities	Cal/lb./min burn	Activities	Cal/lb./min burn
Rowing	.090	–50 yards per min	.070
Skating	.038	Table Tennis	.030
Skiing		Tennis	
–Downhill	.060	–Moderate	.045
–5 mph on flat surface	.078	–Competition	.064
Soccer	.059	Volleyball	.030
Stationary Cycling		Walking	.045
–Moderate	.055	–4.5 mph	
–Vigorous	.070	Wrestling	.085
Strength Training	.050	Zumba	
Swimming (crawl)		–Moderate	.065
–20 yards per min	.031	–Vigorous	.095
–25 yards per min	.040		
–45 yards per min	.057		

Lab 6: Are You Ready to Begin an Exercise Program?

Name: _____   Date: _____

Gender: _____   Age: _____   Section: _____

Read each statement, then circle which number best describes how you feel. For accurate results, please be honest with your answers.

	Strongly Agree	Mildly Agree	Mildly Disagree	Strongly Disagree
1. I am able to walk, ride a bike, swim, or walk in a shallow pool.	4	3	2	1
2. I enjoy exercising.	4	3	2	1
3. I believe that exercise can lower my risk for disease and premature death.	4	3	2	1
4. I believe that exercising overall contributes to better health.	4	3	2	1
5. I have previously participated in an exercise program.	4	3	2	1
6. I have experienced the feeling of being physically fit.	4	3	2	1
7. I can imagine myself exercising.	4	3	2	1
8. I am currently thinking about starting an exercise program.	4	3	2	1
9. I am willing to move past thinking about starting and giving exercise a try for a few weeks.	4	3	2	1
10. I am willing to plan time to exercise at least three days a week.	4	3	2	1
11. I am able to find a place to exercise (Fitness center, outside, at home, etc.)	4	3	2	1
12. I am able to find others who would join me in exercising.	4	3	2	1
13. I will not let external factors prevent me from exercising (fatigue, moody, job, finances, bad weather, etc.)	4	3	2	1
14. I am willing to spend a small amount of money for proper exercise clothing.	4	3	2	1
15. If I am concerned about my current health, I will see my primary care physician prior to starting an exercise program.	4	3	2	1
16. I believe exercise will make me feel better and improve my quality of life.	4	3	2	1

Score Your Test:

This questionnaire evaluates four categories—mastery (self-control), attitude, health, and commitment—that predict how ready you are to begin exercising. Mastery involves whether you can be in control of your exercise program. Attitude evaluates your perception toward exercise. Health measures how much you attribute health benefits/quality of life to exercise. Commitment assesses your dedication to fulfill the exercise program.

Write the numbers you circled above to the corresponding question numbers in spaces below. Add the scores for each line to get your totals. Scores may vary from four to 16. A score of 12 and higher indicates that that factor is important to you, eight and below is low. If you score 12 or more in each category, then your chances of initiating and adhering to an exercise program are good. If you fail to score at least 12 points in three categories, your chances of succeeding at exercise are slim.

Mastery: 1. [   ] + 5. [   ] + 6. [   ] + 9. [   ] = [   ]

Attitude: 2. [   ] + 7. [   ] + 8. [   ] + 13. [   ] = [   ]

Health: 3. [   ] + 4. [   ] + 15. [   ] + 16. [   ] = [   ]

Commitment: 10. [   ] + 11. [   ] + 12. [   ] + 14. [   ] = [   ]

Lab 7: VO$_{2Max}$ Using the 1.5-Mile Run

Name: _____   Date: _____

Gender: _____   Age: _____   Section: _____

Participation

You do not have to run <u>the entire</u> 1.5 miles; you must, however, try your hardest to complete the 1.5 miles as quickly as you can to get an accurate time. Everyone is required to run throughout (not consistently) the lab unless a doctor's excuse is provided. If no attempt is made at running, five points will automatically be deducted from the lab, and therefore, the highest grade available to make will be a D.

Preparation

You may want to practice pacing yourself prior to taking the test to avoid going too fast at the start and becoming prematurely fatigued. Allow yourself a day or two to recover from your practice run before taking the test.

Instructions

1. Break up into pairs. One partner will run while the other counts laps and times the partner running.

2. On a four-lap-per-mile track, six laps = 1.5 miles on the outside track (18 = 1.5 on the inside track). **To warm up, the partner going first must walk/lightly jog one lap before starting.** This one lap **does NOT count** as part of the total. Once everyone completes their warm-up lap, the Instructor will send runners off to begin their timed run in small groups.

3. Try to cover the distance as fast as possible without overexerting yourself. If possible, monitor your own time, or have someone call out your time at various intervals of the test to determine whether your pace is correct.

4. Record the amount of time, in minutes and seconds, it takes you to complete the 1.5-mile distance.

   Running time: _____ min _____ sec

5. Everyone must also complete a cool-down lap after completing their six laps for the test by walking or jogging slowly. This lap should not be timed or counted. The stopwatch should end when

each partner finishes their sixth lap. Everyone will be doing a total of eight laps (outside) or 20 laps (inside); this includes the warm-up and cool-down laps.

I. Determining Maximal Oxygen Consumption

1. Convert your running time from minutes and seconds to a decimal figure. ***This is the only part you will round to the nearest tenth.*** For example, a time of 14 minutes and 25 seconds would be $14 + (25 \div 60) = 14.41$, rounded to the nearest tenth = **14.4 minutes.**

Running time: _____ min + (_____ sec ÷ 60 sec/min) = _____ min

2. Insert your running time into the equation below, where

T = running time (in minutes)

$$VO_{2max} = (483 \div T) + 3.5$$

For example, a person who completes 1.5 miles in 14.4 minutes would calculate maximal oxygen consumption as follows:

$VO_{2max} = (483 \div 14.4) + 3.5 = 37.04 =$ **37 ml/kg/min** (round to the nearest whole number).

$VO_{2max} = (483 \div$ _____) + 3.5 = _____ ml/kg/min
                                              run time in min.

3. Use the chart below to locate your VO_{2max} score and Fitness Rating and copy these values from the chart into the appropriate place in the table.

TABLE

	VO_{2max}	Cardiovascular Fitness Rating
1.5-mile run test		

CHART

Women	Very Poor	Poor	Fair	Good	Excellent	Superior
Age: 18–29	Below 31.6	31.6–35.4	35.5–39.4	39.5–43.9	44.0–50.1	Above 50.1
30–39	Below 29.9	29.9–33.7	33.8–36.7	36.8–40.9	41.0–46.8	Above 46.8
40–49	Below 28.0	28.0–31.5	31.6–35.0	35.1–38.8	38.9–45.1	Above 45.1
50–59	Below 25.5	25.5–28.6	28.7–31.3	31.4–35.1	35.2–39.8	Above 39.8
Men						
Age: 18–29	Below 38.1	38.1–42.1	42.2–45.6	45.7–51.0	51.1–56.1	Above 56.1
30–39	Below 36.7	36.7–40.9	41.0–44.3	44.4–48.8	48.9–54.2	Above 54.2
40–49	Below 34.6	34.6–38.3	38.4–42.3	42.4–46.7	46.8–52.8	Above 52.8
50–59	Below 31.1	31.1–35.1	35.2–38.2	38.3–43.2	43.3–49.6	Above 49.6

II. Using Your Results, Answer All Parts in DETAIL

1. How did you score? Are you surprised by your rating for cardiovascular fitness? Are you satisfied with your **current rating?**

2. Are you satisfied with your **current level** of cardiovascular fitness as evidenced in your daily life—your ability to walk, run, bicycle, climb stairs, do yard work, or engage in recreational activities? If not, why?

3. What cardiorespiratory fitness category would you like to achieve by the end of the semester? **Explain in detail how** you plan to reach this goal.

Lab 8: Assessing Muscular Strength

Name: _____   Date: _____

Gender: _____   Age: _____   Section: _____

I. Hand Grip Strength

A. Using your dominant hand to grip the dynamometer, wrap your fingers around the pulling mechanism until the bones in the middle of your finger are gripping it comfortably. Adjust the dynamometer handle for a firm fit.

B. Move your elbow to be at 90 degrees. Hold the arm two to three inches away from the side of your body.

C. Keeping the rest of your body motionless, tighten your grip as hard as you can for a few seconds.

D. Write down the score reached, usually in pounds if in America; if it is metric only and in kilograms, then multiply by 2.2046.

E. Attempt three trials and record the highest of the three. Then compare to the percentile rank below in Table 1.

F. In Table 2, note the category that corresponds to the percentile rank and write it down.

II. Hand Chosen (please circle)

Right or Left

III. Grip Assessment

Score recorded in pounds: _____

Percentile Rank (Table 1):_____

Category (Table 2):_____

Table 1: Percentile Ranking for Grip Strength and Gender

Percentile Ranking	Women (lbs)	Male (lbs)
99	101	153
95	94	145
90	91	141
80	86	139
70	80	132
60	78	124
50	74	122
40	71	114
30	66	110
20	64	100
10	60	91
5	58	76

Table 2: Percentile Rank and Category

Percentile Rank	Category
≥90	Excellent
70–78	Good
50–60	Average
30–40	Fair
≤20	Poor

Lab 9: Assessing Muscular Flexibility

Name: _____   Date: _____

Gender: _____   Age: _____   Section: _____

> Please refer to the last page for directions for each: sit and reach, total body/trunk rotation, and shoulder rotation starting on page 4. Please use Tables 1, 2, 3, 4, and 5 to complete the chart below and learn what your category rating is for each exercise as well as your overall flexibility rating.

Assessment	Inches	Percentile Rank	Category	Points
Modified Sit-and-Reach				
Total Body Rotation O Right O Left				
Shoulder Rotation				

Overall Points: _____

Overall Category: _____

Table 1: Percentile Ranks for Sit-and-Reach in Inches

Percentile Rank	Age: Men				Percentile Rank	Age: Women			
	≤18	19–35	36–49	≥50		≤18	19–35	36–49	≥50
99	20.8	20.1	18.9	16.2	99	22.6	21.0	19.8	17.2
95	19.6	18.9	18.2	15.8	95	19.5	19.3	19.2	15.7
90	18.2	17.2	16.1	15.0	90	18.7	17.9	17.4	15.0
80	17.8	17.0	14.6	13.3	80	17.8	16.7	16.2	14.2
70	16.0	15.8	13.9	12.3	70	16.5	16.2	15.2	13.6
60	15.2	15.0	13.4	11.5	60	16.0	15.8	14.5	12.3
50	14.5	14.4	12.6	10.2	50	15.2	14.8	13.5	11.1
40	14.0	13.5	11.6	9.7	40	14.5	14.5	12.8	10.1
30	13.4	13.0	10.8	9.3	30	13.7	13.7	12.2	9.2

(Continued)

Percentile Rank	Age: Men				Percentile Rank	Age: Women			
	≤18	19–35	36–49	≥50		≤18	19–35	36–49	≥50
20	11.8	11.6	9.9	8.8	20	12.6	12.6	11.0	8.3
10	9.5	9.2	8.3	7.8	10	11.4	10.1	9.7	7.5
05	8.4	7.9	7.0	7.2	05	9.4	8.1	8.5	3.7
01	7.2	7.0	5.1	4.0	01	6.5	2.6	2.0	1.5

▨ High physical fitness standard　　　Health fitness standard

Table 2: Total Body Rotation in Inches

	Percentile Rank	Age: Left Rotation				Percentile Rank	Age: Right Rotation			
		<18	19–35	36–49	>50		<18	19–35	36–49	>50
MEN	99	29.1	28.0	26.6	21.0	99	28.2	27.8	25.2	22.2
	95	26.6	24.8	24.5	20.0	95	25.5	25.6	23.8	20.7
	90	25.0	23.6	23.0	17.7	90	24.3	24.1	22.5	19.3
	80	22.0	22.0	21.2	15.5	80	22.7	22.3	21.0	16.3
	70	20.9	20.3	20.4	14.7	70	21.3	20.7	18.7	15.7
	60	19.9	19.3	18.7	13.9	60	19.8	19.0	17.3	14.7
	50	18.6	18.0	16.7	12.7	50	19.0	17.2	16.3	12.3
	40	17.0	16.8	15.3	11.7	40	17.3	16.3	14.7	11.5
	30	14.9	15.0	14.8	10.3	30	15.1	15.0	13.3	10.7
	20	13.8	13.3	13.7	9.5	20	12.9	13.3	11.2	8.7
	10	10.8	10.5	10.8	4.3	10	10.8	11.3	8.0	2.7
	05	8.5	8.9	8.8	0.3	05	8.1	8.3	5.5	0.3
	01	3.4	1.7	5.1	0.0	01	6.6	2.9	2.0	0.0
WOMEN	99	29.3	28.6	27.1	23.0	99	19.6	29.4	27.1	21.7
	95	26.8	24.8	25.3	21.4	95	27.6	25.3	25.9	19.7
	90	25.5	23.0	23.4	20.5	90	25.8	23.0	21.3	19.0
	80	23.8	21.5	20.2	19.1	80	23.7	20.8	19.6	17.9
	70	21.8	20.5	18.6	17.3	70	22.0	19.3	17.3	16.8
	60	20.5	19.3	17.7	16.0	60	20.8	18.0	16.5	15.6
	50	19.5	18.0	16.4	14.8	50	19.5	17.3	14.6	14.0
	40	18.5	17.2	14.8	13.7	40	18.3	16.0	13.1	12.8
	30	17.1	15.7	13.6	10.0	30	16.3	15.2	11.7	8.5
	20	16.0	15.2	11.6	6.3	20	14.5	14.0	9.8	3.9
	10	12.8	13.6	8.5	3.0	10	12.4	11.1	6.1	2.2
	05	11.1	7.3	6.8	0.7	05	10.2	8.8	4.0	1.1
	01	8.9	5.3	4.3	0.0	01	8.9	3.2	2.8	0.0

Table 3: Shoulder Rotation in Inches

Percentile Rank	Age: Men				Percentile Rank	Age: Women			
	≤18	19–35	36–49	≥50		≤18	19–35	36–49	≥50
99	2.2	–1.0	18.1	21.5	99	2.6	–2.4	11.5	13.1
95	15.2	10.4	20.4	27.0	95	8.0	6.2	15.4	16.5
90	18.5	15.5	20.8	27.9	90	10.7	9.7	16.8	20.9
80	20.7	18.4	23.3	28.5	80	14.5	14.5	19.2	22.5
70	23.0	20.5	24.7	29.4	70	16.1	17.2	21.5	24.3
60	24.2	22.9	26.6	29.9	60	19.2	18.7	23.1	25.1
50	25.4	24.4	28.0	30.5	50	21.0	20.0	23.5	26.2
40	26.3	25.7	30.0	31.0	40	22.2	21.4	24.4	28.1
30	28.2	27.3	31.9	31.7	30	23.2	24.0	25.9	29.9
20	30.0	30.1	33.3	33.1	20	25.0	25.9	29.8	31.5
10	33.5	31.8	36.1	37.2	10	27.2	29.1	31.1	33.1
05	34.7	33.5	37.8	38.7	05	28.0	31.3	33.4	34.1
01	40.8	42.6	43.0	44.1	01	32.5	37.1	34.9	35.4

▨ High physical fitness standard   ▨ Health fitness standard

Table 4: Category Ratings

Percentile Rank	Flexibility Category	Points
≥90	Excellent	5
70–89	Good	4
50–69	Average	3
30–49	Fair	2
≤20	Poor	1

Table 5: Overall Flexibility Rating

Overall Points	Overall Flexibility Category
≥13	Excellent
10–12	Good
7–9	Average
4–6	Fair
≤3	Poor

Directions

Sit and Reach

Equipment needed: Acuflex 1 – Modified Sit and Reach Box, or a yardstick on top of a 12" high box.

1. Always warm up properly before doing any flexibility exercise.

2. Remove shoes, sit on the floor with your hips, back, and head against a wall with your legs fully extended (you may have a partner help hold your knees in place). The bottom of your feet should be against the Accuflex 1 or box.

3. Place your hands with one on top of the other and reach forward as far as possible, keeping your back and head against the wall. A partner then needs to slide the reach indicator on the Acuflex 1 (or yardstick) along the top until the indicator touches your fingers.

4. Your head and back at this time may now come off the wall. Gradually reach forward three times with the third time stretching as far as you can and holding the position for at least 2 seconds.

5. Write down your final number rounded to the nearest half inch. You may do this test twice and average both scores for a final result. Refer to Table 1 for the percentile ranks and fitness categories.

Total Body/Trunk Rotation

Equipment needed: Acuflex II Trunk Rotation Test or measuring tape to build your own scale.

1. If you are using measuring tape, you may tape two measuring tapes to the wall. One measuring tape will be upside down for participants who want to rotate to their left. Note that if you are using measuring tape, participants must line their toes up with the 15" marker on the tape, it is recommended that masking tape be put on the floor and centered with the 15" marker on both measuring tapes.

2. Warm up appropriately.

3. First decide which way you want to rotate, right or left. Then use the correct measuring tape (if you are using the Acuflex II panel it does not matter which way you want to rotate). You should be about an arm's length away from the wall, with your feet/toes pointing straight ahead. Your feet should be separated slightly, about shoulder width apart and your toes should be touching the center of the line on the floor (15" marker). Hold out your arm horizontally, away from the wall and make a fist. Make sure the measuring tapes and Acuflex are at shoulder height.

4. Rotate your trunk with your extended arm going backwards, you can slightly bend your knees during this test however the feel cannot be moved or rotated. As you rotate and make contact with the Acuflex the panel will slide and you may see your result. If you are using the measuring tapes you will need to hold your final position for at least 2 seconds, with the little finger side forward during the sliding movement, and have a partner read your result. You must utilize proper

hand position, the hand may not be open, and you must use your fist to slide the panel, not our fingers or knuckles. The body must be kept as straight as possible during the test.

5. Perform two attempts with your chosen side and record the farthest amount achieved. Then do the test again with another two attempts and writing down the larger result. You will then average both for your final result. Refer to Table 2 for percentile ranks and categories.

Shoulder Rotation

Equipment needed: Acuflex III Shoulder Rotation Test

1. Warm up properly.

2. Using the shoulder caliper, the first thing you need to do is measure your biacromial width (this is the distance between the outer edges of the acromion processes of the shoulders). Write this measurement down somewhere.

3. Place the Acuflex III behind the back, using a reverse grip (thumbs out) to hold the device. Place your index finger of the right hand next to the zero point of the scale (lower scale on the Acuflex III) and hold it firmly in place throughout the test. Then place your left hand on the other end of the device, wherever is most comfortable.

4. Standing straight up, extend both arms to full length with your elbows locked. Slowly bring the Acuflex III over your head until it reaches about the forehead level. The goal is to be able to reach about the forehead level with your hands as close together as possible on the measuring device. Therefore, after your first successful rotation, return to the starting position with your arms down, your right hand stays in place, slide your left hand in towards your right slightly and repeat the task. Continue to do this until you are no longer successful at getting your arms above your forehead level and measure your last successful trial, to do this you will measure the inner edge of the left hand on the side of the little finger.

5. To determine your final score you will first need to subtract your biacromial width from your best score during your trial (shortest distance measured). Use Table 3 for percentile ranks and fitness categories.

Adapted from:

1. Franklin Community School (2015). Retrieved from http://www2.fcsconline.org/staff/ferrisa/Kinesiology/Goniometer%20LAB-Flexibility.pdf

2. Top End Sports (2015). Retrieved from http://www.topendsports.com/testing/tests/trunk-rotation.htm

3. Top End Sports (2015). Retrieved from http://www.topendsports.com/testing/tests/shoulder-flex.htm

Lab 10: Assessing Range of Motion

Name: _____   Date: _____

Gender: _____   Age: _____   Section: _____

Directions: Use a goniometer to measure each joints range of motion. Place the circular portion of the goniometer over the joint that is being measured. Have the individual then rotate their joint, then rotate the straight potion on the goniometer to match their limb and read the degree amount they achieved. Make sure they did not use any muscle or move, stretch, or rotate their body. Note that the degrees listed for each joint below are the expected range majority of people are able to achieve. Some people can be under (injury) or may go over (great flexibility or genetics).

1. Shoulder Flexion _____
   180° Raise arm straight forward.

2. Shoulder Extension _____
   60° Raise arm straight backward.

3. Shoulder Abduction _____
   180° Bring arm up sideways.

4. Elbow Flexion _____
   150° Bring lower arm to the biceps (bicep curl).

5. Hip Flexion (with knee flexed) _____
   110–130° Lay down on back, flex knee, bring thigh close to abdomen.

6. Hip Extension (with knee extended) _____
   30° Lay down on stomach, keep knee straight, move thigh backward without moving the pelvis.

7. Knee Flexion _____
   130° Lay down on stomach, touch calf to hamstring.

8. Hip Abduction _____
   45–50° Raise thigh away from midline without leaning.

9. Hip Adduction _____
   20–30° Bring thigh toward and across the midline without rotating hips.

10. Hip Outward/External Rotation _____
    45° Sit on the edge of a chair, have knee flexed and swing lower leg toward midline.

11. Hip Inward/Internal Rotation _____
    40° Sit on the edge of a chair, have knee flexed and swing lower leg away from midline.

Adapted from the CDC and MIT

http://www.cdc.gov/ncbddd/jointrom/documents/normal-rom-data-description-and-sample-tables.pdf

http://web.mit.edu/tkd/stretch/stretching_1.html

Lab 11: Creating a Personal Fitness Plan

Name: _____   Date: _____

Gender: _____   Age: _____   Section: _____

For this lab, you will be utilizing the "FITT" concept and creating your very own fitness program by following the ACSM guidelines. If you currently do not take part in any type of exercise/fitness program, this is your chance to create a plan for you. If you currently have an exercise plan, you may use it; however, you must make sure you meet the ACSM guidelines. If you do not, then you need to adjust your current plan for this lab. Refer to Chapter 5 on Muscular Strength and Endurance and Chapter 6 on Flexibility. Please see pages __x__ for muscular strength and endurance exercises and pages __x__ for flexibility exercises. Note that on page __x__, there are multiple flexibility exercises shown that are no longer considered standard in use; you cannot use these options for your flexibility exercises. For ACSM guidelines, please see pages __x__.

First, create a goal you would like to meet for each part (Cardio, Muscular, and Flexibility); then continue on creating your fitness program. Keep in mind a reward is not "I will look good or feel better"; this is a benefit. A reward is something positive that you do for yourself that is extra, such as buying new sneakers for meeting your goal, etc.

I. Cardiorespiratory Endurance   GOAL:

A. Frequency (How often each week):

_____

B. Intensity (Moderate or vigorous and what percent of your MHR, HRR, or VO2 max):

_____

C. Time (How long will each session be):

_____

D. Type (Aerobic activities):

_____

E. Facility (Where will these exercises take place):

_____

F. What time of day will you exercise?

_____

G. Reward:

_____

II. Muscular Strength and Endurance   GOAL:

A. Frequency:

_____

B. Intensity (Resistance or pounds used for each exercise or percent RM):

_____

C. Type (List all exercises that will be used):

_____

_____

D. Time (List sets and reps for each exercise):

_____

_____

_____

_____

E. Facility:

_____

F. Reward:

_____

III. Muscular Flexibility   GOAL:

Frequency:

_____

Intensity:

_____

Type (Exercises used):

_____

_____

Time (Reps for each exercise, length of each stretch, and length of final hold for each stretch):

_____

_____

_____

_____

Facility:

_____

Reward:

_____

Lab 12: How Stressed are You?

Name: _____   Date: _____

Gender: _____   Age: _____   Section: _____

Using the list below, please identify which stressful life events, within the past 12 months, that may be having an effect on your mental and physical health. Use Table 1 below for scoring each stressor that applies to you, with +3 being the highest positive stress score and -3 being the lowest negative stress score. Note that 0 is to be used on stressors that are not affecting you and that the '–' sign **does not indicate a negative number**, only that that stressor was a negative stress for you.

Table 1: Scoring for Stress

Positive Effect	Not Affecting	Negative Effect
+3 Jubilant	0	–3 Shocked
+2 Delighted		–2 Dismayed
+1 Pleased		–1 Dissatisfied

I. Stress Items and Events

A. General Stress

Event	Stress Score	Event	Stress Score
Substance Abuse		Can't Afford "Needs"	
Imprisonment		Increasing/Decreasing Income	
Marriage		Mortgage Loans	
Sexual Intimacy		Vehicle Loans	
Pregnancy		Student Loans	
Family Death		New Job	
Friend/Acquaintance Death		Job Loss	
Your Divorce		Altering of Job Responsibilities	

(*Continued*)

Event	Stress Score	Event	Stress Score
Parent Divorce		Relationship with Boss	
Divorce by Friend or Family		Relationship with Coworkers	
Boyfriend/Girlfriend		Time Management Skills	
Relationship with Family		Personal Accomplishment?	
Personal Health		Vacation	
Personal Fitness		Spirituality	
Family/Friend Health		Other:	
Sleeping Behavior		Other:	
Nutritional Behavior		Other:	
Study Behavior		Other:	
Acceptance by Peers		Other:	
Social Activities		Other:	
Recreational Activities		Other:	
Transportation		Other:	
Friendship(s)		Other:	
Ability to Relax and Laugh		Other:	

B. Education

Event	Stress Score	Event	Stress Score
School Choice		Exams	
School Change		Assignments	
Loneliness		Class Workload	
Privacy		Instructors	
Military Obligations		Fraternity/Sorority	
Change of Major		Decent Housing	
Missing Classes		Roommate(s) Relationships	
Grades		Change of Roommate	
Academic Probation		Removal from Housing	
Courses		Moving	
Graduation		Career Options	

II. Scoring and Interpretations

A. Add the numbers for the negative score by themselves to reach a total (ignore the minus sign to do this). Write your total negative stress score in the appropriate column under Table 3. Find your total score in Table 2 and fill in your category in the corresponding column.

B. Add all the positive stress scores together and write in your total in the appropriate box below in Table 3. Then, add your negative stress total to your positive stress total to receive an overall stress total score. Use your overall total stress score to find in Table 2 and write the correct category in the corresponding box in Table 3.

Table 2: Stress Categories

Stress Category	Negative Score	Total Scores
Poor	≥15	≥30
Fair	9–14	20–29
Average	6–8	15–19
Good	1–5	6–14
Excellent	0	1–5

Table 3: Stress Scale Comparisons

	Calculated Points	Related Stress Category
Negative Scores		
Positive Scores		N/A
Total Scores		

Lab 13: How at Risk are You for Developing Stress?

Name: _____   Date: _____

Gender: _____   Age: _____   Section: _____

Respond to the survey below; note SA = Strongly Agree, MA = Mildly Agree, MD = Mildly Disagree, SD = Strongly Disagree.

I. Stress Risk

	SA	MA	MD	SD
1. I try to include physical activity in my daily routines.	1	2	3	4
2. I use aerobic exercise three or more times a week, 10 minutes each.	1	2	3	4
3. I usually sleep seven to eight hours a night.	1	2	3	4
4. I usually eat one warm and nutritionally balanced meal a day.	1	2	3	4
5. I drink two or fewer cups of coffee a day.	1	2	3	4
6. I am at a recommended body comp.	1	2	3	4
7. I enjoy good health.	1	2	3	4
8. I do not use any form of tobacco.	1	2	3	4
9. I drink at or fewer than one (women) or two (men) drinks per day.	1	2	3	4
10. I do not use recreational drugs.	1	2	3	4
11. I have someone I love and trust for when I have problems.	1	2	3	4
12. I regularly receive and return affection.	1	2	3	4
13. My family loves one another.	1	2	3	4
14. My personal relationships provide me emotional security.	1	2	3	4
15. When stressed, I have people I can ask advice from.	1	2	3	4
16. I feel free to discuss my emotions, problems, and feelings people close to me.	1	2	3	4
17. People rely on me for help.	1	2	3	4
18. I am able to control my anger and aggression.	1	2	3	4
19. I have a strong group of friends that I do activities with.	1	2	3	4
20. I usually do something fun once a week.	1	2	3	4

	SA	MA	MD	SD
21. My spiritual beliefs provide strength and guide my life.	1	2	3	4
22. I help provide service to others.	1	2	3	4
23. I enjoy my job/school.	1	2	3	4
24. I am good at my job/coursework.	1	2	3	4
25. I manage my time well.	1	2	3	4
26. My income meets my needs.	1	2	3	4
27. I get along well with my coworkers/classmates.	1	2	3	4
28. I know how to say no to additional work or commitments when there is not time.	1	2	3	4
29. I make time every day for quiet contemplation.	1	2	3	4
30. I work on stress management when my stress increases.	1	2	3	4

Add up your points to a total and match it to the corresponding category using Table 1 below.

Stress Risk

Score   ☐

Rating   ☐

Table 1

Total Score	Categories
0–30	Excellent
31–41	Good
41–50	Average
51–60	Fair
≥60	Poor

II. In detail, discuss how current stress and your personality affect you in your daily life.

_____

_____

_____

_____

_____

III. Prioritize two behaviors you would like to change to help decrease your risk of stress.

1. _____

2. _____

IV. List two stress management techniques (as discussed in the textbook) you plan to use to help

change these behaviors.

1. _____

2. _____

V. Discuss how you plan to use these techniques to accomplish changing these behaviors.

_____

_____

_____

_____

Lab 14: Alcohol and Addictive Behavior

Name: _____   Date: _____

Gender: _____   Age: _____   Section: _____

> Responding to the following questions may be helpful in determining if you have tendencies that lead to addictive behavior. Questions like these are often used to determine if there are dependencies on chemical substances. It is not designed to diagnose, but instead raise awareness on certain behavioral traits that you or people you know may have.

I. Acknowledging Addictive Behavior (circle the appropriate response):

Do you depend on others often?	Yes	No
Do you often indulge in anything in excess?	Yes	No
Are you compulsive?	Yes	No
Do you spend time thinking about a specific drug?	Yes	No
Do you use any drugs beyond medical reasons?	Yes	No
Do you misuse prescription drugs?	Yes	No
Can you get beyond a week without misusing drugs?	Yes	No
Has anyone mentioned you might have a drug problem?	Yes	No
Has anyone close to you sought help for themselves for drug issues?	Yes	No
Do you ever lie about drug use?	Yes	No
Do you relate well to others who use the same drug(s) as you?	Yes	No
Do you struggle when trying to stop the use of a drug?	Yes	No
Do you act emotional if people keep you from accessing your drug?	Yes	No
Do you ever suffer from withdrawal?	Yes	No
Have you ever sought help for drug use?	Yes	No
Has any part of your life struggled due to use of a drug?	Yes	No
Have you failed to reduce the amount of drug(s) you use?	Yes	No
Have you ever placed anyone at risk due to misuse of a drug?	Yes	No

Note that if you circled yes to five or more of these questions, then there is a strong chance that you may have addictive behavior and may need to look at a more diagnostic evaluation by a professional. However, depending on which response is circled, fewer than five can still show potential addictive behaviors.

II. Alcohol Use and Addictive Behavior

Have you missed school/work due to drinking?	Yes	No
Does drinking interfere with your school/work?	Yes	No
Have you skipped exercising due to drinking?	Yes	No
Has drinking interfered with your long- or short-term goals?	Yes	No
Have you drank to increase your self-confidence (liquid courage)?	Yes	No
Have you drank to be accepted socially?	Yes	No
Do you drink more than one (for women) or two (for men) drinks per day regularly?	Yes	No
Do you drink alone?	Yes	No
Do you lie about the amount of drinks you have had?	Yes	No
Have you looked for another drink before finishing the one you have?	Yes	No
Do you use drinking to relieve stress, worry, or life?	Yes	No
Do you easily get annoyed when someone comments on your drinking?	Yes	No
Do you participate in binge drinking?	Yes	No
Have you ever missed an appointment due to drinking?	Yes	No
When you pour your own drink, is it a larger amount then others are getting?	Yes	No
Do you need a drink at certain parts of the day?	Yes	No
Have you run low on finances due to drinking?	Yes	No
Do you ever get aggressive when drinking?	Yes	No
Do you ever struggle to remember what you have done while drinking?	Yes	No
Do you ever feel a physical dependency when not drinking?	Yes	No
Do you feel like you need to reduce how much you are drinking?	Yes	No
Have you ever seen a healthcare specialist for drinking?	Yes	No
Have you ever been in the hospital due to drinking?	Yes	No
Do you ever take a drink to kick-start the day?	Yes	No
Have your sleeping patterns been altered by drinking?	Yes	No
Has your reputation changed at all from drinking?	Yes	No
Does drinking affect your relationships?	Yes	No

III. Note that stating yes to any of the above questions may point to potential addictive behavior. Answering yes to multiple items may show alcohol dependency issues, and evaluation by a professional should be considered.

Lab 15: AIDS Awareness

Name: _____   Date: _____

Gender: _____ Age: _____   Section: _____

Circle your responses to the following questions on your AIDS and HIV knowledge.

1. AIDS is the end stage of HIV.	Yes	No
2. HIV is a chronic disease that spreads through risky behavior (like unsafe sex).	Yes	No
3. AIDS is curable.	Yes	No
4. Abstaining from sex is the only guaranteed way to protect against HIV.	Yes	No
5. A person with HIV may look and feel healthy.	Yes	No
6. Condoms are guaranteed to protect you from HIV.	Yes	No
7. Using drugs and alcohol make a person less likely to use a condom.	Yes	No
8. Using latex condoms provide the best protection from HIV.	Yes	No
9. Using drugs and alcohol may make you more likely to have unplanned sex.	Yes	No
10. A pregnant woman with HIV may transmit it to her unborn child.	Yes	No
11. Donating blood can increase your risk of an HIV infection.	Yes	No
12. HIV can be spread among people by touch (holding hands or hugging).	Yes	No
13. An HIV antibody test is the only way we determine if a person has an HIV infection.	Yes	No
14. HIV destroys the immune system.	Yes	No
15. HIV infection can be in the body for 10 years before symptoms from AIDS show.	Yes	No
16. If you have HIV, then you have AIDS.	Yes	No
17. HIV can be prevented.	Yes	No
18. Early treatment for HIV can reduce the symptoms that individuals experience.	Yes	No
19. Pharmaceutical drugs may lengthen the life of someone infected with HIV.	Yes	No
20. Specific drugs are designed to delay HIV infection from progressing and stop AIDS development.	Yes	No

AIDS Awareness Correct Answers

1. True. The HIV disease erodes and ultimately destroys the individuals immune system. AIDs is the term used to describe the end stage of the HIV infection and becomes labelled as a diseases or illness. This is due to the fact that now the individual will have severe symptoms, mainly from a secondary infection, such as pneumonia, which takes advantage of the compromised immune system and can potentially cause death.

2. True. People are only more likely to get HIV because of the behavior and choices they make.

3. False. Although there are drugs that can delay the development of AIDS, there is no cure.

4. True. Abstinence will guarantee no HIV transmission from sex; however, sharing items like previously used needles can be a risk.

5. True. Many times an individual with HIV is asymptomatic and therefore it may be years before realizing they have the infection.

6. False. Only by abstaining from sex can an individual guarantee protection from HIV.

7. True. Young adults especially have shown that alcohol consumption will reduce the use of protection.

8. True. When used correctly, condoms may reduce the risk however there is no guarantee that condoms will protect against HIV infection.

9. True. Even the most controlled individuals will make poor decisions during alcohol and drug consumption.

10. True. HIV can be given to an unborn baby from the mother through the placenta, as well as through breastfeeding.

11. False. HIV is not transmitted from GIVING blood; new needles are used, and bodily fluid is being removed from you.

12. False. HIV is only passed from one individual to another by bodily fluids.

13. True. Only an HIV antibody test is the way to tell if a person has the HIV disease.

14. True. HIV specifically attacks your white blood cells, thereby compromising your immune system.

15. True. It could be 10 or more years before AIDS develops.

16. False. Having HIV does not mean you also have AIDS; this could occur much later during the HIV disease.

17. True. It can be prevented as long as individuals choose low risk lifestyle behaviors as well as use protection when engaging in sexual activity.

18. True. The quicker treatment is started, the better the chance for quantity and quality of life.

19. True. Drugs have been developed that can lengthen the life of those suffering from HIV.

20. True. Development of antiretroviral drugs allow for longer lifespans with a reduction of symptoms for those who have HIV. However, it does not cure or make the disease completely symptom-free.

CPSIA information can be obtained
at www.ICGtesting.com
Printed in the USA
BVHW062336050522
636133BV00005B/331